Abbreviations

ant.	=	anterior	obl.	=	oblique
a. or aa.	=	artery or arteries	post.	=	posterior
art.	=	articulation	proc. or procc.	=	process or processes
br. or brr.	=	branch or branches	prot.	=	protuberance
caud.	=	caudal	prox.	=	proximal
cran.	=	cranial	r. or rr.	=	ramus or rami
dist.	=	distal	sup.	=	superior
div. or divv.	=	division or divisions	superf.	=	superficial
dors.	=	dorsal	surf.	=	surface
ext.	=	external	sut.	=	suture
exten.	=	extensor	transv.	=	transverse
flex.	=	flexor	tuberc.	=	tubercle
inf.	=	inferior	tuberos.	=	tuberosity
int.	=	internal	v. or vv.	=	vein or veins
intermed.	=	intermediate	var.	=	variant
inteross.	=	interosseous	vent.	=	ventral
lat.	=	lateral	vert. or vertt.	=	vertebra or vertebrae
lig. or ligg.	=	ligament or ligaments			
lumbr.	=	lumbrical			
m. or mm.	=	muscle or muscles	♀	=	female
med.	=	medial	♂	=	male
n. or nn.	=	nerve or nerves			

Note: Square brackets [ ] are used for alternative terms denoted as such in the 6th edition of the *Nomina Anatomica* (1989). Round brackets ( ) are used to denote other alternative terms, not necessarily in the *Nomina Anatomica*. Round brackets are also used to indicate the percentage reduction or magnification of structure(s) illustrated in the figures; because of the great variability in individual body size, these percentages should only be considered as approximate values.

Sobotta

Atlas of Human Anatomy

Volume 1
Head, Neck, Upper Limb

Sobotta

Atlas of Human Anatomy

Volume 1
Head, Neck, Upper Limb

Edited by

Professor Dr. med. R. Putz
Vorstand des Anatomischen Instituts
der Ludwig-Maximilians-Universität
München, Germany

Professor Dr. med. R. Pabst
Leiter der Abteilung für
Funktionelle und Angewandte Anatomie
der Medizinischen Hochschule
Hannover, Germany

12th English Edition
Nomenclature in English

Translated and edited by

Anna N. Taylor, Ph.D.
Professor of Neurobiology
University of California at Los Angeles School of Medicine
Research Career Scientist
Department of Veterans Affairs
West Los Angeles Medical Center
Los Angeles, California

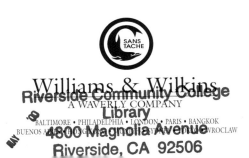

Williams & Wilkins
A WAVERLY COMPANY
BALTIMORE • PHILADELPHIA • LONDON • PARIS • BANGKOK
BUENOS AIRES • MUNICH • TOKYO • SYDNEY • WROCLAW

Printer and Binder: ~~~~~

A translation of Sobotta Atlas der Anatomie des Menschen, 20. Auflage,
Urban & Schwarzenberg, München, Copyright © 1993.

Landwehrstraße 61
D-80336 München
Germany

Copyright © 1997 Williams & Wilkins

351 West Camden Street
Baltimore, Maryland 21201-2436 USA

Rose Tree Corporate Center
1400 North Providence Road
Building II, Suite 5025
Media, Pennsylvania 19063-2043 USA

Library of Congress Cataloging-in-Publication Data

Atlas der Anatomie des Menschen. English.
    Sobotta atlas of human anatomy.—12th English ed., nomenclature in
English / edited by R. Putz and R. Pabst; translated and edited by Anna N.
Taylor.
      p. cm.
    Translation of: Atlas der Anatomie des Menschen. 20. Aufl. 1993.
Includes index.
    Contents: v. 1. Head, neck, upper limbs—v. 2. Thorax, abdomen,
pelvis, lower limb.
    ISBN 0-683-18209-9 (V.1).—ISBN 0-683-18210-2 (V.2).—ISBN 0-683-
30047-4 (set)
    1. Human anatomy—Atlases. I. Sobotta, Johannes, 1869-1845. II. Putz,
Reinhard. III. Pabst, Reinhard, Dr. med. IV. Taylor, Anna N. V. Title.
    [DNLM: 1. Anatomy, Regional—atlases. QS 17 A88125 1996a]
QM25.A7913 1996
611'.0022'2—dc20
DNLM/DLC
for Library of Congress   96-10269
                                                              CIP

The atlas consists of two separate volumes:
    Vol. 1: Head, Neck, Upper Limb   ISBN 0-683-18209-9
    Vol. 2: Thorax, Abdomen, Pelvis, Lower Limb   ISBN 0-683-18210-2

To purchase additional copies of this book, call our customer service department at **(800) 638-0672** or fax orders to **(800) 447-8438.** For other book
services, including chapter reprints and large quantity sales, ask for the
Special Sales department.

Customers in Canada should call **(800) 268-4178** or fax **(905) 470-6780**.
For all other calls originating outside of the United States, please call **(410)
528-4223** or fax **(410) 528-8550**.

Visit Williams & Wilkins on the Internet: **http://www.wwilkins.com** or
contact our customer service department at custserv@wwilkins.com.
Williams & Wilkins customer service representatives are available from 8:30
am to 6:00 pm, EST, Monday through Friday, for telephone access.

This atlas was founded by Johannes Sobotta, former Professor of Anatomy
and Director of the Anatomical Institute of the University of Bonn, Germany.

German Edition:
Editorial: Dr. med. Dorothea Schneiderbanger, Eva Zielonka
Production: Renate Hausdorf, Peter Mazzetti
Cover Design: Dieter Vollendorf
Cover Illustration: Ulrike Brugger

German Editions:
1st Edition: 1904-1907 J. F. Lehmanns Verlag, München
2nd–11th Editions: 1913-1944 J. F. Lehmanns Verlag, München
12th Edition: 1948 and following editions: Urban & Schwarzenberg,
    München
13th Edition: 1953
14th Edition: 1956
15th Edition: 1957
16th Edition: 1967 (Vol. 1: ISBN 3-541-02816-5)
               (Vol. 2: ISBN 3-541-02826-2)
17th Edition: 1972 (Vol. 1: ISBN 3-541-02817-3)
               (Vol. 2: ISBN 3-541-02827-0)
18th Edition: 1982 (Vol. 1: ISBN 3-541-02818-1)
               (Vol. 2: ISBN 3-541-02828-9)
19th Edition: 1988 (Vol. 1: ISBN 3-541-02819-X)
               (Vol. 2: ISBN 3-541-02829-7)
20th Edition: 1993 (Vol. 1: ISBN 3-541-17360-2)
               (Vol. 2: ISBN 3-541-17370-X)

Foreign Editions:
Arabic Edition: Modern Technical Center, Damascus

Previous English Edition (with nomenclature in English): Urban &
Schwarzenberg, Baltimore

English Edition (with nomenclature in Latin): Urban & Schwarzenberg,
München

French Edition: Atlas d'Anatomie Humaine, Tec & Doc Lavoisier, Paris

Greek Edition: Gregory Parissianos, Athens

Indonesian Edition: Atlas Anatomi Manusia, Penerbit Buku Kedokteran EGC,
Jakarta

Italian Edition: Atlante di Anatomia Umana, UTET, Torino

Korean Edition: Panmun Book Company, Seoul

Japanese Edition: Igaku Shoin Ltd., Tokyo

Portuguese Edition (with nomenclature in Portuguese): Atlas de Anatomie
Humana, Editora Guanabara Koogan, Rio de Janeiro

Portuguese Edition (with nomenclature in Latin): Atlas de Anatomie
Humana, Editora Guanabara Koogan, Rio de Janeiro

Spanish Edition: Atlas de Anatomia Humana, Editorial Medica
Panamericana, Buenos Aires/Madrid

Turkish Edition: Insan Anatomisi Atlasi, Beta Basim Yayim Dagitim, Istanbul

96 97 98 99 00
1 2 3 4 5 6 7 8 9 10

Contents

Preface

In 1903, J. Sobotta set out to create an atlas designed for practical use by both medical students and physicians. With the first edition, he presented a series of topographic overviews, supplemented with tables, that facilitated recognition at a glance of anatomical relationships in dissected specimens. Prof. Sobotta's original goal remained that of the atlas's subsequent editors, H. Becher, H. Ferner, and J. Staubesand, thereby assuring that "Sobotta" would become the basic teaching atlas for generations of medical students and the definitive anatomical reference work for physicians.

The original concept—still valid today—has further developed its teaching component with strong emphasis on current methodology and on depiction of the direct relationship of anatomy to clinical practice. This intention is exemplified by this edition's numerous functional schematics of joints, its considerable increase in the illustration of sectional anatomy, and the many illustrations produced by modern imaging techniques (ultrasound, computed tomography, magnetic resonance imaging). Clinically important variations of arteries are demonstrated both with anatomic diagrams and with arteriograms. Endoscopic surveys and color photographs of surgical procedures expand many of the illustrations of organs, thereby permitting comparison with operative sites in live subjects. Taken together, the illustrations of surface anatomy and the numerous references in captions and text to practical usage and to clinical terminology advance the concept of the "interlocking" of preclinical and clinical subject matter that is called for in today's medical curricula.

A new opening chapter entitled "General Anatomy" provides a survey of the essentials of anatomical organization. While this predominantly schematic presentation is intended to be a learning aid, it is also intended to help maintain a sense of the organism as a whole, despite the considerable anatomical detail.

For ease in orientation, captioning has been standardized; leader lines for many illustrations have also been revised. The atlas now includes a total of 1495 illustrations. The 6th edition of the *Nomina Anatomica* (1989) has formed the basis for the illustration labeling, and its nomenclature has been adopted as much as possible.

With the exception of discussions about the general concept of the atlas and mutual correction of one another's efforts, the editors have worked separately on individual chapters, with the work divided as follows:

R. Putz: General anatomy, upper limb, brain, eye, ear, back, lower limb;
R. Pabst: Head, neck, thoracic and abdominal walls, thoracic, abdominal, and pelvic viscera.

The inclusion of the large number of new figures is the result of the extraordinary capability of the following medical illustrators: Ulrike Brugger, Rüdiger Himmelhan, Sonja Klebe, and Horst Ruß. Many innovative ideas incorporated in the atlas originated from their suggestions, and it is also to their credit that the classic quality of the illustrations has been retained. We also owe a debt of gratitude to a number of colleagues who made clinical illustrations available to us (see Acknowledgments).

It is not possible in the space of this Preface to acknowledge the many ideas shared with us by colleagues, both anatomists and clinicians, as well as those coming from our medical students. Nor is it possible to acknowledge individually the contributions of all those at our respective institutes and at the publishers who have been involved with this 20th edition. Nonetheless, everyone who helped—whether by specimen preparation, manuscript preparation, or proofreading—has our heartfelt thanks. We also wish to thank our families for their forebearance during this time-consuming project.

A standard work such as "Sobotta" lives from its dialogue with the reader. We therefore make a request of all users of this edition—medical students, clinicians, and especially academic anatomists—that they pass on to us critiques or suggestions on the new format of this atlas.

Munich and Hanover, September 1993
R. PUTZ AND R. PABST

Preface to the 12th English Edition

As a research scientist, it has been my privilege to translate both the previous English edition and the present edition of this seminal work. Knowledge of anatomical structure forms the basis for advances in biomedical sciences and clinical medicine. At all levels of scientific inquiry, from the cellular and molecular to the organismic, the organizational principles of anatomy are essential. Though as scientists in this last decade of the 20th century we are blessed with an ever increasing array of new imaging and communication techniques which facilitate the comprehension of anatomy, it is my opinion that an anatomical atlas of the quality of "Sobotta" is irreplaceable in the learning process. Terminology also evolves—as is apparent in the increasing anglicization of Latin terms for modern English usage. With the 6th edition of the *Nomina Anatomica* (Churchill Livingstone, 1989) and Professor Carmine Clemente's edition of *Gray's Anatomy* (Lea & Febiger, 1985) and his atlas *Anatomy* (Urban & Schwarzenberg, 1987), as sources, I have striven to continue to standardize and yet modernize the terminology.

I am grateful to my colleagues in the Department of Neurobiology at UCLA for their knowledgeable input. In particular, I owe special thanks to Professors Clemente and Ynez O'Neill. Once again I must express my appreciation to the publishers, first Lea & Febiger and then Williams & Wilkins, for entrusting me with this project and to their excellent staff, in particular, Ms. Harriet Felscher, the superb editor, who assisted in its completion. I am eternally grateful to my parents for maintaining a bilingual home and for their encouragement in the pursuit of foreign languages in the Cleveland public school system's model program.

Translation of this edition would not have been possible without the invaluable contributions of Kenneth C. Taylor, my husband and partner in all aspects of this project.

Anna Newman Taylor
Los Angeles, California

Illustrations and Artists

The basis for the use of four-color illustrations in this atlas is educational: color is used to strengthen contrast and to differentiate structures otherwise difficult to isolate visually. Thus, color for the various tissue types (tendons, cartilage, bones, muscle) and vessels (arteries, veins, lymphatics) and nerves are different in appearance from living or dead tissue and from that of the preserved cadaver. Here arteries are red, veins are blue, nerves yellow; lymphatic vessels and nodes are generally shown as green.

This edition consists of illustrations created by K. Hajek, Prof. E. Lepier, H. v. Eickstedt, K. Endtresser, J. Kosanke, J.v. Marchtaler, J. Dimes, U. Brugger, N. Lechenbauer, L. Schnellbächer, and K. Schuhmacher whose original collaboration under Prof. Sobotta and under the book's later editors, Profs. Becher, Ferner, and Staubesand laid the groundwork for the entire illustrative body of the book. Carrying on this tradition with new illustrations for the present edition are illustrators Ulrike Brugger, Rüdiger Himmelhan, Sonja Klebe, and Horst Ruß.

The following figure numbers list new illustrations developed for this edition as well as new drawings

of existing illustrations that incorporate important updates:

U. Brugger
1a-c, 2 a and b, 11a-d, 18-24, 28, 29, 30, 37-44, 46, 47, 48, 49, 143a-c, 145a-d, 263, 268, 269a-f, 271a-d, 282, 289, 293, 295, 297, 308, 312, 316, 318, 319, 325, 328, 331, 336, 370, 371a-d, 382, 383, 384, 385, 386, 415a-d, 418a-c, 432, 434, 437 444, 446, 447, 474, 451-460, 465, 469, 470a-c, 432, 434, 437, 444, 446, 447, 474, 451-460, 465, 469, 470a-g, 474, 475, 478-482, 491-496, 499, 506, 508, 509, 511, 515, 516, 517, 520, 521, 536, 539, 540, 545-559, 574, 576, 578, 579, 637, 638, 653, 660, 675, 676, 677
Diagrams for Figures 424, 425, 499, 515, 544-562, 564, 655, 656, 661, 662 and 663
R. Himmelhan
340-343, 362-365
S. Klebe
77, 122, 125, 126, 153, 157, 188, 212, 213, 231a-d, 256a and b, 276-279
Diagrams for Figures 101, 102, 103, 158/159, 212, 213, 275, 276, 278, 279
H. Ruß
473

Acknowledgments

We are extremely grateful to the following clinical colleagues who contributed the ultrasound, computed tomography, and magnetic resonance images as well as the endoscopic photographs and color photographs of surgical operations:

Prof. Altaras, Center for Radiology, University of Giessen
(Figs. 934, 948, 949)
Dr. Baumeister, Division of Radiology, University of Freiburg
(Fig. 1063)
Prof. Daniel, Division of Cardiology, Hannover Medical School
(Figs. 838, 839, 840, 903)
Prof. Düker, Radiology Division of the Dental, Oral, and Facial Clinic, University of Freiburg
(Fig. 175)
Dr. Ehrenheim, Nuclear Medicine, Hannover Medical School
(Figs. 906, 1114a, b, 1124a, b)
Prof. Galanski, Dr. Schäfer, Diagnostic Radiology I, Hannover Medical School
(Figs. 75, 76, 813a, b, 864, 899, 928, 1109, 1117, 1120, 1122)
Prof. Gebel, Division of Gastroenterology and Hepatology, Hannover Medical School
(Figs. 264a, b, 881, 908, 919a, b, 929, 936a, 944, 945, 950, 959, 960, 995, 1012, 1054)
Dr. Goei, Radiology, Heerlen, Netherlands
(Figs. 1080, 1081) (with permission: Radiology 1989;173:137–141)
Dr. Greeven, St. Elisabeth Hospital, Neuwied
(Figs. 158, 159, 1151)
Prof. von der Hardt, Children's Clinic, Hannover Medical School
(Fig. 868b)
Dr. Hennig, Radiology Division, University of Freiburg
(Fig. 519)
Prof. Jonas, Urology, Hannover Medical School
(Figs. 1019a, b, 1020)
Prof. Kunze, Children's Polyclinic, University of Münich
(Figs. 14-17)
Dr. Laubert, ENT Clinic, Hannover Medical School
(Figs. 160, 205, 206)
Prof. Pfeifer, Radiology Division of the City Surgical Clinic, University of Münich
(Figs. 299, 300, 311, 313, 725-728, 764-767, 1168, 1199, 1200, 1229, 1230)

Prof. Ravelli, Emeritus, Institute for Anatomy, University of Innsbruck
(Fig. 723)
Dr. Rau, Emeritus, Radiology Division, University of Freiburg
(Figs. 851, 852, 863)
Prof. Reich, Clinic for Oral-Facial Surgery, University of Bonn
(Figs. 128, 129)
Dr. B. Sommer and M. Bauer, PD, Radiologists, Munich
(Figs. 560-564, 628, 748, 1203-1205, 1333)
Dr. Scheibe, Surgical Division, Rosman Hospital, Breisach
(Figs. 1202a-c)
Prof. Schillinger, Women's Clinic, University of Freiburg
(Figs. 1041, 1042, 1043)
Prof. Schlösser, Center for Women's Medicine, Hannover Medical School
(Figs. 1040a, b, 1049, 1051a, b, 1088b)
Prof. Schumacher, Neuroradiology, Radiology Division, University of Freiburg
(Fig. 438)
Prof. Stotz, Inner City Orthopedic Polyclinic, University of Münich
(Fig. 1162)
Prof. Emer.Vogel, Inner City Radiologic Polyclinic, University of Münich
(Figs. 431, 433, 609, 610)
Prof. Vollrath, ENT Clinic, Monchengladbach
(Fig. 239, 240, 241)
Prof. Wagner †, Diagnostic Radiology II, Hannover Medical School
(Figs. 889, 983, 986, 989, 992, 1058)
Prof. Wenz, Radiology Division, University of Freiburg
(Fig. 724)
Dr. Willfür, Abdominal and Transplant Surgery, Hannover Medical School
(Fig. 970)
Dr. Wimmer, Radiology Division, University of Freiburg
(Fig. 755)

Additional illustrations were obtained from the following texts:

Birkner R. Typical Radiographs of the Skeleton. Munich, Vienna, Baltimore: U&S, 1990.
(Fig. 1169)
Wicke L. Atlas of Radiologic Anatomy, 3rd Ed. Munich, Vienna, Baltimore: U&S, 1985.
(Figs. 880a, b)

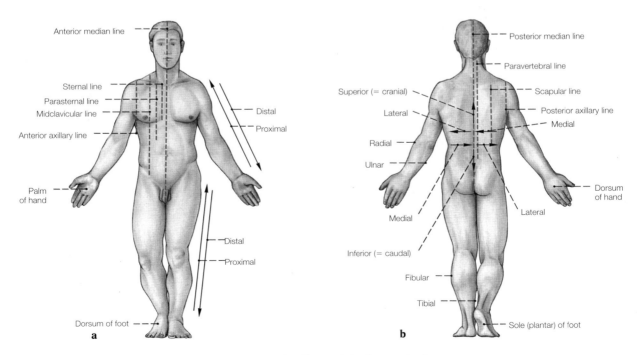

1 Sagittal plane
2 Median plane
3 Coronal (frontal) plane
4 Horizontal (transverse) plane

5 Sagittal axis
6 Transverse axis
7 Longitudinal axis

Fig. 1 a–c Planes and axes of the human body.

a Sagittal plane, sagittal and longitudinal axes
b Horizontal plane (= transverse plane), transverse and sagittal axes

c Coronal plane (= frontal plane), longitudinal and transverse axes

Anterior median line

Sternal line
Parasternal line
Midclavicular line
Anterior axillary line

Palm of hand

Distal
Proximal

Distal
Proximal

Dorsum of foot

a

Posterior median line
Paravertebral line
Scapular line
Posterior axillary line
Medial

Superior (= cranial)
Lateral

Radial
Ulnar

Medial

Inferior (= caudal)

Fibular

Tibial

Dorsum of hand

Lateral

Sole (plantar) of foot

b

Fig. 2 a, b Orientation lines of the human body and terms of direction and position.
a Anterior (= ventral) view.
b Posterior (= dorsal) view.

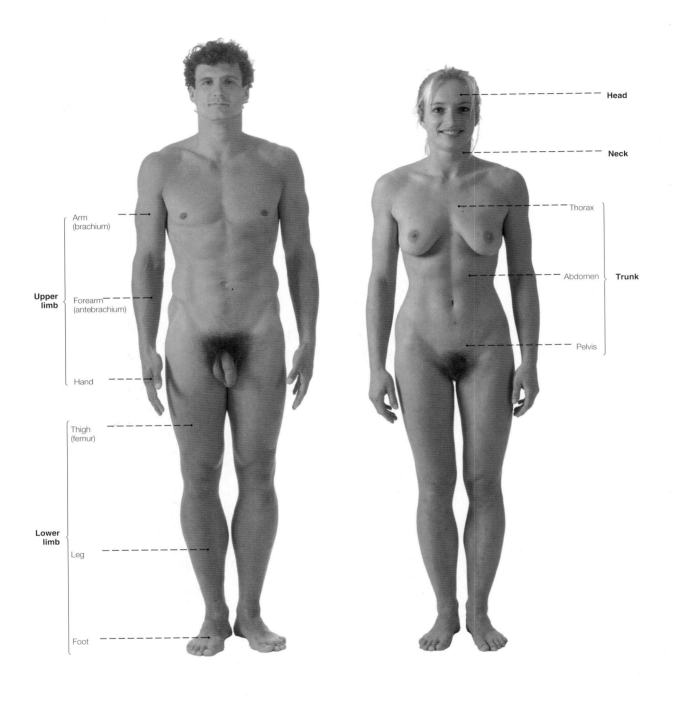

Fig. 3 Surface anatomy of the male, anterior view.

Fig. 4 Surface anatomy of the female, anterior view.

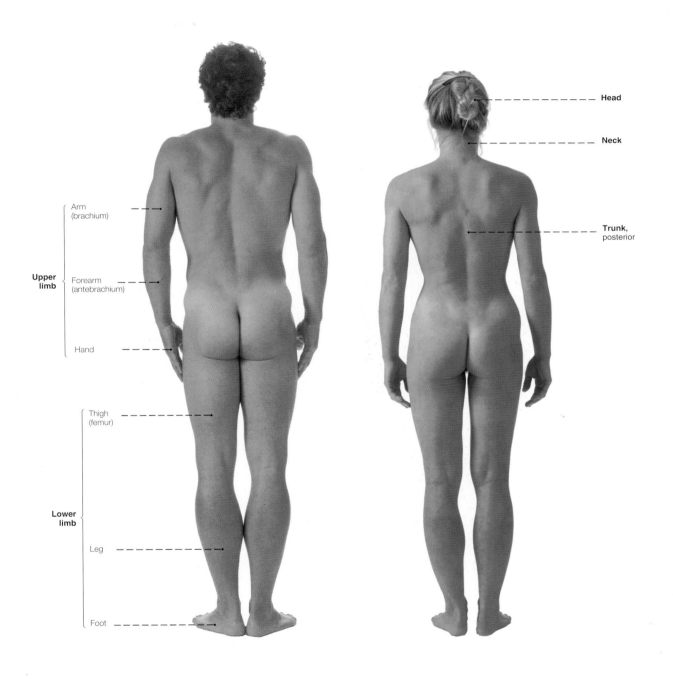

Fig. 5 Surface anatomy of the male, posterior view.

Fig. 6 Surface anatomy of the female, posterior view.

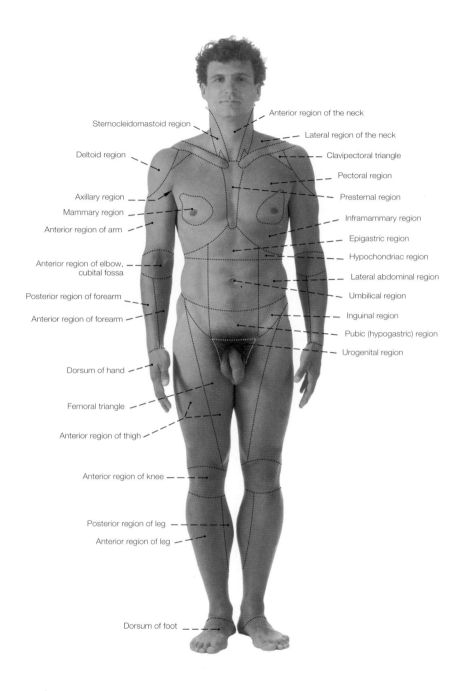

Sternocleidomastoid region

Deltoid region

Axillary region

Mammary region

Anterior region of arm

Anterior region of elbow, cubital fossa

Posterior region of forearm

Anterior region of forearm

Dorsum of hand

Femoral triangle

Anterior region of thigh

Anterior region of knee

Posterior region of leg

Anterior region of leg

Dorsum of foot

Anterior region of the neck

Lateral region of the neck

Clavipectoral triangle

Pectoral region

Presternal region

Inframammary region

Epigastric region

Hypochondriac region

Lateral abdominal region

Umbilical region

Inguinal region

Pubic (hypogastric) region

Urogenital region

Fig. 7 Regions of the human body, anterior view.

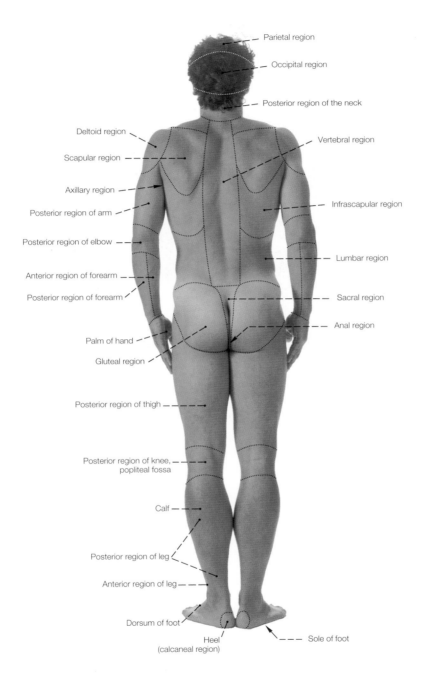

Fig. 8 Regions of the human body, posterior view.

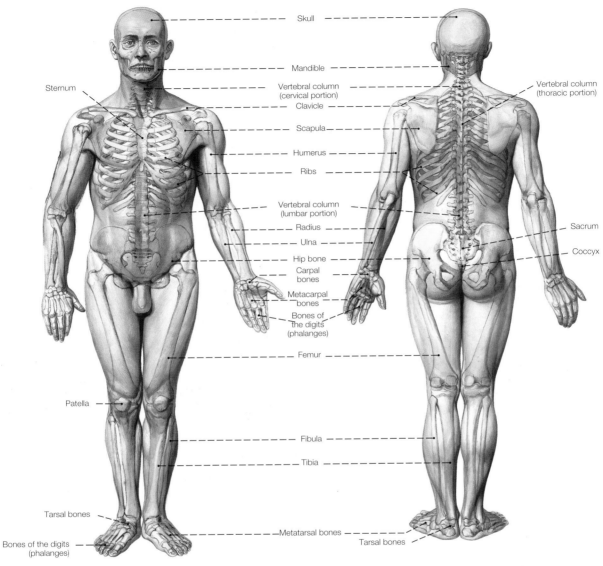

Fig. 9 The skeleton, anterior view.

Fig. 10 The skeleton, posterior view.

Regions of the human body

> **Head**
>
> **Neck**
>
> **Trunk**
> Thorax
> Abdomen
> Pelvis
>
> **Upper limb**
> Shoulder girdle
> Arm
>
> **Lower limb**
> Pelvic girdle
> Leg

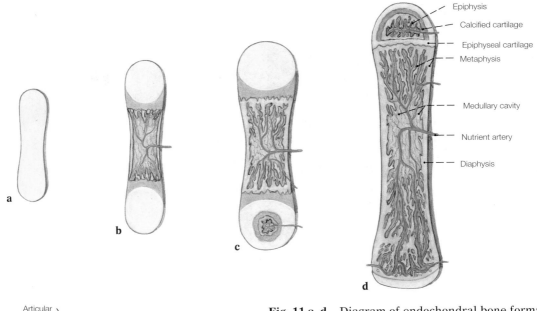

Epiphysis

Calcified cartilage

Epiphyseal cartilage

Metaphysis

Medullary cavity

Nutrient artery

Diaphysis

Fig. 11 a–d Diagram of endochondral bone formation
a Cartilage precursor of the later bone
b Formation of a periosteal bone collar and subsequent penetration of the calcified cartilage matrix of the diaphysis by vascular mesenchyme, appearance of the center of ossification in the diaphysis
c Age-dependent appearance of endochondral ossification centers in the epiphyses and formation of cartilaginous epiphyseal growth plates (see Fig. 331)
d Age-dependent synostosis of the epiphyseal plates (see Fig. 331)

◀ **Fig. 12** Structure of a long bone, exemplified in a longitudinal section of the humerus. The epiphyseal lines are barely visible.

Articular cartilage

Head of humerus; Spongy (cancellous) bone; Red bone marrow

(Proximal extremity)

Epiphyseal line

Metaphysis (proximal)

Shaft of humerus; Compact bone

Nutrient artery

Nutrient canal

Shaft

Periosteum

Medullary cavity; Yellow bone marrow

Metaphysis (distal)

Olecranon fossa

Lateral epicondyle

(Distal extremity)

Articular cartilage

Spongy (cancellous) bone; Red bone marrow

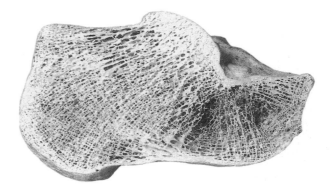

Fig. 13 The spongiform architecture of bone, exemplified in a longitudinal section of the calcaneus. The arch-like configuration of the trabeculae is indicative of flexing capability.

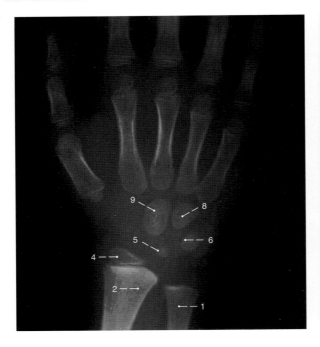

Fig. 14 Radiograph of the right hand of a 4½-year-old male child, dorsopalmar (PA) projection.

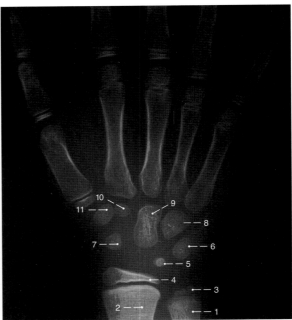

Fig. 15 Radiograph of the right hand of a 7-year-old male child, dorsopalmar (PA) projection.

1 Ulna, diaphysis
2 Radius, diaphysis
3 Ulna, distal epiphysis

4 Radius, distal epiphysis
5 Lunate bone
6 Triquetral bone

7 Scaphoid bone
8 Hamate bone
9 Capitate bone

10 Trapezoid bone
11 Trapezium bone

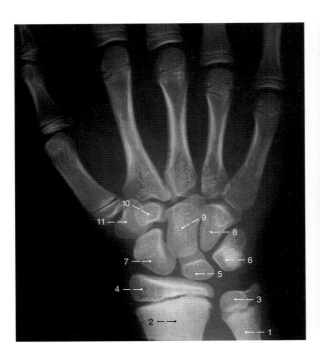

Fig. 16 Radiograph of the right hand of an 11-year-old female adolescent, dorsopalmar (PA) projection.

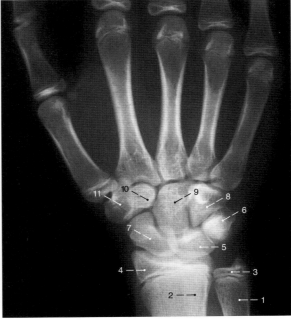

Fig. 17 Radiograph of the right hand of a 13-year-old male adolescent, dorsopalmar (PA) projection.

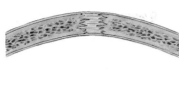

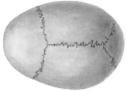

Fig. 18 Fibrous joint, exemplified by the sutures of the skull.

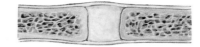

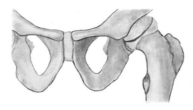

Fig. 19 Cartilaginous joint, exemplified by the pubic symphysis.

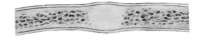

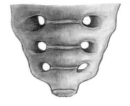

Fig. 20 Osseous joint, exemplified by the sacrum.

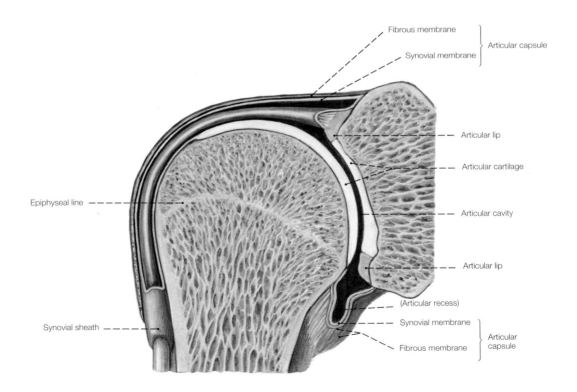

Fig. 21 Synovial joint, exemplified by the shoulder joint. Section in the scapular plane.

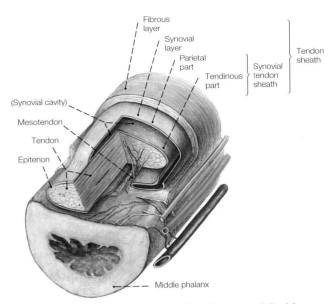

1 Line of muscle action
2 Lever arm of muscle
3 Axis of rotation of joint

(Origin)
Fascia
Head
1
Belly
Tendon (Insertion)
2
3

Fig. 22 Organizational principle of skeletal muscle, exemplified by the brachialis muscle.

Fibrous layer
Synovial layer
Parietal part
Tendinous part
Synovial tendon sheath
Tendon sheath
(Synovial cavity)
Mesotendon
Tendon
Epitenon
Middle phalanx

Fig. 23 Structure of a tendon sheath, exemplified by a finger.

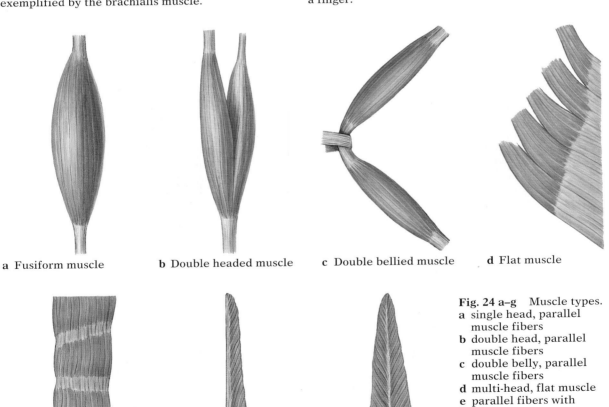

a Fusiform muscle   **b** Double headed muscle   **c** Double bellied muscle   **d** Flat muscle

e Intersected muscle   **f** Unipennate muscle   **g** Bipennate muscle

Fig. 24 a–g Muscle types.
a single head, parallel muscle fibers
b double head, parallel muscle fibers
c double belly, parallel muscle fibers
d multi-head, flat muscle
e parallel fibers with tendinous intersections, multi-belly muscle
f unipennate muscle
g bipennate muscle

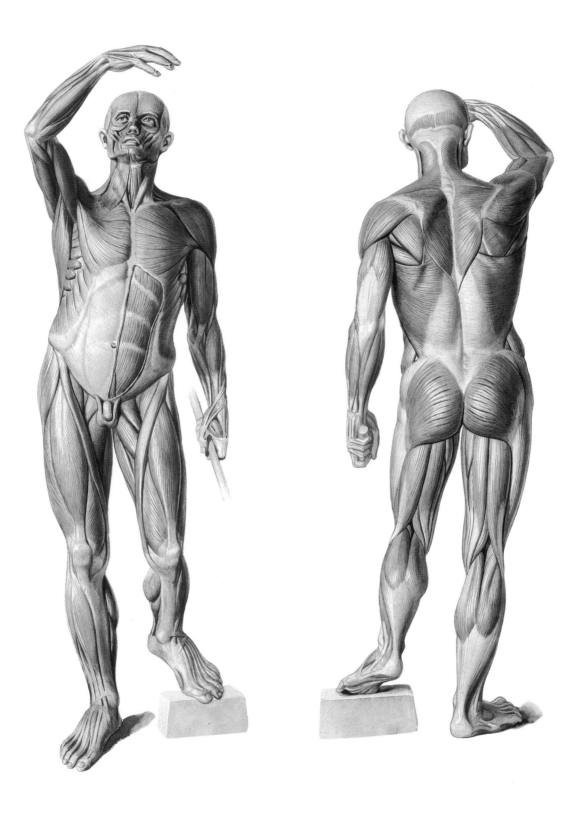

Fig. 25 Survey of the skeletal musculature, anterior view.

Fig. 26 Survey of the skeletal musculature, posterior view.

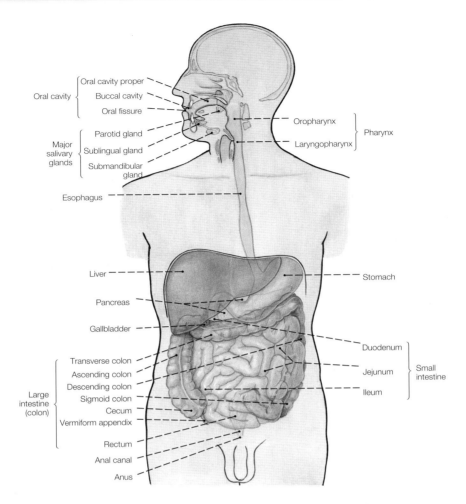

Fig. 27 Survey of the digestive system, medial and anterior aspects.

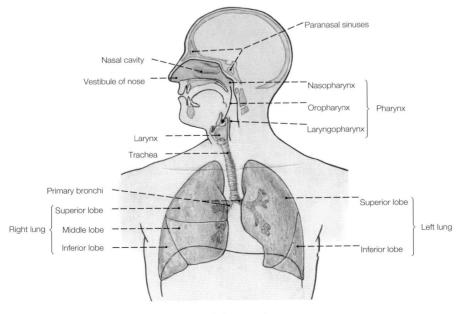

Fig. 28 Survey of the respiratory system, medial and anterior aspects.

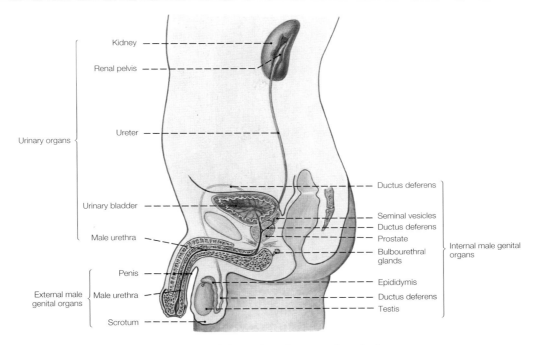

Fig. 29 Survey of the male urinary and genital organs, medial aspect.

Kidney

Renal pelvis

Urinary organs

Ureter

Urinary bladder

Male urethra

External male genital organs

Penis

Male urethra

Scrotum

Ductus deferens

Seminal vesicles

Ductus deferens

Prostate

Bulbourethral glands

Internal male genital organs

Epididymis

Ductus deferens

Testis

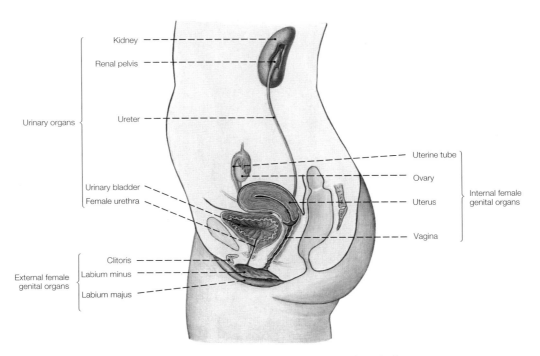

Fig. 30 Survey of the female urinary and genital organs, medial aspect.

Kidney

Renal pelvis

Urinary organs

Ureter

Urinary bladder

Female urethra

External female genital organs

Clitoris

Labium minus

Labium majus

Uterine tube

Ovary

Internal female genital organs

Uterus

Vagina

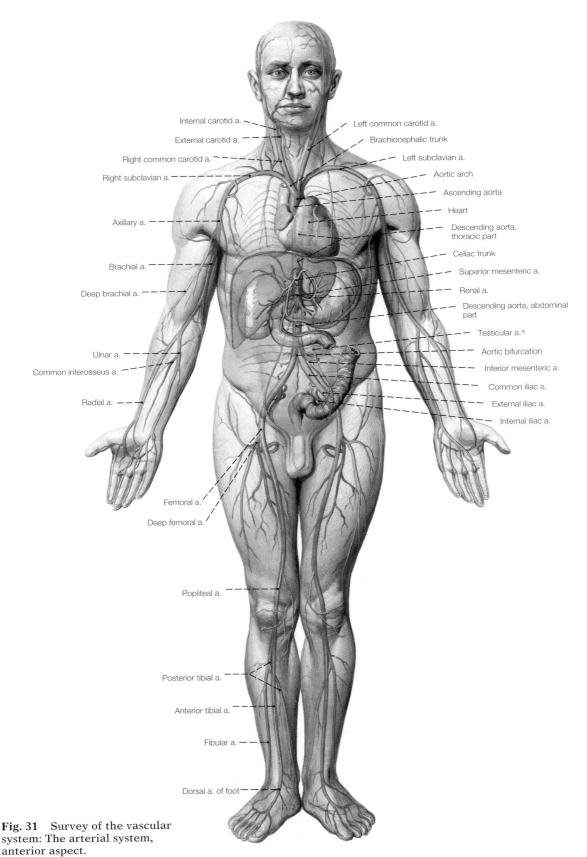

Internal carotid a.
External carotid a.
Right common carotid a.
Right subclavian a.
Axillary a.
Brachial a.
Deep brachial a.
Ulnar a.
Common interosseus a.
Radial a.
Femoral a.
Deep femoral a.
Popliteal a.
Posterior tibial a.
Anterior tibial a.
Fibular a.
Dorsal a. of foot

Left common carotid a.
Brachiocephalic trunk
Left subclavian a.
Aortic arch
Ascending aorta
Heart
Descending aorta, thoracic part
Celiac trunk
Superior mesenteric a.
Renal a.
Descending aorta, abdominal part
Testicular a.*
Aortic bifurcation
Inferior mesenteric a.
Common iliac a.
External iliac a.
Internal iliac a.

Fig. 31 Survey of the vascular system: The arterial system, anterior aspect.

* In the female: Ovarian a.

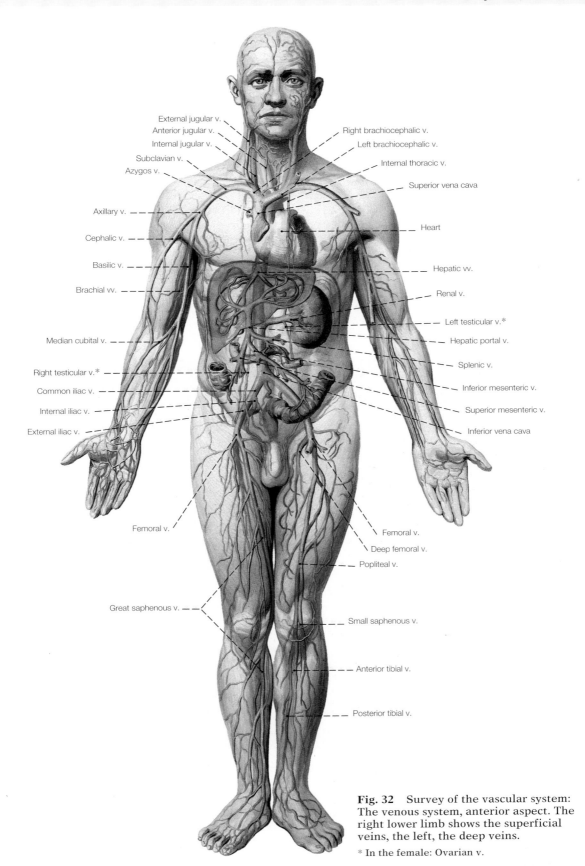

External jugular v.

Anterior jugular v.

Internal jugular v.

Subclavian v.

Azygos v.

Axillary v.

Cephalic v.

Basilic v.

Brachial vv.

Median cubital v.

Right testicular v.*

Common iliac v.

Internal iliac v.

External iliac v.

Femoral v.

Great saphenous v.

Right brachiocephalic v.

Left brachiocephalic v.

Internal thoracic v.

Superior vena cava

Heart

Hepatic vv.

Renal v.

Left testicular v.*

Hepatic portal v.

Splenic v.

Inferior mesenteric v.

Superior mesenteric v.

Inferior vena cava

Femoral v.

Deep femoral v.

Popliteal v.

Small saphenous v.

Anterior tibial v.

Posterior tibial v.

Fig. 32 Survey of the vascular system: The venous system, anterior aspect. The right lower limb shows the superficial veins, the left, the deep veins.

* In the female: Ovarian v.

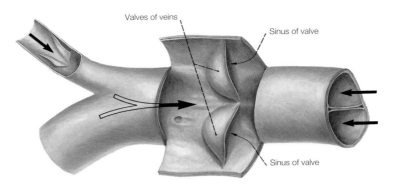

Fig. 33 Function of the venous valves. The arrow pointing to the right indicates the normal direction of blood flow. Regurgitation (arrows pointing to the left) causes the valves to close.

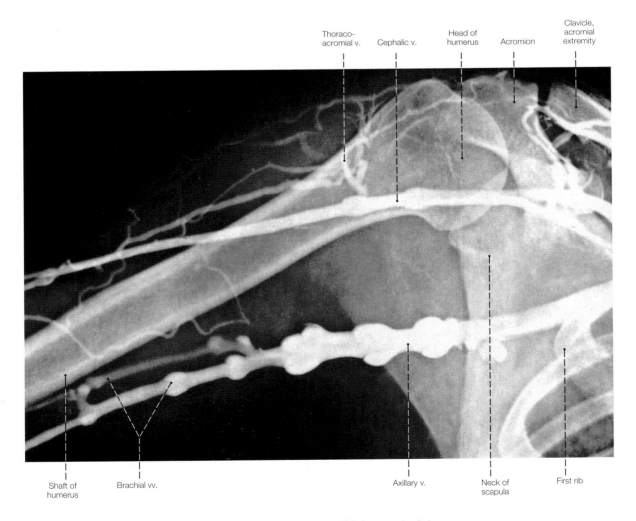

Fig. 34 Radiograph (veno- or phlebogram) of the brachial, axillary, and cephalic veins and some of their tributaries, AP projection. Note the succession of valvular segments clearly visible in the axillary vein.

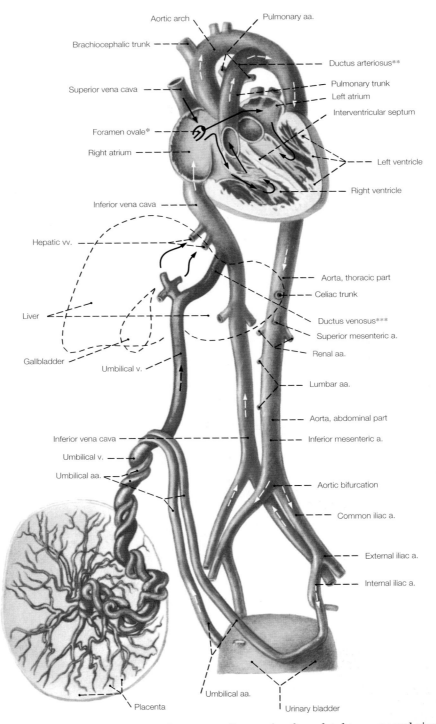

Aortic arch

Brachiocephalic trunk

Superior vena cava

Foramen ovale*

Right atrium

Inferior vena cava

Hepatic vv.

Liver

Gallbladder

Umbilical v.

Inferior vena cava

Umbilical v.

Umbilical aa.

Pulmonary aa.

Ductus arteriosus**

Pulmonary trunk

Left atrium

Interventricular septum

Left ventricle

Right ventricle

Aorta, thoracic part

Celiac trunk

Ductus venosus***

Superior mesenteric a.

Renal aa.

Lumbar aa.

Aorta, abdominal part

Inferior mesenteric a.

Aortic bifurcation

Common iliac a.

External iliac a.

Internal iliac a.

Umbilical aa.

Placenta

Urinary bladder

Fig. 35 Schema of the fetal circulation. Vessels carrying mixed arterial and venous blood are colored violet. Arrows indicate the direction of blood flow (cf. C.D. CLEMENTE. *Gray's Anatomy*. Lea & Febiger, 1985:619–621).

* Communication between right and left atria
** Communication between the pulmonary trunk and arch of aorta
*** Communication between umbilical v. and inferior vena cava

Conversion from fetal to postnatal circulation:

* The valve-like connection between the right and left atria via the foramen ovale is passively closed when breathing commences.

** The ductus arteriosus (BOTALLI), on the other hand, closes only during the first month of life as its lumen gradually becomes obliterated.

*** The ductus venous (ARANTI) is obliterated after birth and becomes the lig. venosum in the portal area of the liver.

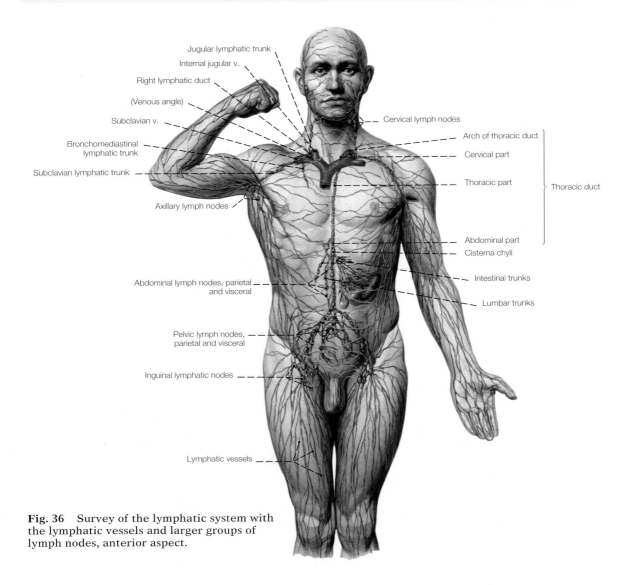

Jugular lymphatic trunk

Internal jugular v.

Right lymphatic duct

(Venous angle)

Subclavian v.

Bronchomediastinal lymphatic trunk

Subclavian lymphatic trunk

Axillary lymph nodes

Abdominal lymph nodes, parietal and visceral

Pelvic lymph nodes, parietal and visceral

Inguinal lymphatic nodes

Lymphatic vessels

Cervical lymph nodes

Arch of thoracic duct

Cervical part

Thoracic part

Thoracic duct

Abdominal part

Cisterna chyli

Intestinal trunks

Lumbar trunks

Fig. 36 Survey of the lymphatic system with the lymphatic vessels and larger groups of lymph nodes, anterior aspect.

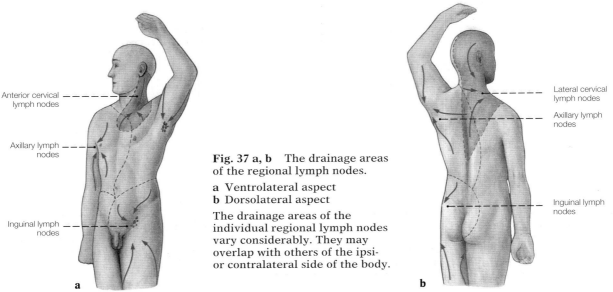

Anterior cervical lymph nodes

Axillary lymph nodes

Inguinal lymph nodes

Lateral cervical lymph nodes

Axillary lymph nodes

Inguinal lymph nodes

Fig. 37 a, b The drainage areas of the regional lymph nodes.

a Ventrolateral aspect
b Dorsolateral aspect

The drainage areas of the individual regional lymph nodes vary considerably. They may overlap with others of the ipsi- or contralateral side of the body.

a

b

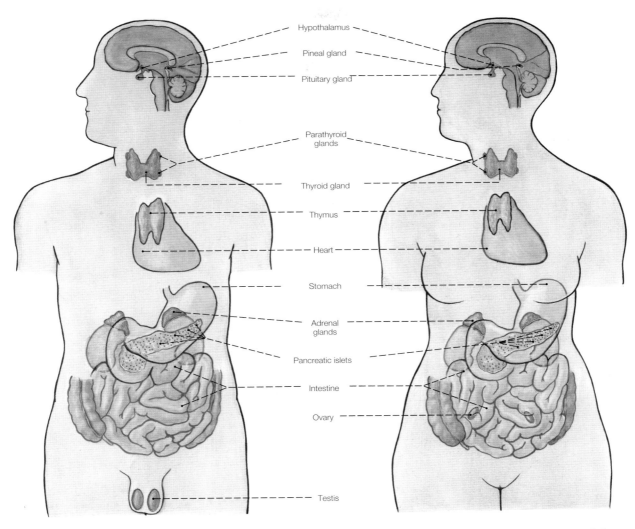

Hypothalamus

Pineal gland

Pituitary gland

Parathyroid glands

Thyroid gland

Thymus

Heart

Stomach

Adrenal glands

Pancreatic islets

Intestine

Ovary

Testis

Fig. 38 The endocrine system of the male, anterior aspect.

Fig. 39 The endocrine system of the female, anterior aspect.

In addition to those endocrine organs (i.e., pituitary, pineal, thyroid, and parathyroid glands, pancreatic islets and testis/ovary) whose primary function is hormone production, other organs are also endocrinologically active. Among the latter are the gastrointestinal mucosa (APUD cells), the kidneys, the right atrium of the heart, etc. Strictly speaking, hormones are produced by virtually all organs.

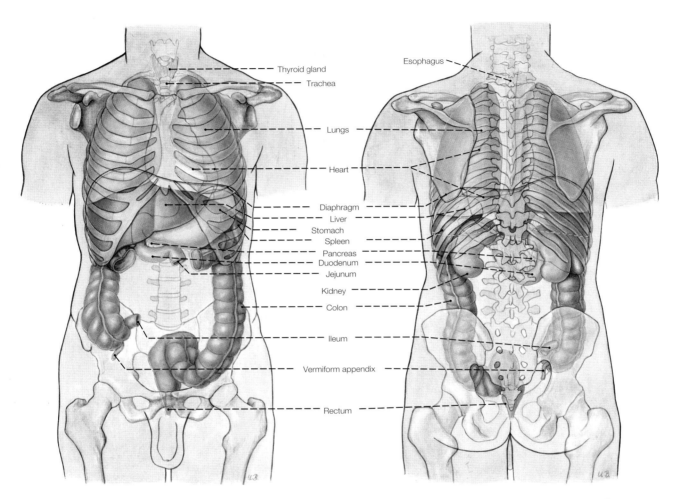

Fig. 40   Projection of the viscera onto the surface of the body, anterior aspect.

Fig. 41   Projection of the viscera onto the surface of the body, posterior aspect.

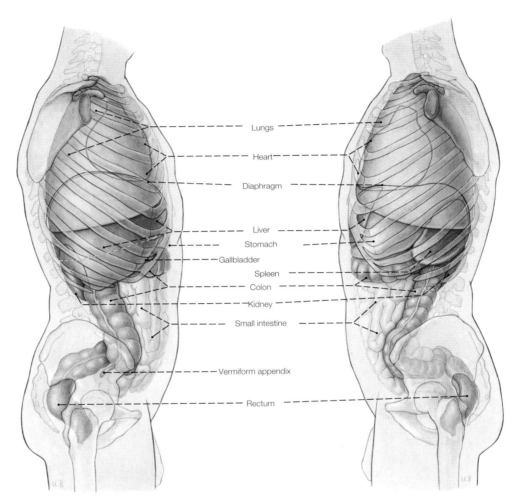

Lungs

Heart

Diaphragm

Liver

Stomach

Gallbladder

Spleen

Colon

Kidney

Small intestine

Vermiform appendix

Rectum

Fig. 42   Projection of the internal organs onto the body surface, viewed from the right side.

Fig. 43   Projection of the internal organs onto the body surface, viewed from the left side.

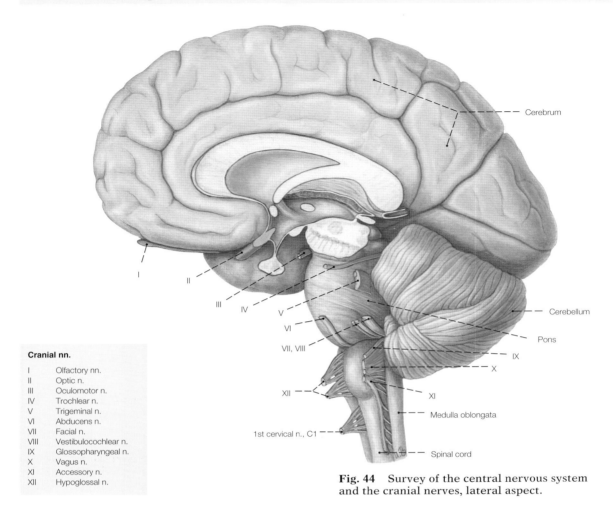

Cranial nn.

I	Olfactory nn.
II	Optic n.
III	Oculomotor n.
IV	Trochlear n.
V	Trigeminal n.
VI	Abducens n.
VII	Facial n.
VIII	Vestibulocochlear n.
IX	Glossopharyngeal n.
X	Vagus n.
XI	Accessory n.
XII	Hypoglossal n.

Fig. 44 Survey of the central nervous system and the cranial nerves, lateral aspect.

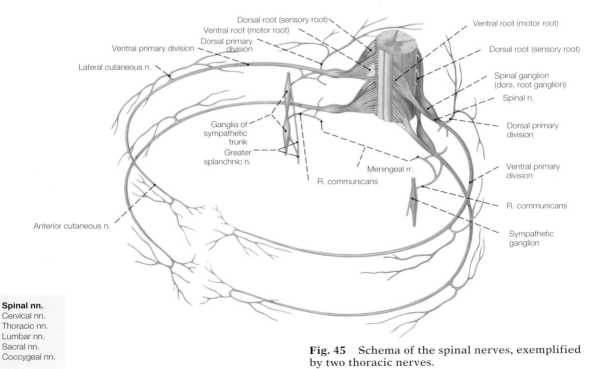

Spinal nn.
Cervical nn.
Thoracic nn.
Lumbar nn.
Sacral nn.
Coccygeal nn.

Fig. 45 Schema of the spinal nerves, exemplified by two thoracic nerves.

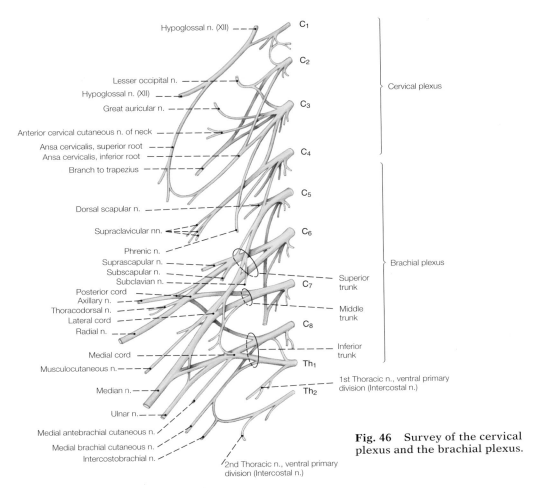

Hypoglossal n. (XII)
C_1
C_2
Lesser occipital n.
Hypoglossal n. (XII)
C_3
Great auricular n.
Anterior cervical cutaneous n. of neck
Ansa cervicalis, superior root
Ansa cervicalis, inferior root
C_4
Branch to trapezius
C_5
Dorsal scapular n.
C_6
Supraclavicular nn.
Phrenic n.
Suprascapular n.
Subscapular n.
Subclavian n.
C_7
Superior trunk
Posterior cord
Axillary n.
Thoracodorsal n.
Lateral cord
Radial n.
C_8
Middle trunk
Medial cord
Musculocutaneous n.
Th_1
Inferior trunk
Median n.
Th_2
1st Thoracic n., ventral primary division (Intercostal n.)
Ulnar n.
Medial antebrachial cutaneous n.
Medial brachial cutaneous n.
Intercostobrachial n.
2nd Thoracic n., ventral primary division (Intercostal n.)

Cervical plexus
Brachial plexus

Fig. 46 Survey of the cervical plexus and the brachial plexus.

Branches of the Cervical Plexus and the Brachial Plexus

Cervical Plexus (Cervical nn. C1–C4, ventral primary divisions)	Brachial Plexus (Cervical nn. C4/5–thoracic n. T1, ventral primary divisions)
Ansa cervicalis 　Superior root 　Inferior root Cutaneous branches 　Lesser occipital n. 　Great auricular n. 　Anterior cutaneous n. of neck 　Supraclavicular nn., medial, intermediate 　　and lateral Muscular branches (longus colli m., longus capitis m., rectus capitis anterior and lateralis mm., intertransversarii mm., trapezius m., levator scapulae m., scalenus medius m.) Phrenic n.	Supraclavicular part: 　Superior trunk → 　Middle trunk　→　} Anterior and posterior divisions 　Inferior trunk　→ 　Dorsal scapular n. 　Suprascapular n. 　Subscapular nn. (Frequently from post. cord) 　Subclavian n. 　Long thoracic n. 　Pectoral nn. (frequently from lat. and med. cords) 　Thoracodorsal n. (frequently from post. cord) 　Muscular branches (Longus colli m., Scalenus mm.) Infraclavicular part 　Lateral cord (←Anterior division) 　　Musculocutaneous n. 　　Median n., lateral root 　Medial cord (←Anterior division) 　　Median n., medial root 　　Ulnar n. 　　Medial brachial cutaneous n. 　　Medial antebrachial cutaneous n. 　Posterior cord (←Posterior division) 　　Axillary n. 　　Radial n.

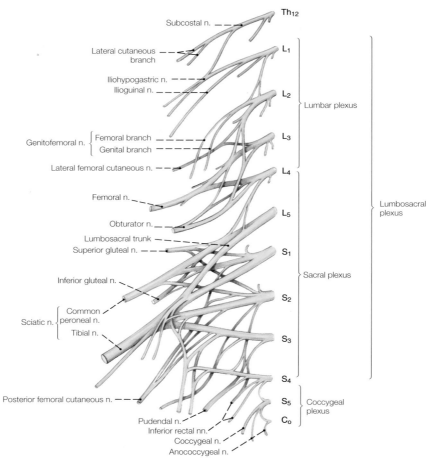

Fig. 47 Survey of the lumbosacral plexus: Lumbar plexus, sacral plexus and coccygeal plexus.

Branches of the Lumbosacral Plexus

Lumbar Plexus (Lumbar nn. L1–L4, ventral primary divisions)	Sacral Plexus (Lumbar nn. L4–Sacral nn. S3, ventral primary divisions)
Iliohypogastric n. Ilioinguinal n. Lateral femoral cutaneous n. Femoral n. Genitofemoral n. Obturator n.	Superior gluteal n. Inferior gluteal n. Sciatic n. Posterior femoral cutaneous n. Pudendal n. Muscular branches (Gemelli mm., quadratus femoris m., obturator mm., piriformis m., levator ani m.) **Coccygeal Plexus** **(Sacral nn., S4, S5, ventral primary divisions)** Coccygeal n., anterior root Anococcygeal n.

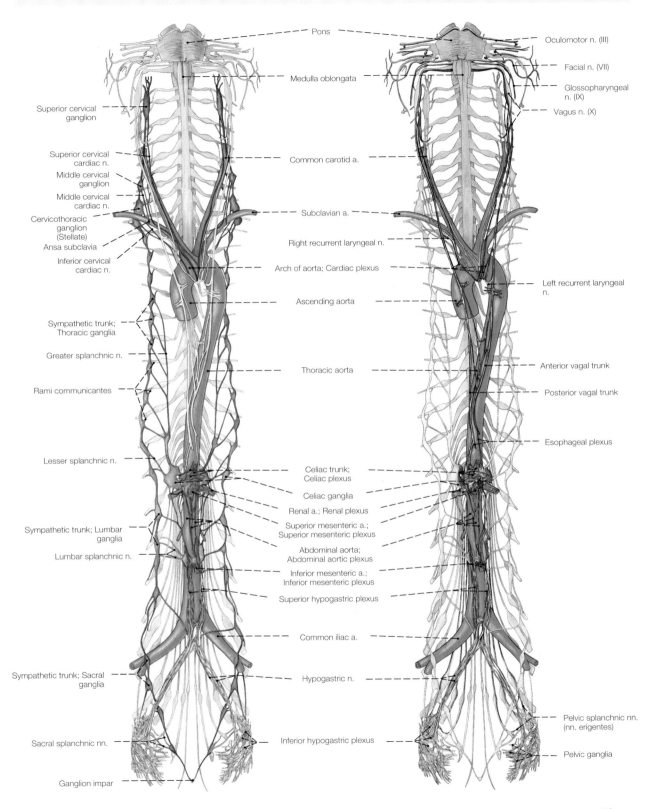

Pons

Medulla oblongata

Superior cervical ganglion

Superior cervical cardiac n.

Middle cervical ganglion

Middle cervical cardiac n.

Cervicothoracic ganglion (Stellate)

Ansa subclavia

Inferior cervical cardiac n.

Common carotid a.

Subclavian a.

Right recurrent laryngeal n.

Arch of aorta; Cardiac plexus

Ascending aorta

Sympathetic trunk; Thoracic ganglia

Greater splanchnic n.

Rami communicantes

Thoracic aorta

Lesser splanchnic n.

Celiac trunk; Celiac plexus

Celiac ganglia

Renal a.; Renal plexus

Superior mesenteric a.; Superior mesenteric plexus

Sympathetic trunk; Lumbar ganglia

Lumbar splanchnic n.

Abdominal aorta; Abdominal aortic plexus

Inferior mesenteric a.; Inferior mesenteric plexus

Superior hypogastric plexus

Common iliac a.

Sympathetic trunk; Sacral ganglia

Hypogastric n.

Sacral splanchnic nn.

Inferior hypogastric plexus

Ganglion impar

Oculomotor n. (III)

Facial n. (VII)

Glossopharyngeal n. (IX)

Vagus n. (X)

Left recurrent laryngeal n.

Anterior vagal trunk

Posterior vagal trunk

Esophageal plexus

Pelvic splanchnic nn. (nn. erigentes)

Pelvic ganglia

Fig. 48 Survey of the visceral nervous system: The sympathetic system. The entire system of sympathetic ganglia that lie along the vertebral column and their connections is known as the sympathetic trunk (green).

Fig. 49 Survey of the visceral nervous system: The parasympathetic system. The parasympathetic fibers (violet) generally course together with other nerve fibers.

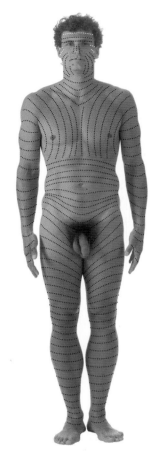

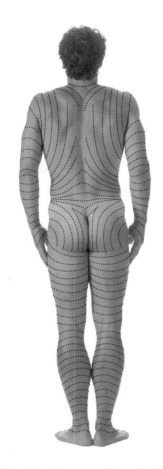

Fig. 50   Cleavage lines of the skin, anterior aspect.

Fig. 51   Cleavage lines of the skin, posterior aspect.

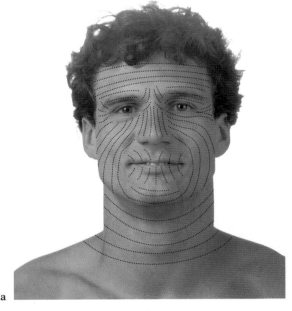

Fig. 52 a, b   Cleavage lines of the skin of the head and neck:
a Anterior aspect;
b Lateral aspect.

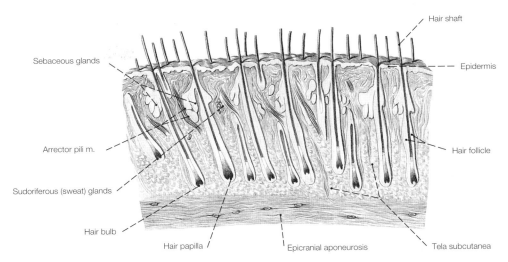

Sebaceous glands

Arrector pili m.

Sudoriferous (sweat) glands

Hair bulb

Hair papilla

Epicranial aponeurosis

Hair shaft

Epidermis

Hair follicle

Tela subcutanea

Fig. 53   Section through the
scalp, ca. 8-fold magnification.

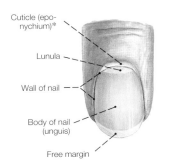

Cuticle (epo-
nychium)*

Lunula

Wall of nail

Body of nail
(unguis)

Free margin

Fig. 54   Terminal phalanx of
digit with fingernail, dorsal view.

* The epidermis of the nail is also
known as the cuticle.

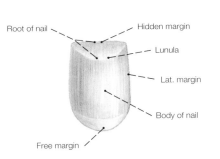

Root of nail

Hidden margin

Lunula

Lat. margin

Body of nail

Free margin

Fig. 55   Fingernail, dorsal view.

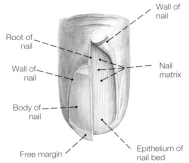

Wall of
nail

Root of
nail

Wall of
nail

Body of
nail

Free margin

Nail
matrix

Epithelium of
nail bed

Fig. 56   Terminal phalanx
of digit with fingernail
partially removed, dorsal
view.

The skin or integument covering the outer surface of
the body (ca. 1.7 m²) consists of several layers. The **skin
proper,** consists of an external covering of stratified
epithelium, the **epidermis,** that varies in thickness and
texture in different parts of the body (e.g., on the
palms of the hands and soles of the feet, it is thick,
hard, and horny in texture.) Below the epidermis is the
dermis, a layer of dense connective tissue formed of
collagenous and elastic fibers and embedded with numerous capillaries and nerve terminals. The space between the dermis and the fascial lining of the body contains the **tela subcutanea,** a loose fibrous envelope beneath the skin, containing fat within its meshes in addition to the cutaneous vessels and nerves. Numerous
small fibrous strands attach the dermis to the underlying tela subcutanea and give it its shape.
The appendages of the skin are the nails of the fingers
and toes, the hairs, and the various glands (sweat or
sudoriferous, sebaceous, and mammary glands) with
their ducts.

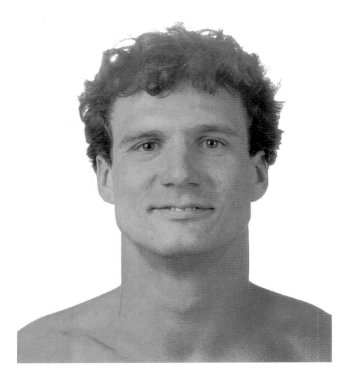

Fig. 57 The head and neck, anterior view (30%).

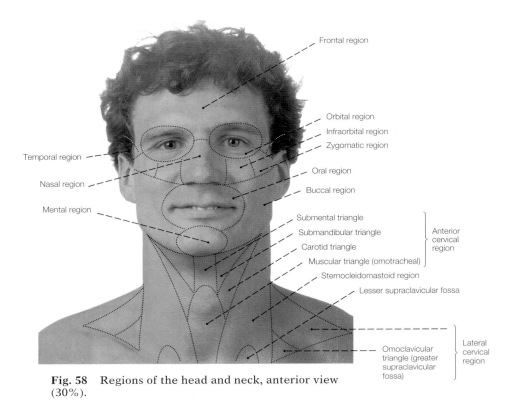

Frontal region

Orbital region

Infraorbital region

Zygomatic region

Temporal region

Oral region

Nasal region

Buccal region

Mental region

Submental triangle

Submandibular triangle

Anterior cervical region

Carotid triangle

Muscular triangle (omotracheal)

Sternocleidomastoid region

Lesser supraclavicular fossa

Omoclavicular triangle (greater supraclavicular fossa)

Lateral cervical region

Fig. 58 Regions of the head and neck, anterior view (30%).

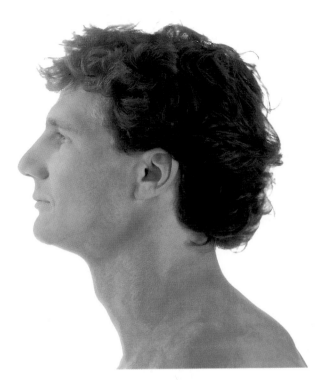

Fig. 59 The head and neck, lateral view (30%).

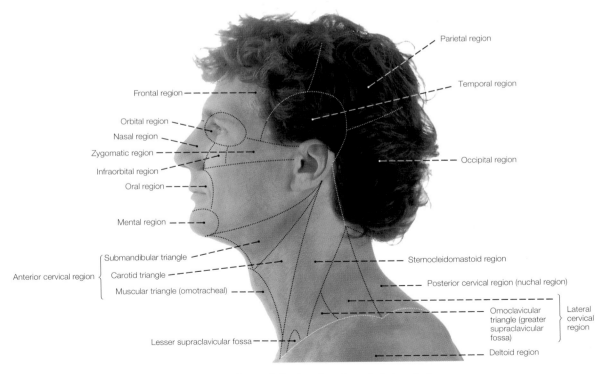

Parietal region

Temporal region

Frontal region

Orbital region

Nasal region

Zygomatic region

Infraorbital region

Oral region

Occipital region

Mental region

Submandibular triangle

Carotid triangle

Anterior cervical region

Muscular triangle (omotracheal)

Sternocleidomastoid region

Posterior cervical region (nuchal region)

Omoclavicular triangle (greater supraclavicular fossa)

Lateral cervical region

Lesser supraclavicular fossa

Deltoid region

Fig. 60 Regions of the head and neck, lateral view (30%).

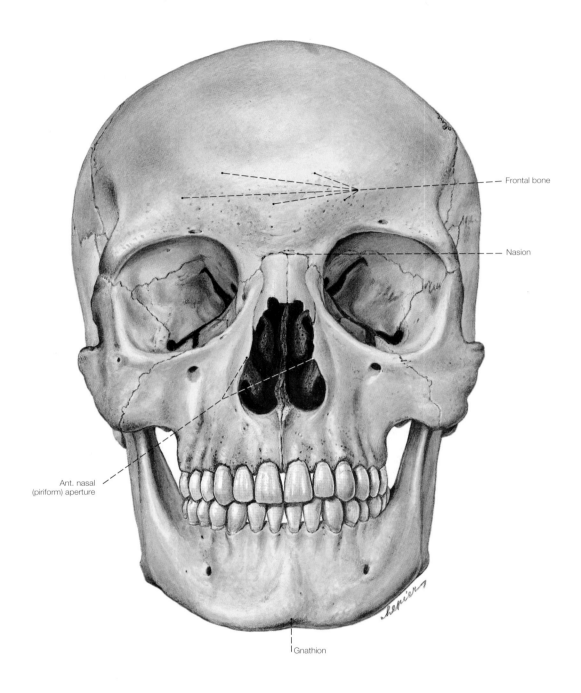

Frontal bone

Nasion

Ant. nasal
(piriform) aperture

Gnathion

Fig. 61 The skull from the front (Norma frontalis) (70%).

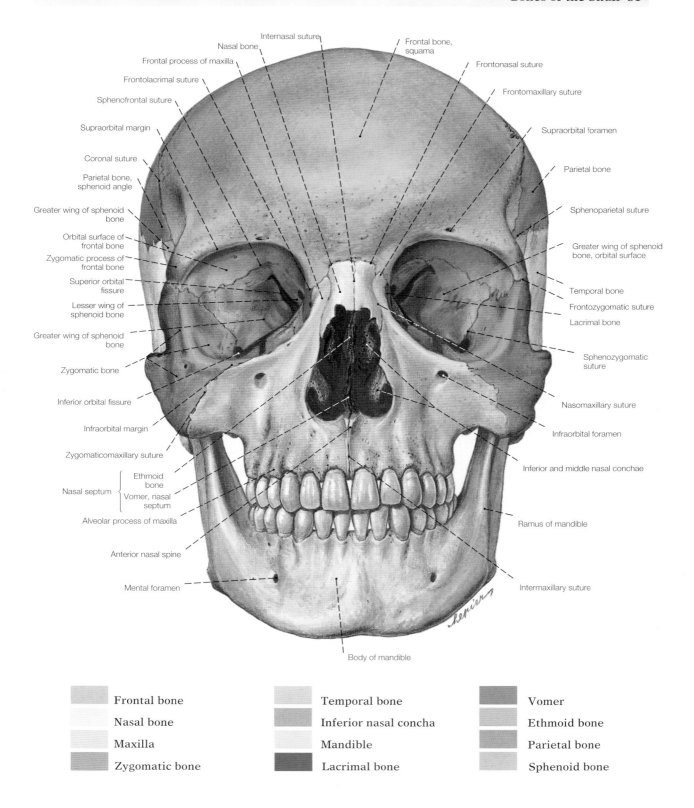

Internasal suture

Nasal bone

Frontal process of maxilla

Frontolacrimal suture

Sphenofrontal suture

Supraorbital margin

Coronal suture

Parietal bone, sphenoid angle

Greater wing of sphenoid bone

Orbital surface of frontal bone

Zygomatic process of frontal bone

Superior orbital fissure

Lesser wing of sphenoid bone

Greater wing of sphenoid bone

Zygomatic bone

Inferior orbital fissure

Infraorbital margin

Zygomaticomaxillary suture

Nasal septum { Ethmoid bone / Vomer, nasal septum

Alveolar process of maxilla

Anterior nasal spine

Mental foramen

Frontal bone, squama

Frontonasal suture

Frontomaxillary suture

Supraorbital foramen

Parietal bone

Sphenoparietal suture

Greater wing of sphenoid bone, orbital surface

Temporal bone

Frontozygomatic suture

Lacrimal bone

Sphenozygomatic suture

Nasomaxillary suture

Infraorbital foramen

Inferior and middle nasal conchae

Ramus of mandible

Intermaxillary suture

Body of mandible

Frontal bone

Nasal bone

Maxilla

Zygomatic bone

Temporal bone

Inferior nasal concha

Mandible

Lacrimal bone

Vomer

Ethmoid bone

Parietal bone

Sphenoid bone

Fig. 62 The skull, or cranium, anterior aspect (Norma frontalis) (70%). The bones of the skull are identified by color as in the color key above.

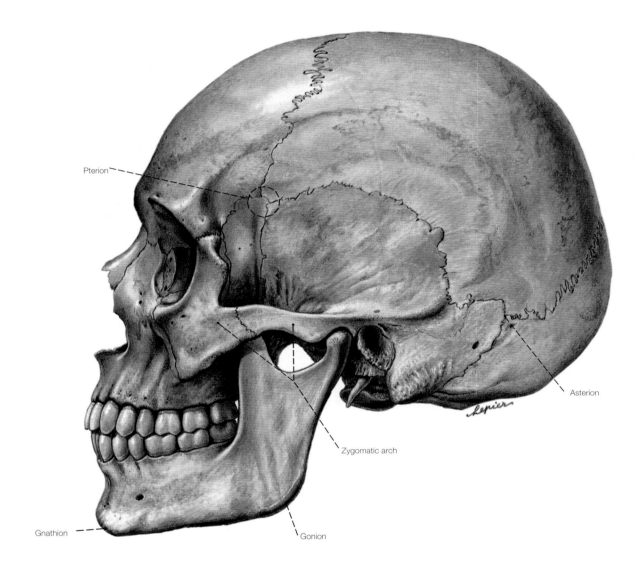

Pterion

Asterion

Zygomatic arch

Gnathion

Gonion

Fig. 63 The skull, lateral aspect (Norma lateralis)
(80%).

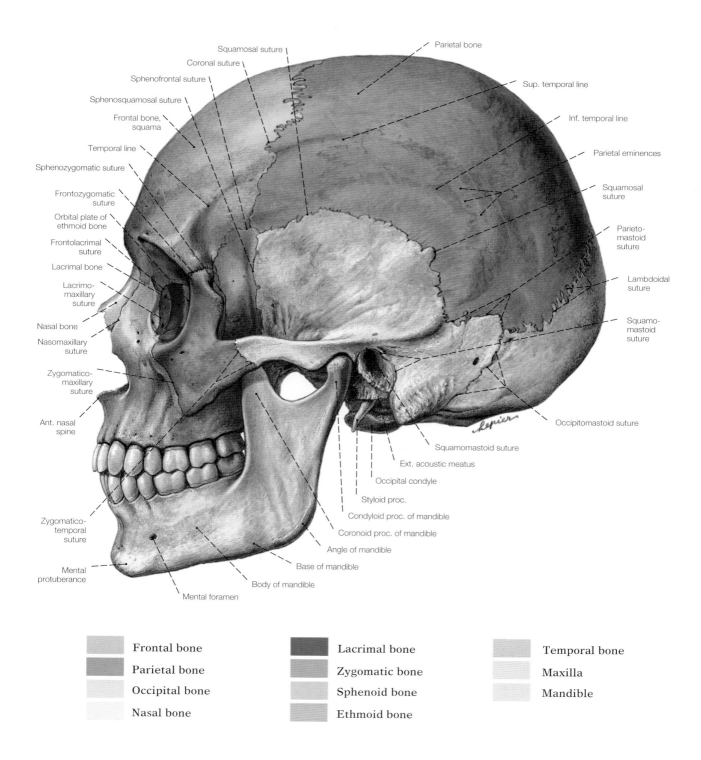

Squamosal suture

Coronal suture

Sphenofrontal suture

Sphenosquamosal suture

Frontal bone, squama

Temporal line

Sphenozygomatic suture

Frontozygomatic suture

Orbital plate of ethmoid bone

Frontolacrimal suture

Lacrimal bone

Lacrimo-maxillary suture

Nasal bone

Nasomaxillary suture

Zygomatico-maxillary suture

Ant. nasal spine

Zygomatico-temporal suture

Mental protuberance

Parietal bone

Sup. temporal line

Inf. temporal line

Parietal eminences

Squamosal suture

Parieto-mastoid suture

Lambdoidal suture

Squamo-mastoid suture

Occipitomastoid suture

Squamomastoid suture

Ext. acoustic meatus

Occipital condyle

Styloid proc.

Condyloid proc. of mandible

Coronoid proc. of mandible

Angle of mandible

Base of mandible

Body of mandible

Mental foramen

Frontal bone

Parietal bone

Occipital bone

Nasal bone

Lacrimal bone

Zygomatic bone

Sphenoid bone

Ethmoid bone

Temporal bone

Maxilla

Mandible

Fig. 64 The skull, lateral aspect (Norma lateralis) (80%). The bones of the skull are identified by color as in the color key above.

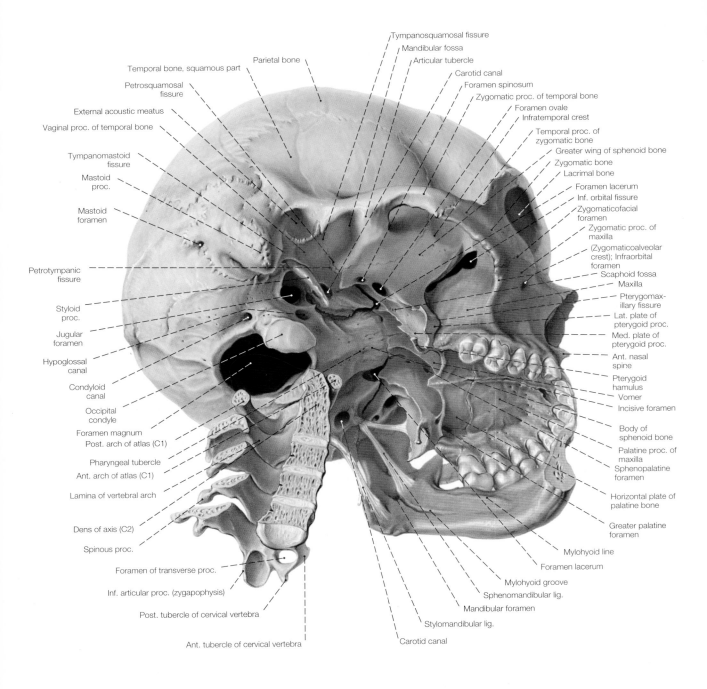

Tympanosquamosal fissure
Mandibular fossa
Articular tubercle
Carotid canal
Foramen spinosum
Zygomatic proc. of temporal bone
Foramen ovale
Infratemporal crest
Temporal proc. of zygomatic bone
Greater wing of sphenoid bone
Zygomatic bone
Lacrimal bone
Foramen lacerum
Inf. orbital fissure
Zygomaticofacial foramen
Zygomatic proc. of maxilla
(Zygomaticoalveolar crest); Infraorbital foramen
Scaphoid fossa
Maxilla
Pterygomaxillary fissure
Lat. plate of pterygoid proc.
Med. plate of pterygoid proc.
Ant. nasal spine
Pterygoid hamulus
Vomer
Incisive foramen
Body of sphenoid bone
Palatine proc. of maxilla
Sphenopalatine foramen
Horizontal plate of palatine bone
Greater palatine foramen
Mylohyoid line
Foramen lacerum
Mylohyoid groove
Sphenomandibular lig.
Mandibular foramen
Stylomandibular lig.
Carotid canal

Parietal bone
Temporal bone, squamous part
Petrosquamosal fissure
External acoustic meatus
Vaginal proc. of temporal bone
Tympanomastoid fissure
Mastoid proc.
Mastoid foramen
Petrotympanic fissure
Styloid proc.
Jugular foramen
Hypoglossal canal
Condyloid canal
Occipital condyle
Foramen magnum
Post. arch of atlas (C1)
Pharyngeal tubercle
Ant. arch of atlas (C1)
Lamina of vertebral arch
Dens of axis (C2)
Spinous proc.
Foramen of transverse proc.
Inf. articular proc. (zygapophysis)
Post. tubercle of cervical vertebra
Ant. tubercle of cervical vertebra

Fig. 65 The skull, lateral view from below (80%). The mandible and upper cervical vertebral column have been bisected.

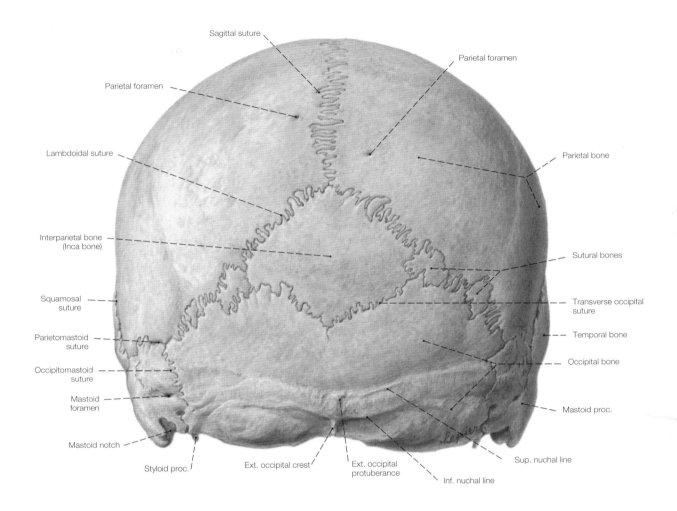

Sagittal suture

Parietal foramen

Parietal foramen

Lambdoidal suture

Parietal bone

Interparietal bone
(Inca bone)

Sutural bones

Squamosal
suture

Transverse occipital
suture

Parietomastoid
suture

Temporal bone

Occipitomastoid
suture

Occipital bone

Mastoid
foramen

Mastoid proc.

Mastoid notch

Styloid proc.

Ext. occipital crest

Ext. occipital
protuberance

Inf. nuchal line

Sup. nuchal line

Fig. 66 The skull, posterior
aspect (Norma occipitalis)
(70%).

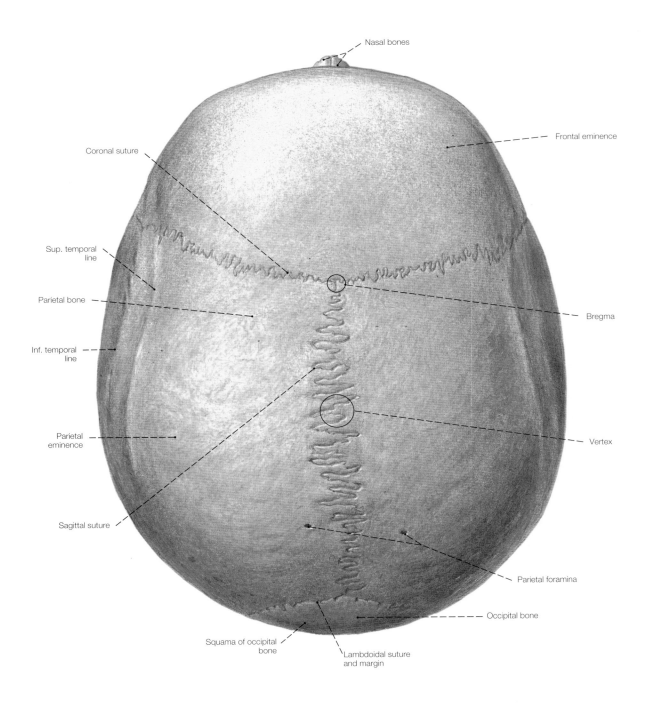

Nasal bones

Frontal eminence

Coronal suture

Sup. temporal line

Parietal bone

Bregma

Inf. temporal line

Parietal eminence

Vertex

Sagittal suture

Parietal foramina

Occipital bone

Squama of occipital bone

Lambdoidal suture and margin

Fig. 67 The skull, viewed from above (Norma verticalis) (80%).

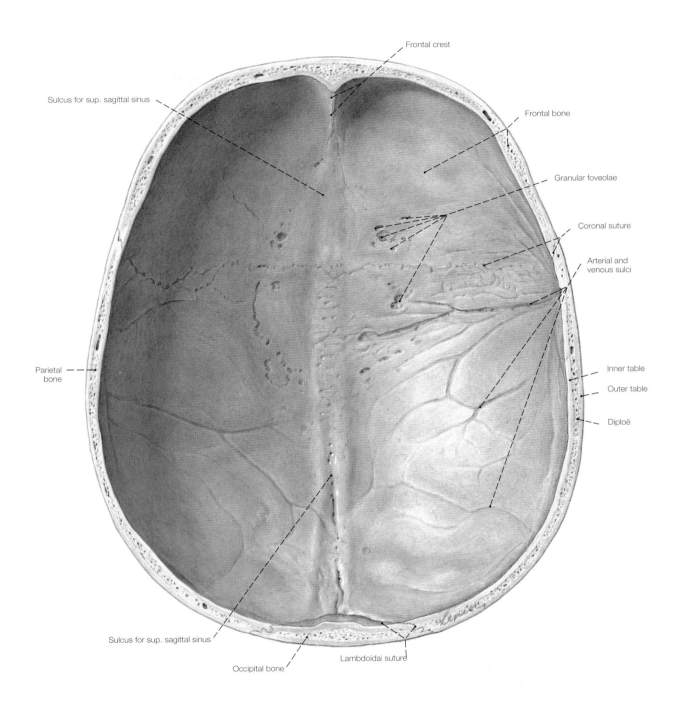

Frontal crest

Sulcus for sup. sagittal sinus

Frontal bone

Granular foveolae

Coronal suture

Arterial and
venous sulci

Parietal
bone

Inner table

Outer table

Diploë

Sulcus for sup. sagittal sinus

Lambdoidal suture

Occipital bone

Fig. 68 The calvaria, internal
aspect (80%).

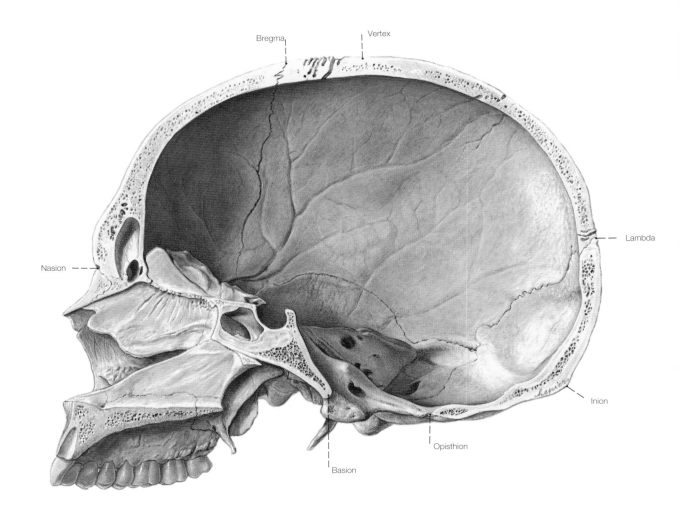

Fig. 69 The skull, paramedian section, medial aspect (80%).

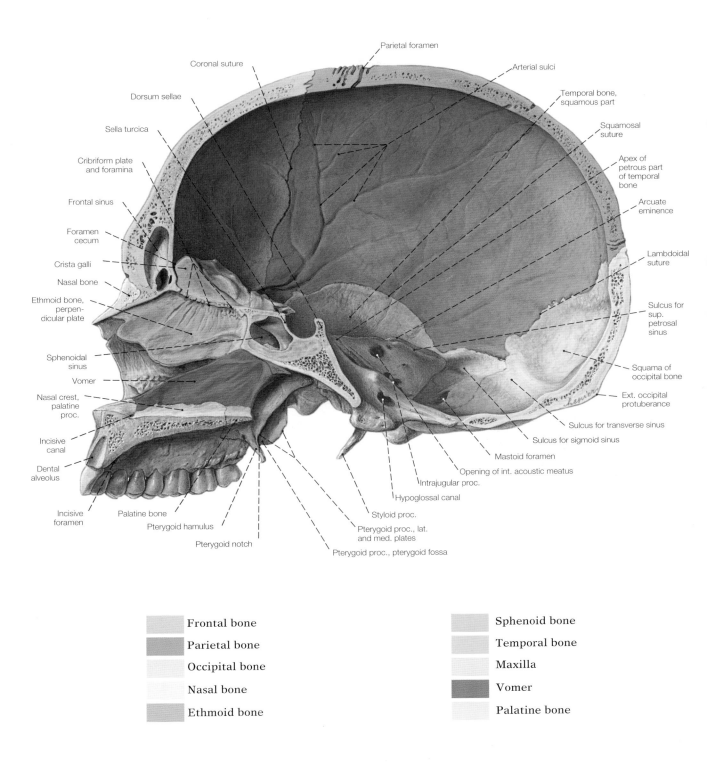

Parietal foramen

Coronal suture

Arterial sulci

Dorsum sellae

Temporal bone, squamous part

Sella turcica

Squamosal suture

Cribriform plate and foramina

Apex of petrous part of temporal bone

Frontal sinus

Arcuate eminence

Foramen cecum

Lambdoidal suture

Crista galli

Nasal bone

Sulcus for sup. petrosal sinus

Ethmoid bone, perpendicular plate

Sphenoidal sinus

Squama of occipital bone

Vomer

Ext. occipital protuberance

Nasal crest, palatine proc.

Sulcus for transverse sinus

Incisive canal

Sulcus for sigmoid sinus

Mastoid foramen

Dental alveolus

Opening of int. acoustic meatus

Intrajugular proc.

Hypoglossal canal

Incisive foramen

Palatine bone

Styloid proc.

Pterygoid hamulus

Pterygoid proc., lat. and med. plates

Pterygoid notch

Pterygoid proc., pterygoid fossa

Frontal bone

Sphenoid bone

Parietal bone

Temporal bone

Occipital bone

Maxilla

Nasal bone

Vomer

Ethmoid bone

Palatine bone

Fig. 70   The skull, paramedian section, medial aspect (80%). The bones of the skull are identified by color as in the color key above.

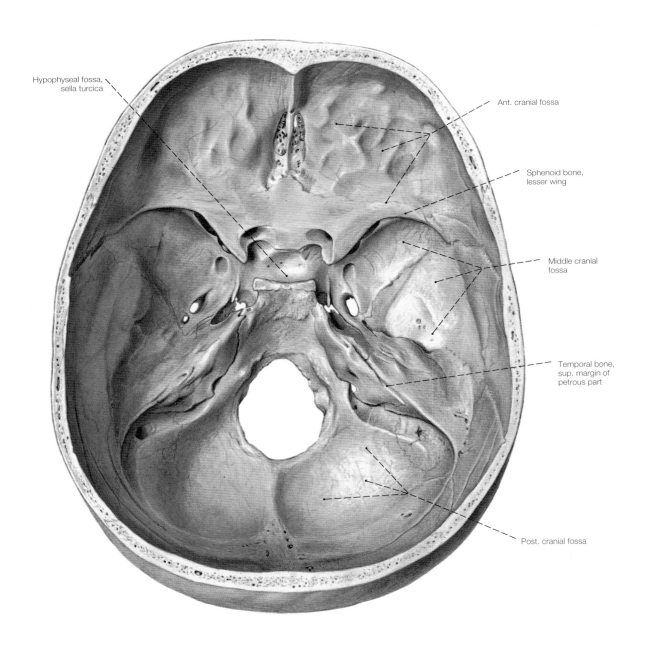

Hypophyseal fossa, sella turcica

Ant. cranial fossa

Sphenoid bone, lesser wing

Middle cranial fossa

Temporal bone, sup. margin of petrous part

Post. cranial fossa

Fig. 71 The internal surface of the base of the skull (80%).

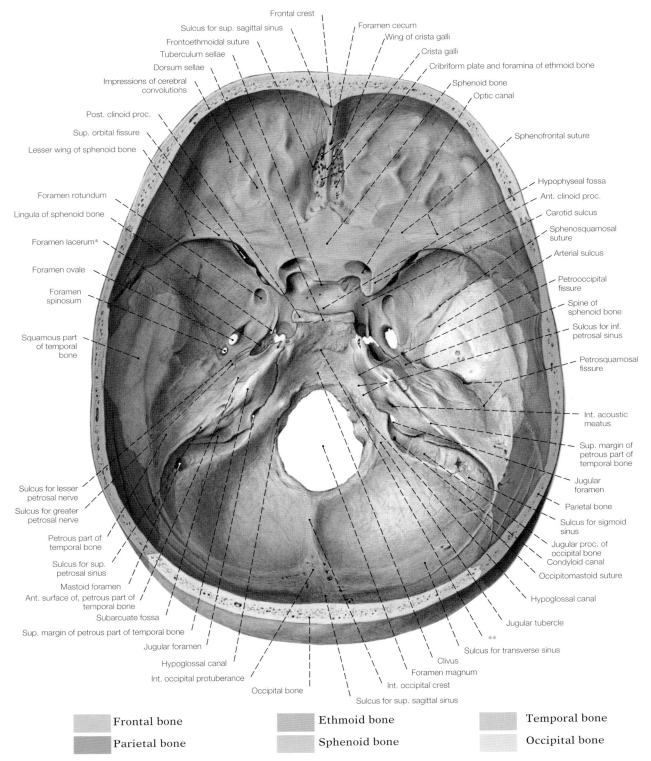

Frontal crest
Sulcus for sup. sagittal sinus
Frontoethmoidal suture
Tuberculum sellae
Dorsum sellae
Impressions of cerebral convolutions
Post. clinoid proc.
Sup. orbital fissure
Lesser wing of sphenoid bone
Foramen rotundum
Lingula of sphenoid bone
Foramen lacerum*
Foramen ovale
Foramen spinosum
Squamous part of temporal bone
Sulcus for lesser petrosal nerve
Sulcus for greater petrosal nerve
Petrous part of temporal bone
Sulcus for sup. petrosal sinus
Mastoid foramen
Ant. surface of, petrous part of temporal bone
Subarcuate fossa
Sup. margin of petrous part of temporal bone
Jugular foramen
Hypoglossal canal
Int. occipital protuberance

Foramen cecum
Wing of crista galli
Crista galli
Cribriform plate and foramina of ethmoid bone
Sphenoid bone
Optic canal
Sphenofrontal suture
Hypophyseal fossa
Ant. clinoid proc.
Carotid sulcus
Sphenosquamosal suture
Arterial sulcus
Petrooccipital fissure
Spine of sphenoid bone
Sulcus for inf. petrosal sinus
Petrosquamosal fissure
Int. acoustic meatus
Sup. margin of petrous part of temporal bone
Jugular foramen
Parietal bone
Sulcus for sigmoid sinus
Jugular proc. of occipital bone
Condyloid canal
Occipitomastoid suture
Hypoglossal canal
Jugular tubercle
**
Sulcus for transverse sinus

Occipital bone
Sulcus for sup. sagittal sinus
Clivus
Foramen magnum
Int. occipital crest

| | Frontal bone | | Ethmoid bone | | Temporal bone |
| | Parietal bone | | Sphenoid bone | | Occipital bone |

Fig. 72 The internal surface of the base of the skull (80%). The bones of the skull are identified by color as in the color key above.

* The foramen lacerum is covered by a layer of fibrocartilage.
** During growth of the skull, these two bones are separated by the sphenooccipital synchrondrosis.

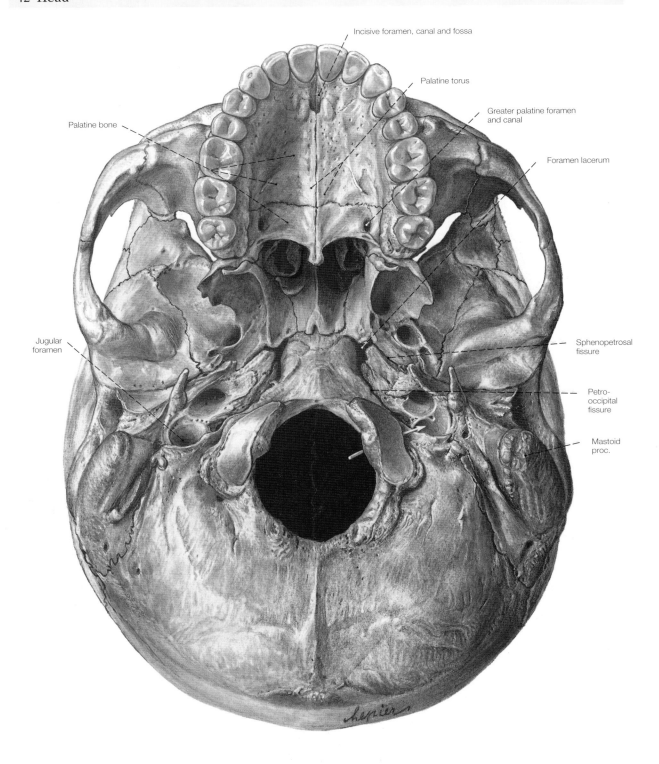

Incisive foramen, canal and fossa

Palatine torus

Greater palatine foramen
and canal

Foramen lacerum

Palatine bone

Jugular
foramen

Sphenopetrosal
fissure

Petro-
occipital
fissure

Mastoid
proc.

Fig. 73 The external surface of the base of the
skull (Norma basalis) (90%). The arrow is in the
left hypoglossal canal.

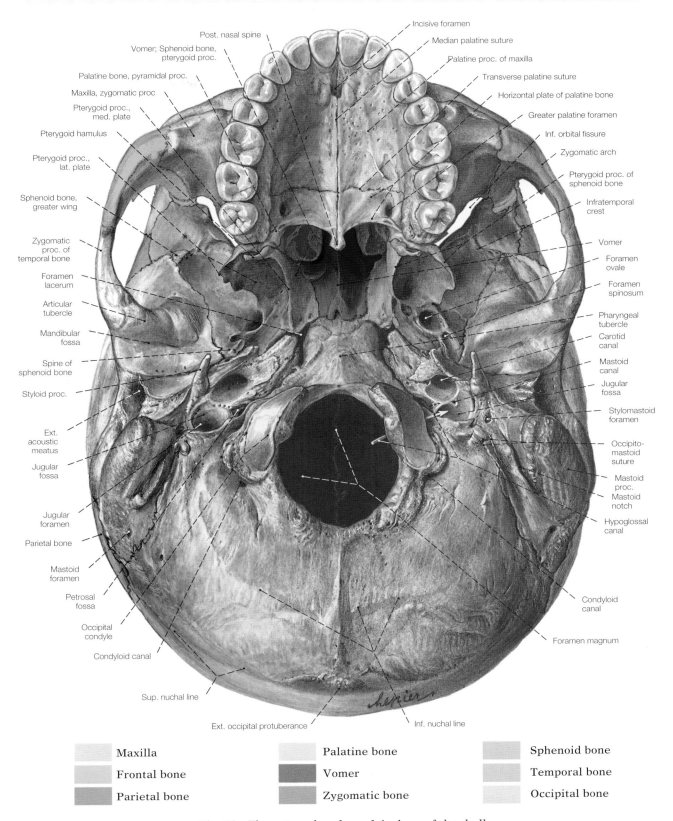

Post. nasal spine

Vomer; Sphenoid bone, pterygoid proc.

Palatine bone, pyramidal proc.

Maxilla, zygomatic proc

Pterygoid proc., med. plate

Pterygoid hamulus

Pterygoid proc., lat. plate

Sphenoid bone, greater wing

Zygomatic proc. of temporal bone

Foramen lacerum

Articular tubercle

Mandibular fossa

Spine of sphenoid bone

Styloid proc.

Ext. acoustic meatus

Jugular fossa

Jugular foramen

Parietal bone

Mastoid foramen

Petrosal fossa

Occipital condyle

Condyloid canal

Sup. nuchal line

Ext. occipital protuberance

Incisive foramen

Median palatine suture

Palatine proc. of maxilla

Transverse palatine suture

Horizontal plate of palatine bone

Greater palatine foramen

Inf. orbital fissure

Zygomatic arch

Pterygoid proc. of sphenoid bone

Infratemporal crest

Vomer

Foramen ovale

Foramen spinosum

Pharyngeal tubercle

Carotid canal

Mastoid canal

Jugular fossa

Stylomastoid foramen

Occipito-mastoid suture

Mastoid proc.

Mastoid notch

Hypoglossal canal

Condyloid canal

Foramen magnum

Inf. nuchal line

Maxilla

Frontal bone

Parietal bone

Palatine bone

Vomer

Zygomatic bone

Sphenoid bone

Temporal bone

Occipital bone

Fig. 74 The external surface of the base of the skull (Norma basalis) (90%). The arrow is in the hypoglossal canal. The bones of the skull are identified by color as in the color key above.

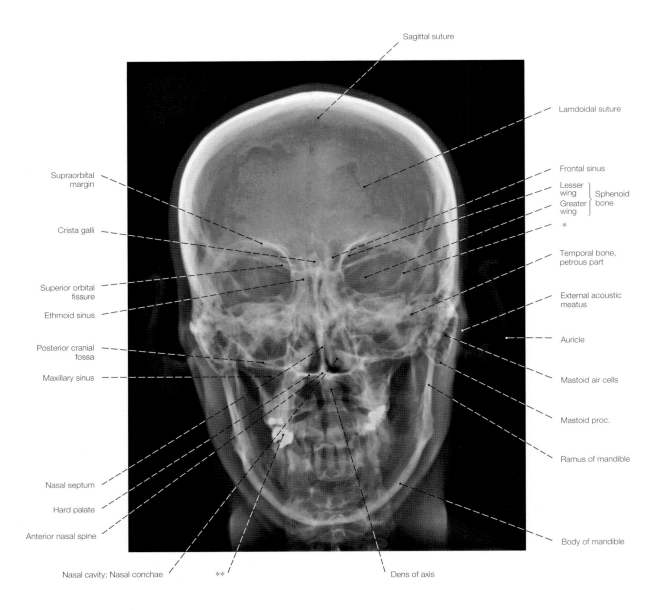

Sagittal suture

Lamdoidal suture

Frontal sinus

Lesser wing ⎱ Sphenoid
Greater wing ⎰ bone

*

Temporal bone, petrous part

External acoustic meatus

Auricle

Mastoid air cells

Mastoid proc.

Ramus of mandible

Body of mandible

Supraorbital margin

Crista galli

Superior orbital fissure

Ethmoid sinus

Posterior cranial fossa

Maxillary sinus

Nasal septum

Hard palate

Anterior nasal spine

Nasal cavity; Nasal conchae

**

Dens of axis

Fig. 75 Radiograph of the skull, PA projection. The x-ray beam is directed obliquely, slanting from caudal dorsal to ventral. Digital fluoroscopic radiography permits the representation of bones and soft tissues.

* Innominate line, a projection line that has no anatomical correlate
** Dental filling

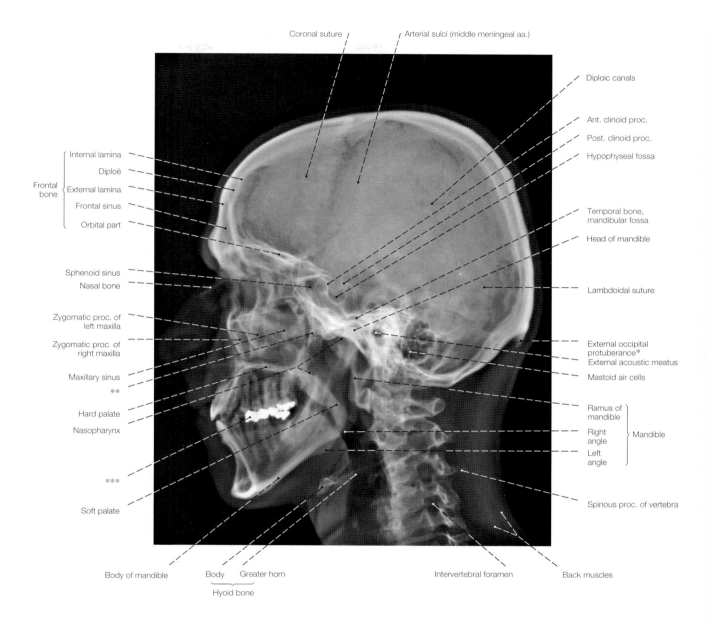

Coronal suture

Arterial sulci (middle meningeal aa.)

Diploic canals

Ant. clinoid proc.

Post. clinoid proc.

Hypophyseal fossa

Internal lamina

Diploë

Frontal bone

External lamina

Frontal sinus

Orbital part

Temporal bone, mandibular fossa

Head of mandible

Sphenoid sinus

Nasal bone

Lambdoidal suture

Zygomatic proc. of left maxilla

Zygomatic proc. of right maxilla

External occipital protuberance*

External acoustic meatus

Maxillary sinus

**

Mastoid air cells

Hard palate

Nasopharynx

Ramus of mandible

Right angle

Mandible

Left angle

***

Soft palate

Spinous proc. of vertebra

Body of mandible

Body   Greater horn

Hyoid bone

Intervertebral foramen

Back muscles

Fig. 76 A digital fluoroscopic radiograph of the skull, lateral projection from the left. The head and cervical vertebral column are turned slightly to the left. The positions of the hyoid bone, the nasal bone, and the vertebral column in the middle of the neck are clearly demarcated by this radiographic technique.

*   Occipital spur (variant)
**   Posterior wall of the maxillary sinus
*** Dental filling

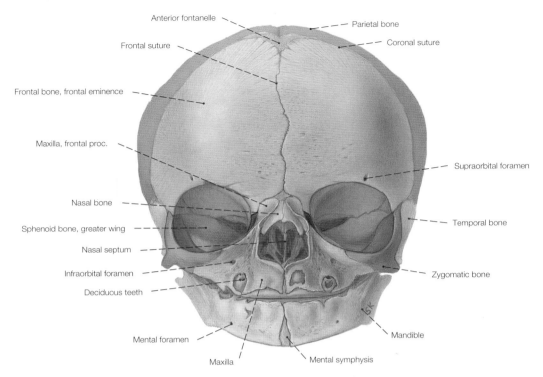

Fig. 77 The skull of a neonate, anterior aspect (80%). The bones of the skull are identified by color as in the color key below.

Lacrimal bone

Frontal bone

Parietal bone

Occipital bone

Maxilla; Incisive bone

Zygomatic bone

Ethmoid bone

Sphenoid bone

Nasal bone; Temporal bone; Mandible

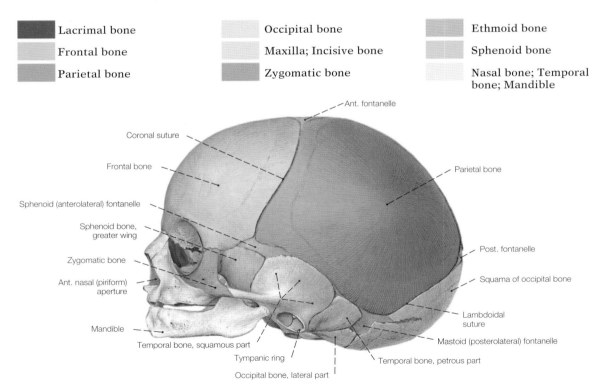

Fig. 78 The skull of a neonate, lateral aspect (80%). The bones of the skull are identified by color as in the color key above.

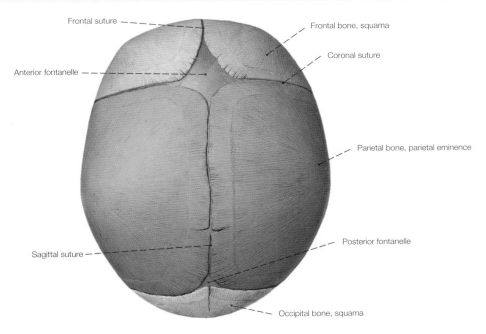

Frontal suture

Frontal bone, squama

Coronal suture

Anterior fontanelle

Parietal bone, parietal eminence

Posterior fontanelle

Sagittal suture

Occipital bone, squama

Fig. 79 The skull of a neonate, superior aspect (80%). The bones of the skull are identified by color as in the color key below.

Vomer

Occipital bone

Maxilla; Incisive bone

Frontal bone

Temporal bone

Zygomatic bone

Parietal bone

Mandible; Palatine bone

Sphenoid bone

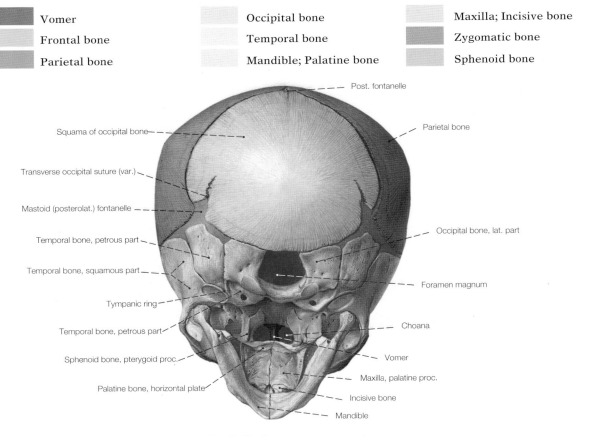

Post. fontanelle

Squama of occipital bone

Parietal bone

Transverse occipital suture (var.)

Mastoid (posterolat.) fontanelle

Occipital bone, lat. part

Temporal bone, petrous part

Temporal bone, squamous part

Foramen magnum

Tympanic ring

Temporal bone, petrous part

Choana

Sphenoid bone, pterygoid proc.

Vomer

Maxilla, palatine proc.

Palatine bone, horizontal plate

Incisive bone

Mandible

Fig. 80 The skull of a neonate, posterior-inferior aspect (80%). The bones of the skull are identified by color as in the color key above.

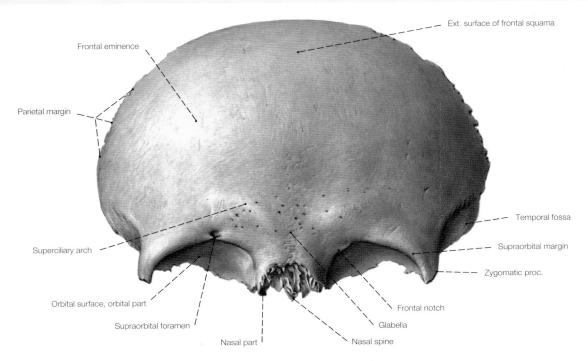

Ext. surface of frontal squama

Frontal eminence

Parietal margin

Temporal fossa

Supraorbital margin

Zygomatic proc.

Superciliary arch

Frontal notch

Orbital surface, orbital part

Glabella

Supraorbital foramen

Nasal part

Nasal spine

Fig. 81 Frontal bone, anterior
view (80%).

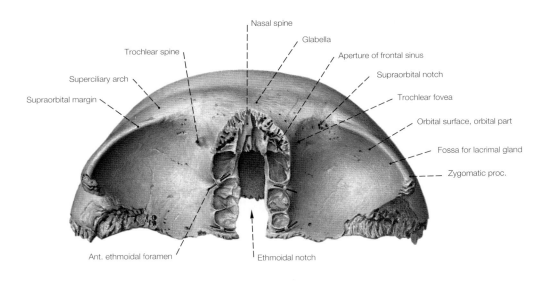

Nasal spine

Glabella

Trochlear spine

Aperture of frontal sinus

Superciliary arch

Supraorbital notch

Supraorbital margin

Trochlear fovea

Orbital surface, orbital part

Fossa for lacrimal gland

Zygomatic proc.

Ant. ethmoidal foramen

Ethmoidal notch

Fig. 82 Frontal bone,
viewed from below (80%).

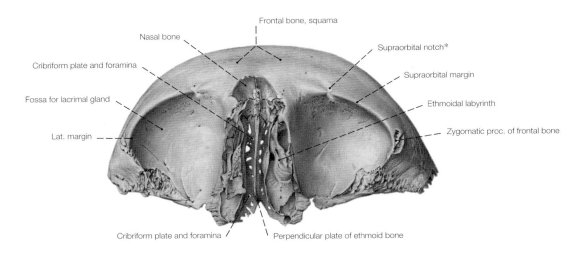

Frontal bone, squama

Nasal bone

Supraorbital notch*

Cribriform plate and foramina

Supraorbital margin

Fossa for lacrimal gland

Ethmoidal labyrinth

Lat. margin

Zygomatic proc. of frontal bone

Cribriform plate and foramina

Perpendicular plate of ethmoid bone

Frontal bone   Ethmoid bone   Nasal bone

Fig. 83 Frontal bone, ethmoid bone, and nasal bones, viewed from below (60%).

* The supraorbital notch may be replaced by a supraorbital foramen.

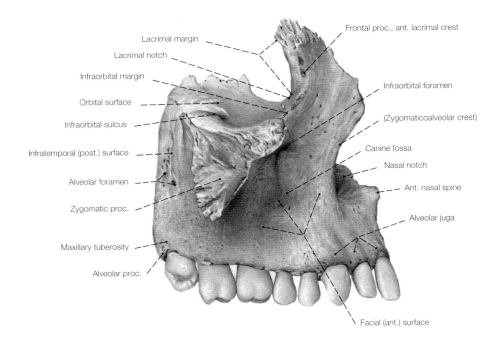

Frontal proc., ant. lacrimal crest

Lacrimal margin

Lacrimal notch

Infraorbital margin

Infraorbital foramen

Orbital surface

(Zygomaticoalveolar crest)

Infraorbital sulcus

Infratemporal (post.) surface

Canine fossa

Nasal notch

Alveolar foramen

Ant. nasal spine

Zygomatic proc.

Alveolar juga

Maxillary tuberosity

Alveolar proc.

Facial (ant.) surface

Fig. 84 The right maxilla, lateral aspect.

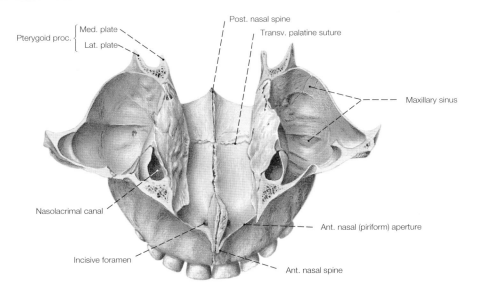

Pterygoid proc. { Med. plate
Lat. plate

Post. nasal spine

Transv. palatine suture

Maxillary sinus

Nasolacrimal canal

Ant. nasal (piriform) aperture

Incisive foramen

Ant. nasal spine

Fig. 85 Hard palate, maxillary sinus, and inferior nasal concha, viewed from above. The maxilla has been sectioned obliquely.

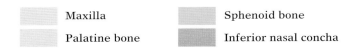

Maxilla

Palatine bone

Sphenoid bone

Inferior nasal concha

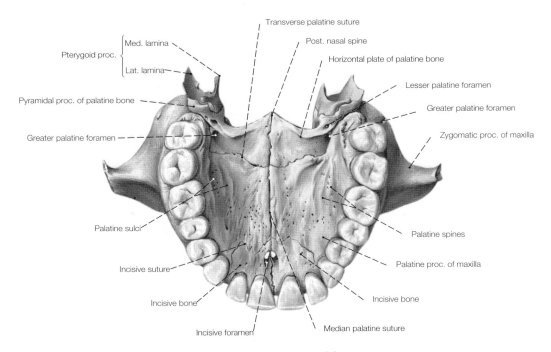

Transverse palatine suture

Post. nasal spine

Horizontal plate of palatine bone

Pterygoid proc. { Med. lamina
Lat. lamina

Lesser palatine foramen

Greater palatine foramen

Pyramidal proc. of palatine bone

Zygomatic proc. of maxilla

Greater palatine foramen

Palatine sulci

Palatine spines

Incisive suture

Palatine proc. of maxilla

Incisive bone

Incisive bone

Incisive foramen

Median palatine suture

Fig. 86 Hard palate, viewed from below.

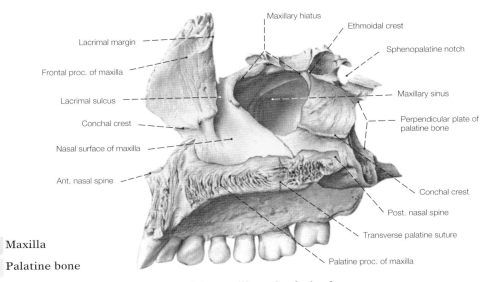

Maxillary hiatus

Ethmoidal crest

Lacrimal margin

Sphenopalatine notch

Frontal proc. of maxilla

Maxillary sinus

Lacrimal sulcus

Perpendicular plate of
palatine bone

Conchal crest

Nasal surface of maxilla

Conchal crest

Ant. nasal spine

Post. nasal spine

Transverse palatine suture

Palatine proc. of maxilla

Maxilla

Palatine bone

Fig. 87 The right maxilla and palatine bone,
medial aspect.

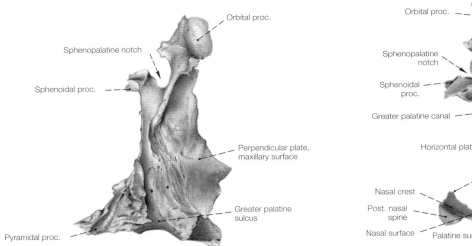

Orbital proc.

Sphenopalatine notch

Sphenoidal proc.

Perpendicular plate,
maxillary surface

Greater palatine
sulcus

Pyramidal proc.

Fig. 88 The right palatine bone,
lateral aspect.

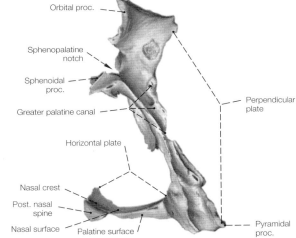

Orbital proc.

Sphenopalatine
notch

Sphenoidal
proc.

Perpendicular
plate

Greater palatine canal

Horizontal plate

Nasal crest

Post. nasal
spine

Nasal surface

Palatine surface

Pyramidal
proc.

Fig. 89 The right palatine bone,
posterior aspect.

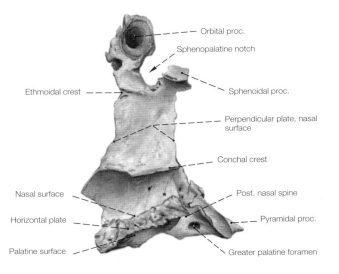

Orbital proc.

Sphenopalatine notch

Ethmoidal crest

Sphenoidal proc.

Perpendicular plate, nasal
surface

Conchal crest

Post. nasal spine

Nasal surface

Pyramidal proc.

Horizontal plate

Greater palatine foramen

Palatine surface

Fig. 90 The right palatine bone,
medial aspect.

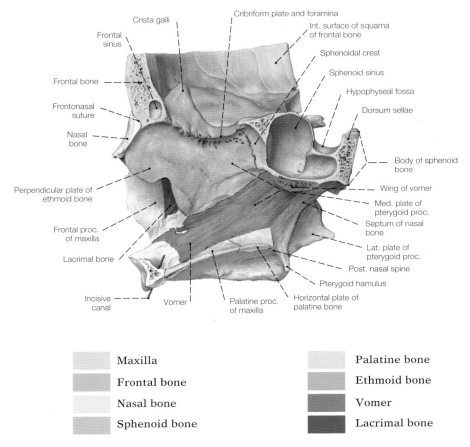

Crista galli

Frontal sinus

Frontal bone

Frontonasal suture

Nasal bone

Perpendicular plate of ethmoid bone

Frontal proc. of maxilla

Lacrimal bone

Incisive canal

Vomer

Palatine proc. of maxilla

Cribriform plate and foramina

Int. surface of squama of frontal bone

Sphenoidal crest

Sphenoid sinus

Hypophyseal fossa

Dorsum sellae

Body of sphenoid bone

Wing of vomer

Med. plate of pterygoid proc.

Septum of nasal bone

Lat. plate of pterygoid proc.

Post. nasal spine

Pterygoid hamulus

Horizontal plate of palatine bone

Maxilla

Frontal bone

Nasal bone

Sphenoid bone

Palatine bone

Ethmoid bone

Vomer

Lacrimal bone

Fig. 91 The nasal septum and adjacent bones of the skull, medial aspect. Paramedian section with the middle nasal concha removed, viewed from the left side.

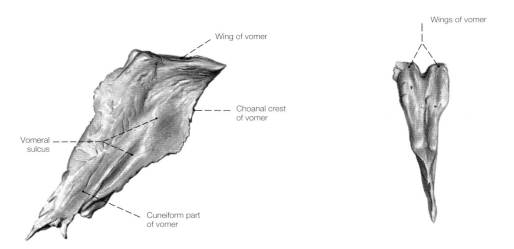

Wing of vomer

Choanal crest of vomer

Vomeral sulcus

Cuneiform part of vomer

Wings of vomer

Fig. 92 Vomer, lateral aspect (140%).

Fig. 93 Vomer, posterior aspect (140%).

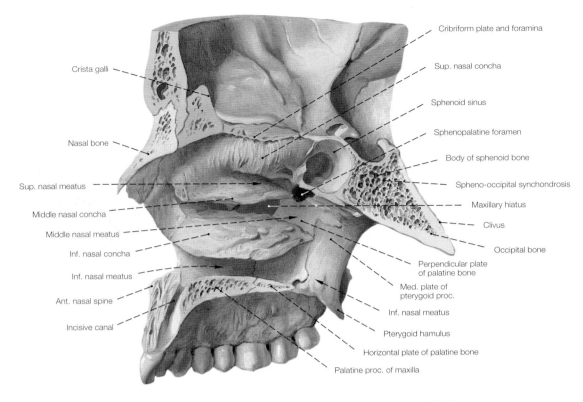

Crista galli

Nasal bone

Sup. nasal meatus

Middle nasal concha

Middle nasal meatus

Inf. nasal concha

Inf. nasal meatus

Ant. nasal spine

Incisive canal

Cribriform plate and foramina

Sup. nasal concha

Sphenoid sinus

Sphenopalatine foramen

Body of sphenoid bone

Spheno-occipital synchondrosis

Maxillary hiatus

Clivus

Occipital bone

Perpendicular plate
of palatine bone

Med. plate of
pterygoid proc.

Inf. nasal meatus

Pterygoid hamulus

Horizontal plate of palatine bone

Palatine proc. of maxilla

Fig. 94 The lateral wall of the right nasal
cavity with adjacent bones. Paramedian
section, medial aspect. Bones are identified
by color as in the color key.

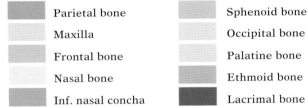

Parietal bone

Maxilla

Frontal bone

Nasal bone

Inf. nasal concha

Sphenoid bone

Occipital bone

Palatine bone

Ethmoid bone

Lacrimal bone

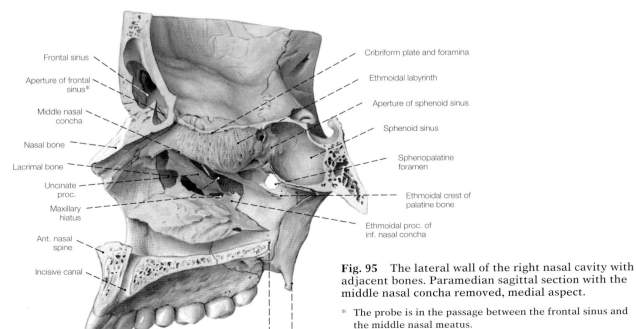

Frontal sinus

Aperture of frontal
sinus*

Middle nasal
concha

Nasal bone

Lacrimal bone

Uncinate
proc.

Maxillary
hiatus

Ant. nasal
spine

Incisive canal

Cribriform plate and foramina

Ethmoidal labyrinth

Aperture of sphenoid sinus

Sphenoid sinus

Sphenopalatine
foramen

Ethmoidal crest of
palatine bone

Ethmoidal proc. of
inf. nasal concha

Post. nasal spine

Pterygoid hamulus

Fig. 95 The lateral wall of the right nasal cavity with
adjacent bones. Paramedian sagittal section with the
middle nasal concha removed, medial aspect.

* The probe is in the passage between the frontal sinus and
the middle nasal meatus.

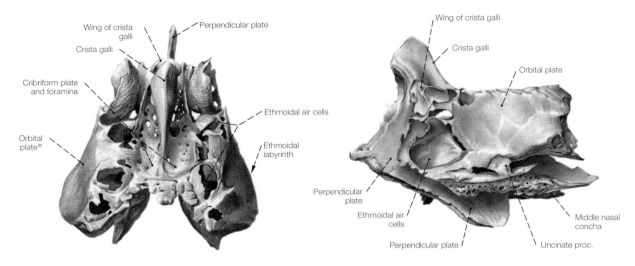

Fig. 96 Ethmoid bone, viewed from above.

* Lamina papyracea, so named because of the paper-thin nature of this bony plate.

Fig. 97 Ethmoid bone, lateral aspect.

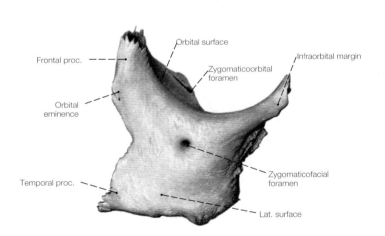

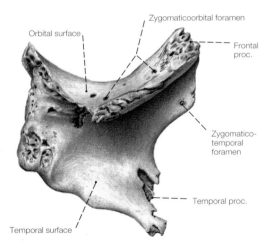

Fig. 98 Right zygomatic bone, lateral aspect.

Fig. 99 Right zygomatic bone, medial aspect viewed from above.

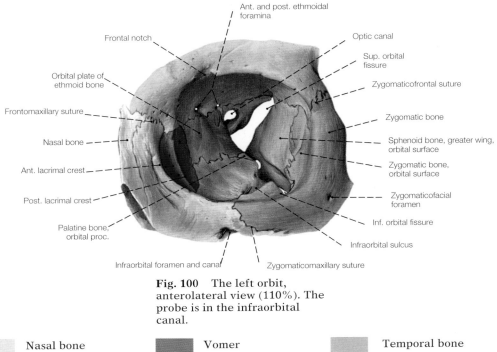

Ant. and post. ethmoidal foramina

Frontal notch

Optic canal

Sup. orbital fissure

Orbital plate of ethmoid bone

Zygomaticofrontal suture

Frontomaxillary suture

Zygomatic bone

Nasal bone

Sphenoid bone, greater wing, orbital surface

Ant. lacrimal crest

Zygomatic bone, orbital surface

Post. lacrimal crest

Zygomaticofacial foramen

Palatine bone, orbital proc.

Inf. orbital fissure

Infraorbital sulcus

Infraorbital foramen and canal

Zygomaticomaxillary suture

Fig. 100 The left orbit, anterolateral view (110%). The probe is in the infraorbital canal.

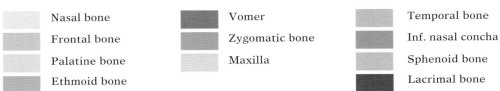

Nasal bone

Frontal bone

Palatine bone

Ethmoid bone

Vomer

Zygomatic bone

Maxilla

Temporal bone

Inf. nasal concha

Sphenoid bone

Lacrimal bone

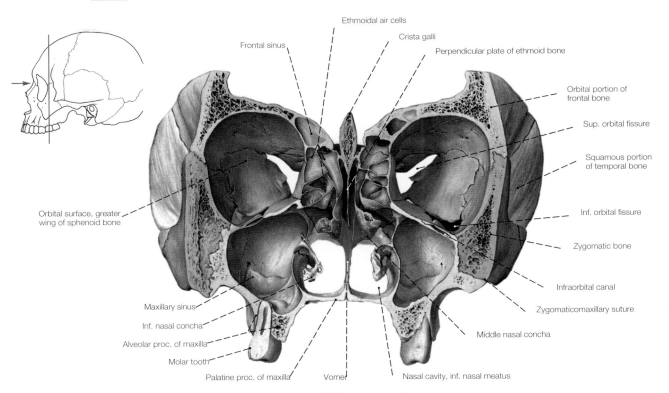

Ethmoidal air cells

Frontal sinus

Crista galli

Perpendicular plate of ethmoid bone

Orbital portion of frontal bone

Sup. orbital fissure

Squamous portion of temporal bone

Orbital surface, greater wing of sphenoid bone

Inf. orbital fissure

Zygomatic bone

Infraorbital canal

Zygomaticomaxillary suture

Maxillary sinus

Inf. nasal concha

Middle nasal concha

Alveolar proc. of maxilla

Molar tooth

Palatine proc. of maxilla

Vomer

Nasal cavity, inf. nasal meatus

Fig. 101 Facial skeleton, anterior aspect (90%). Frontal section through the middle of the orbits.

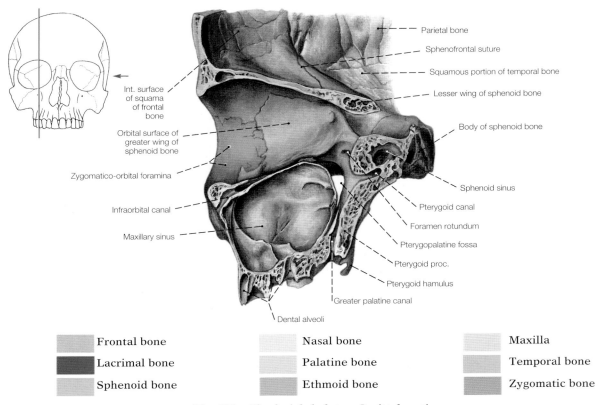

Parietal bone

Sphenofrontal suture

Squamous portion of temporal bone

Lesser wing of sphenoid bone

Body of sphenoid bone

Sphenoid sinus

Pterygoid canal

Foramen rotundum

Pterygopalatine fossa

Pterygoid proc.

Pterygoid hamulus

Greater palatine canal

Dental alveoli

Int. surface of squama of frontal bone

Orbital surface of greater wing of sphenoid bone

Zygomatico-orbital foramina

Infraorbital canal

Maxillary sinus

Frontal bone	Nasal bone	Maxilla
Lacrimal bone	Palatine bone	Temporal bone
Sphenoid bone	Ethmoid bone	Zygomatic bone

Fig. 102 The facial skeleton. Sagittal section through the middle of the right orbit, medial aspect.

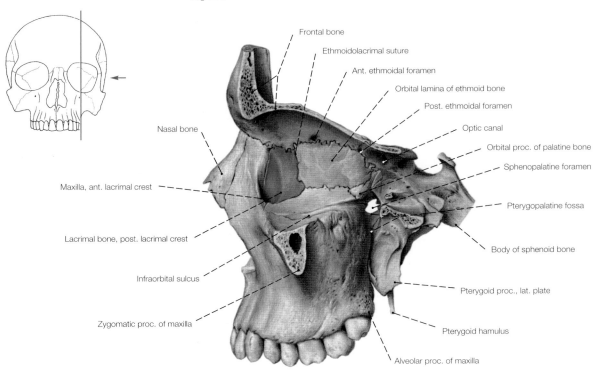

Frontal bone

Ethmoidolacrimal suture

Ant. ethmoidal foramen

Orbital lamina of ethmoid bone

Post. ethmoidal foramen

Optic canal

Orbital proc. of palatine bone

Sphenopalatine foramen

Pterygopalatine fossa

Body of sphenoid bone

Pterygoid proc., lat. plate

Pterygoid hamulus

Alveolar proc. of maxilla

Nasal bone

Maxilla, ant. lacrimal crest

Lacrimal bone, post. lacrimal crest

Infraorbital sulcus

Zygomatic proc. of maxilla

Fig. 103 The facial skeleton. Sagittal section through the middle of the left orbit, lateral aspect.

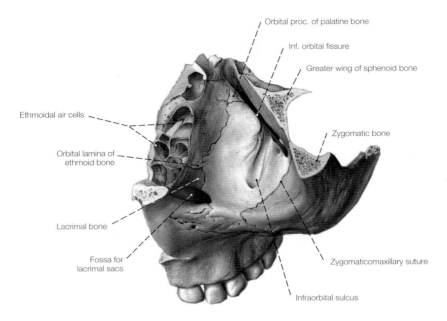

Orbital proc. of palatine bone

Inf. orbital fissure

Greater wing of sphenoid bone

Ethmoidal air cells

Orbital lamina of ethmoid bone

Zygomatic bone

Lacrimal bone

Fossa for lacrimal sacs

Zygomaticomaxillary suture

Infraorbital sulcus

Fig. 104 Facial skeleton. Transverse section through the middle of the left orbit, viewed from above.

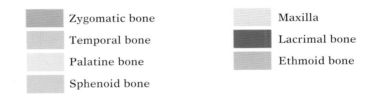

Zygomatic bone

Temporal bone

Palatine bone

Sphenoid bone

Maxilla

Lacrimal bone

Ethmoid bone

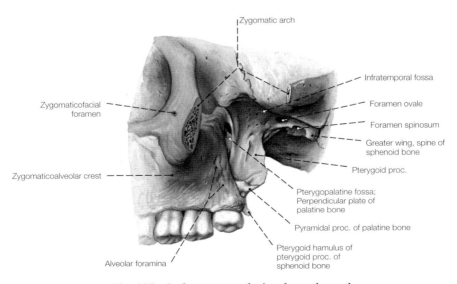

Zygomatic arch

Zygomaticofacial foramen

Infratemporal fossa

Foramen ovale

Foramen spinosum

Greater wing, spine of sphenoid bone

Zygomaticoalveolar crest

Pterygoid proc.

Pterygopalatine fossa; Perpendicular plate of palatine bone

Pyramidal proc. of palatine bone

Pterygoid hamulus of pterygoid proc. of sphenoid bone

Alveolar foramina

Fig. 105 Left pterygopalatine fossa, lateral aspect. The zygomatic arch has been removed.

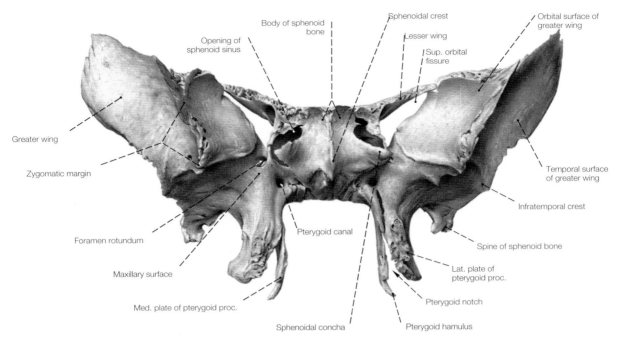

Sphenoidal crest

Body of sphenoid bone

Opening of sphenoid sinus

Lesser wing

Orbital surface of greater wing

Sup. orbital fissure

Greater wing

Zygomatic margin

Temporal surface of greater wing

Infratemporal crest

Foramen rotundum

Pterygoid canal

Spine of sphenoid bone

Maxillary surface

Lat. plate of pterygoid proc.

Med. plate of pterygoid proc.

Pterygoid notch

Sphenoidal concha

Pterygoid hamulus

Fig. 106 Sphenoid bone, anterior aspect.

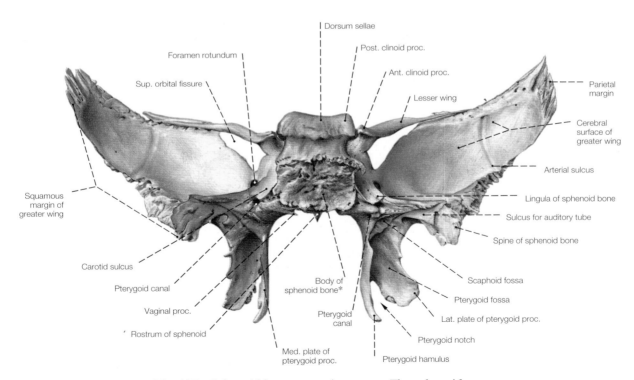

Dorsum sellae

Foramen rotundum

Post. clinoid proc.

Ant. clinoid proc.

Parietal margin

Sup. orbital fissure

Lesser wing

Cerebral surface of greater wing

Arterial sulcus

Squamous margin of greater wing

Lingula of sphenoid bone

Sulcus for auditory tube

Spine of sphenoid bone

Carotid sulcus

Scaphoid fossa

Pterygoid canal

Body of sphenoid bone*

Pterygoid fossa

Vaginal proc.

Pterygoid canal

Lat. plate of pterygoid proc.

Rostrum of sphenoid

Pterygoid notch

Med. plate of pterygoid proc.

Pterygoid hamulus

Fig. 107 Sphenoid bone, posterior aspect. The sphenoid bones in Figs. 106 and 107 are from an adolescent. Therefore, the synchondrosis between the occipital bone and the sphenoid bone has not yet ossified.

* View of the marginal surface of the spheno-occipital synchondrosis.

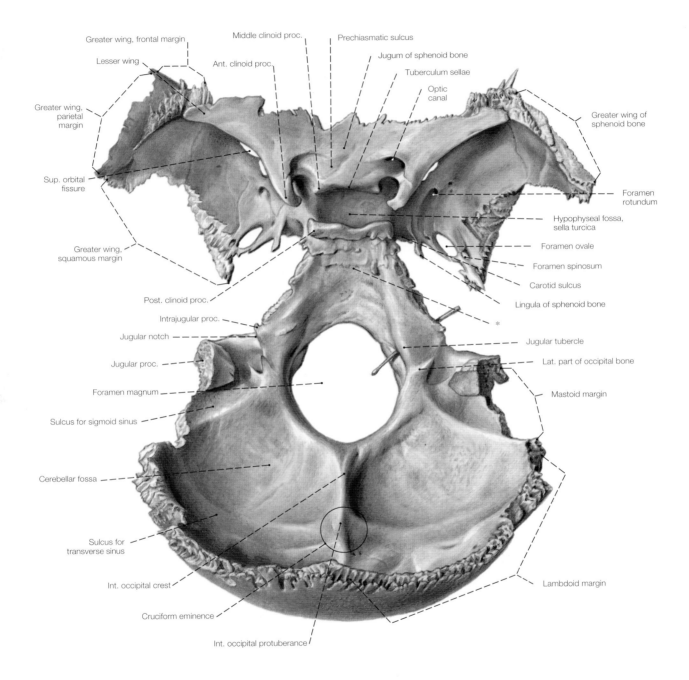

Greater wing, frontal margin

Lesser wing

Greater wing, parietal margin

Sup. orbital fissure

Greater wing, squamous margin

Post. clinoid proc.

Intrajugular proc.

Jugular notch

Jugular proc.

Foramen magnum

Sulcus for sigmoid sinus

Cerebellar fossa

Sulcus for transverse sinus

Int. occipital crest

Cruciform eminence

Int. occipital protuberance

Middle clinoid proc.

Ant. clinoid proc.

Prechiasmatic sulcus

Jugum of sphenoid bone

Tuberculum sellae

Optic canal

Greater wing of sphenoid bone

Foramen rotundum

Hypophyseal fossa, sella turcica

Foramen ovale

Foramen spinosum

Carotid sulcus

Lingula of sphenoid bone

*

Jugular tubercle

Lat. part of occipital bone

Mastoid margin

Lambdoid margin

Fig. 108 The occipital bone and the sphenoid bone of an adult, internal surface. The probe is in the right hypoglossal canal.

* Synostosis of the spheno-occipital synchondrosis occurs toward the end of the second decade of life.

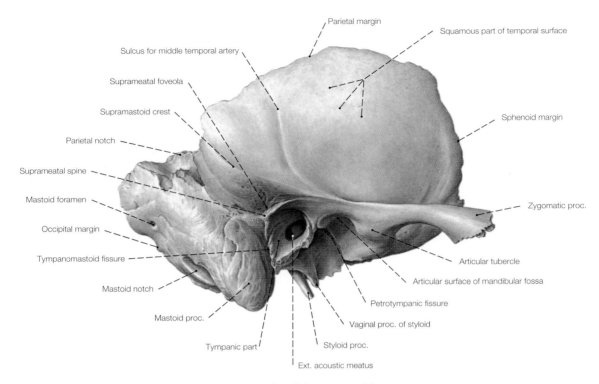

Parietal margin

Squamous part of temporal surface

Sulcus for middle temporal artery

Suprameatal foveola

Supramastoid crest

Sphenoid margin

Parietal notch

Suprameatal spine

Mastoid foramen

Zygomatic proc.

Occipital margin

Tympanomastoid fissure

Articular tubercle

Mastoid notch

Articular surface of mandibular fossa

Mastoid proc.

Petrotympanic fissure

Tympanic part

Vaginal proc. of styloid

Styloid proc.

Ext. acoustic meatus

Fig. 109 The right temporal bone,
lateral aspect (120%).

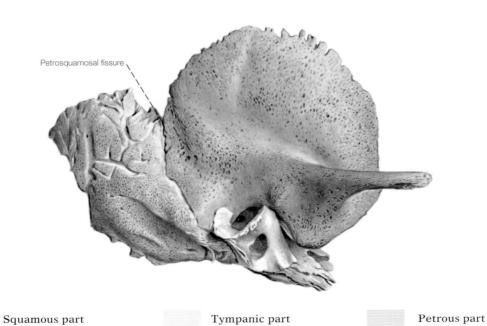

Petrosquamosal fissure

Squamous part   Tympanic part   Petrous part

Fig. 110 The right temporal bone of a neonate,
lateral aspect (240%).

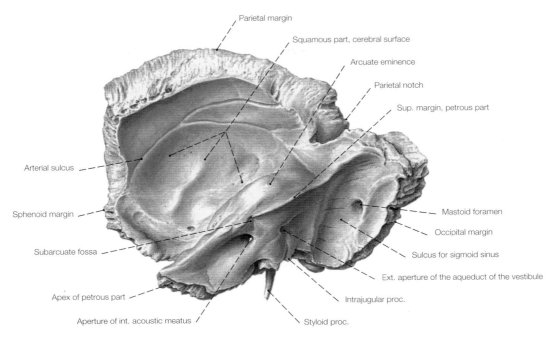

Parietal margin

Squamous part, cerebral surface

Arcuate eminence

Parietal notch

Sup. margin, petrous part

Arterial sulcus

Mastoid foramen

Occipital margin

Sphenoid margin

Subarcuate fossa

Sulcus for sigmoid sinus

Ext. aperture of the aqueduct of the vestibule

Apex of petrous part

Intrajugular proc.

Aperture of int. acoustic meatus

Styloid proc.

Fig. 111   The right temporal bone,
medial aspect (110%).

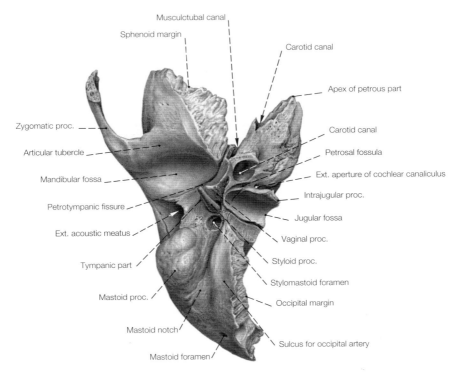

Musculotubal canal

Sphenoid margin

Carotid canal

Apex of petrous part

Zygomatic proc.

Carotid canal

Articular tubercle

Petrosal fossula

Mandibular fossa

Ext. aperture of cochlear canaliculus

Petrotympanic fissure

Intrajugular proc.

Ext. acoustic meatus

Jugular fossa

Tympanic part

Vaginal proc.

Styloid proc.

Mastoid proc.

Stylomastoid foramen

Occipital margin

Mastoid notch

Sulcus for occipital artery

Mastoid foramen

Fig. 112   The right temporal bone,
viewed from below (110%).

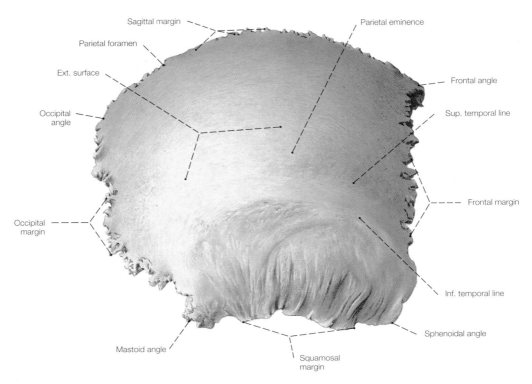

Sagittal margin

Parietal foramen

Ext. surface

Occipital angle

Occipital margin

Mastoid angle

Squamosal margin

Parietal eminence

Frontal angle

Sup. temporal line

Frontal margin

Inf. temporal line

Sphenoidal angle

Fig. 113 The right parietal bone, lateral aspect (80%).

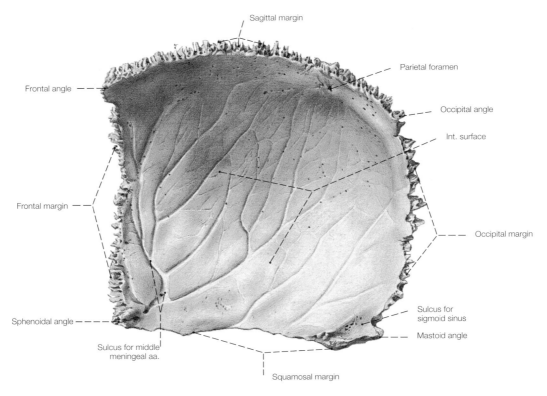

Sagittal margin

Parietal foramen

Frontal angle

Occipital angle

Int. surface

Frontal margin

Occipital margin

Sphenoidal angle

Sulcus for sigmoid sinus

Mastoid angle

Sulcus for middle meningeal aa.

Squamosal margin

Fig. 114 The right parietal bone, medial aspect (80%).

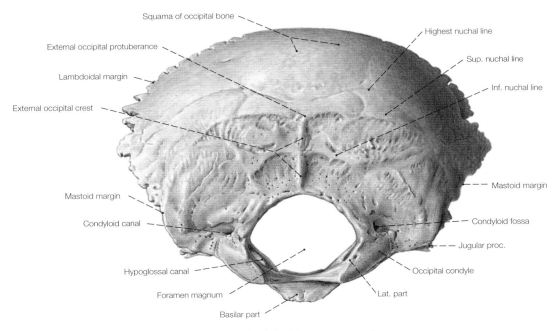

Squama of occipital bone

External occipital protuberance

Lambdoidal margin

External occipital crest

Mastoid margin

Condyloid canal

Hypoglossal canal

Foramen magnum

Basilar part

Highest nuchal line

Sup. nuchal line

Inf. nuchal line

Mastoid margin

Condyloid fossa

Jugular proc.

Occipital condyle

Lat. part

Fig. 115 Occipital bone, external surface viewed from below.

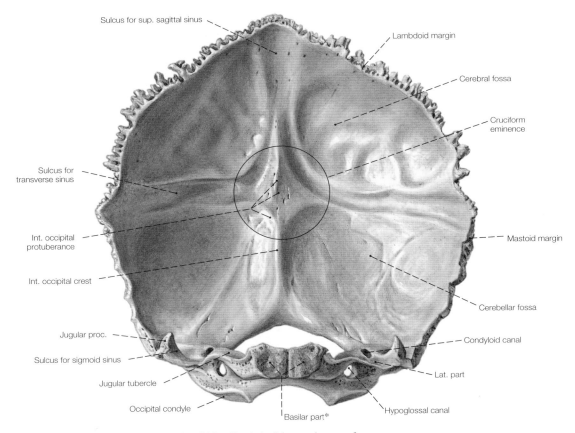

Sulcus for sup. sagittal sinus

Sulcus for transverse sinus

Int. occipital protuberance

Int. occipital crest

Jugular proc.

Sulcus for sigmoid sinus

Jugular tubercle

Occipital condyle

Lambdoid margin

Cerebral fossa

Cruciform eminence

Mastoid margin

Cerebellar fossa

Condyloid canal

Lat. part

Hypoglossal canal

Basilar part*

Fig. 116 Occipital bone, internal surface viewed from anterior (120%).

* View of the surface adjacent to the spheno-occipital synchondrosis.

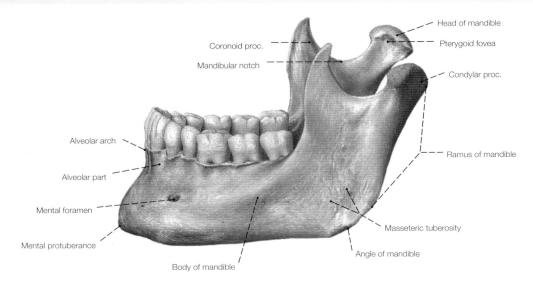

Head of mandible

Coronoid proc.

Pterygoid fovea

Mandibular notch

Condylar proc.

Alveolar arch

Alveolar part

Ramus of mandible

Mental foramen

Mental protuberance

Masseteric tuberosity

Angle of mandible

Body of mandible

Fig. 117 The mandible, lateral aspect viewed from above.

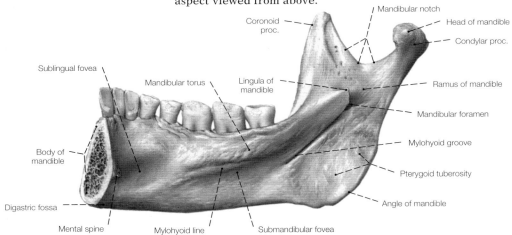

Mandibular notch

Coronoid proc.

Head of mandible

Condylar proc.

Sublingual fovea

Mandibular torus

Lingula of mandible

Ramus of mandible

Mandibular foramen

Body of mandible

Mylohyoid groove

Pterygoid tuberosity

Digastric fossa

Angle of mandible

Mental spine

Mylohyoid line

Submandibular fovea

Fig. 118 The mandible, medial aspect of the right half.

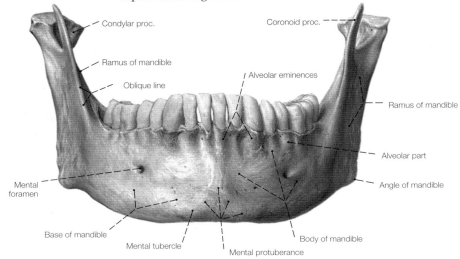

Condylar proc.

Coronoid proc.

Ramus of mandible

Oblique line

Alveolar eminences

Ramus of mandible

Alveolar part

Angle of mandible

Mental foramen

Base of mandible

Mental tubercle

Mental protuberance

Body of mandible

Fig. 119 The mandible, anterior aspect.

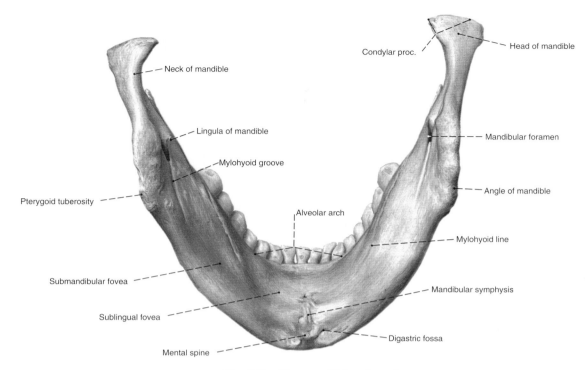

Neck of mandible

Condylar proc.

Head of mandible

Lingula of mandible

Mandibular foramen

Mylohyoid groove

Pterygoid tuberosity

Angle of mandible

Alveolar arch

Mylohyoid line

Submandibular fovea

Mandibular symphysis

Sublingual fovea

Digastric fossa

Mental spine

Fig. 120 The mandible, viewed from below.

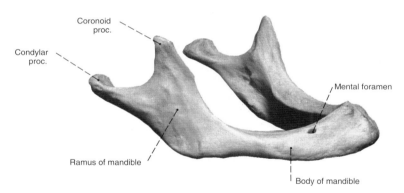

Coronoid proc.

Condylar proc.

Mental foramen

Ramus of mandible

Body of mandible

Fig. 121 The mandible, of an elderly person, viewed laterally from above (80%). The alveolar part is completely atrophied, moving the opening of the mental foramen and the exit of the mental nerve upward.

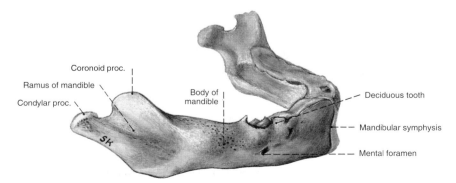

Coronoid proc.

Ramus of mandible

Condylar proc.

Body of mandible

Deciduous tooth

Mandibular symphysis

Mental foramen

SK

Fig. 122 The mandible in the newborn, viewed laterally from above (170%). Compare the ramus of the mandible, body of the mandible, and coronoid process with Figures 117 and 121.

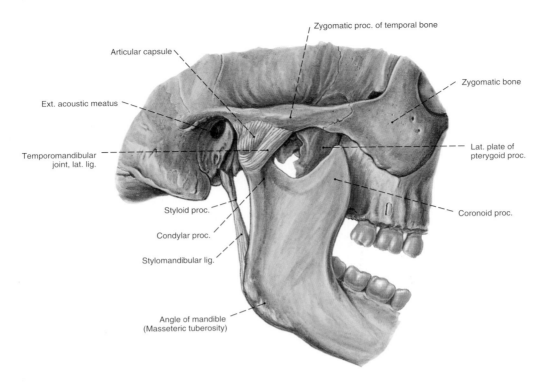

Fig. 123 The temporomandibular joint, lateral aspect.

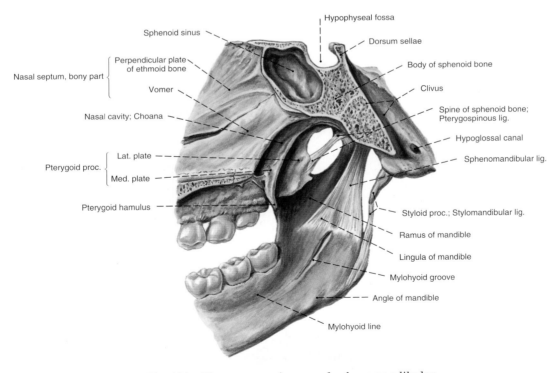

Fig. 124 The pterygospinous and sphenomandibular ligaments. A paramedian section, medial aspect.

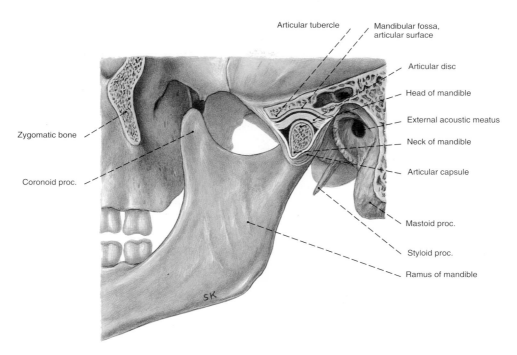

Fig. 125 The temporomandibular joint. Sagittal section, mouth virtually closed, lateral aspect.

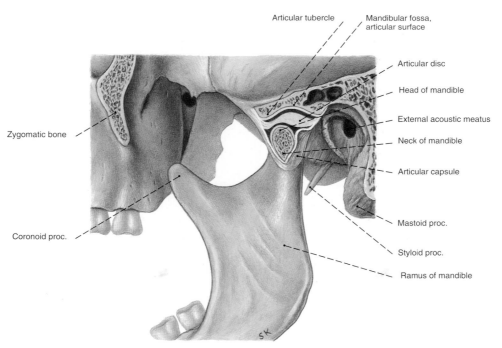

Fig. 126 The temporomandibular joint. Sagittal section, mouth open, lateral aspect.
Compare the positions of the head of the mandible and the articular disc in Figures 125 and 126.

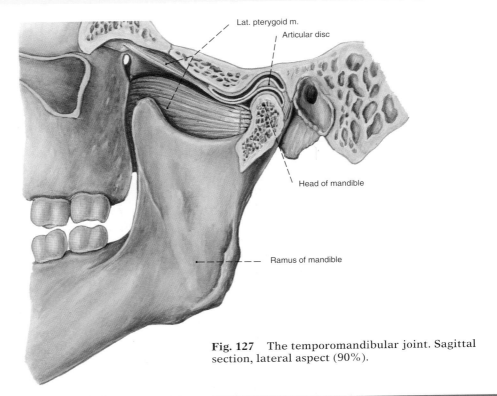

Lat. pterygoid m.

Articular disc

Head of mandible

Ramus of mandible

Fig. 127 The temporomandibular joint. Sagittal section, lateral aspect (90%).

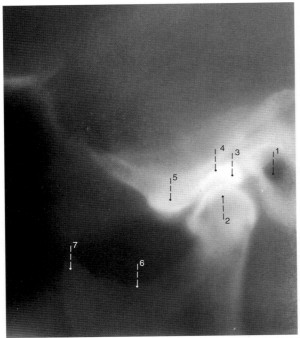

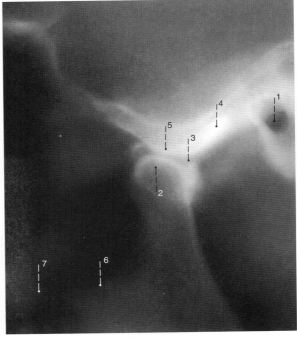

1 External acoustic meatus
2 Condylar proc.
3 Articular disc
4 Temporal bone, mandibular fossa

5 Temporal bone, articular tubercle
6 Mandibular notch
7 Coronoid proc.

Fig. 128 Radiograph of the temporomandibular joint, with the mouth closed. Lateral projection, after injection of the joint with contrast material (arthrography).

Fig. 129 Radiograph of the temporomandibular joint, with the mouth open. Projection as in Figure 128. Compare the different positions of the head of the mandible and the articular disc in Figures 128 and 129. Also refer to Figures 125 and 126.

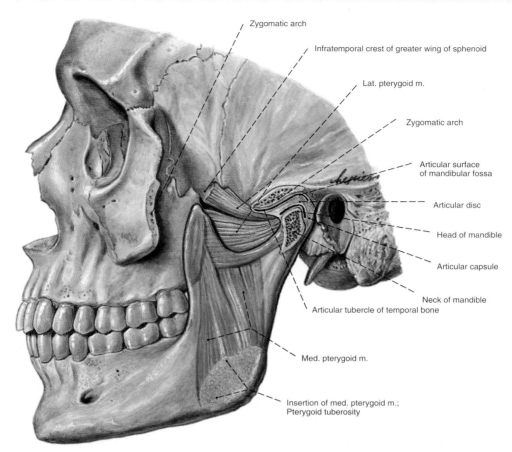

Fig. 130 The temporomandibular joint and the muscles of mastication, lateral aspect.

Sagittal section with the condylar and coronoid processes represented as transparent.

Muscles of Mastication

Name *Innervation*	Origin	Insertion	Function
1. Masseter muscle *Superficial part*	Zygomatic process of max-illa, inferior border of zygomatic arch	Angle and lower half of lateral surface of ramus of mandible	Closes the jaws by elevating the mandible
Intermediate part	Inner surface of zygomatic arch	Ramus of mandible	
Deep part *Masseteric n.* *(Mandibular n., V3)*	Posterior part of inferior border and inner surface of zygomatic arch	Superior half of ramus of mandible and lateral surface of coronoid process of mandible	
2. Temporalis muscle *Deep temporal nn.* *(Mandibular n., V3)*	Temporal fossa and temporal fascia	Coronoid process (medial surface, apex, anterior border) and ramus of mandible (anterior border)	Elevates mandible (closes jaws), posterior fibers retract mandible
3. Lateral pterygoid muscle *Lateral pterygoid n.* *(Mandibular n., V3)*	Superior head: infratemporal crest and lateral surface of greater wing of sphenoid; Inferior head: lateral surface of lateral pterygoid plate	Condyloid process of mandible (neck); temporomandibular joint (articular disc)	Opens the jaws, protrudes mandible, moves mandible side-to-side
4. Medial pterygoid muscle *Medial pterygoid n.,* *(Mandibular n., V3)*	Pterygoid fossa; pyramidal process of palatine bone; lateral pterygoid plate	Medial surface of ramus and angle of mandible opposite the masseter muscle	Closes the jaws; with lateral pterygoid muscle protrudes and moves mandible side-to-side

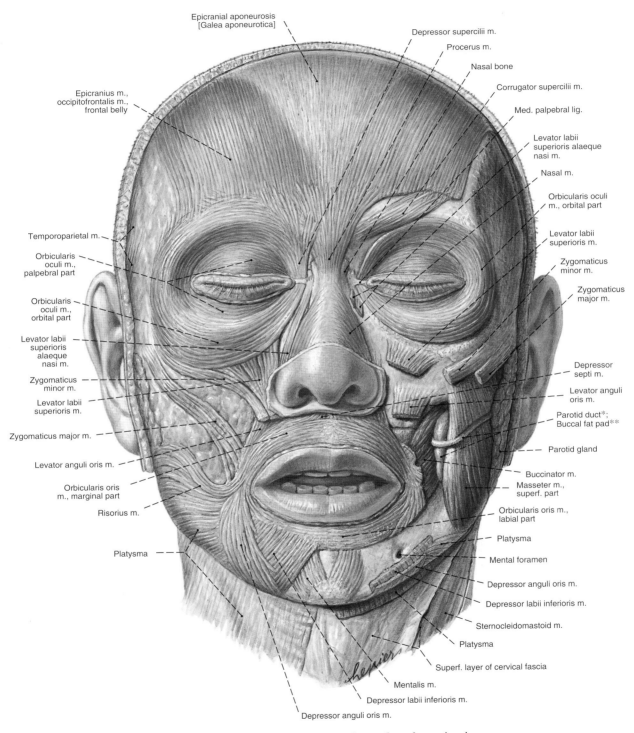

Epicranial aponeurosis [Galea aponeurotica]

Epicranius m., occipitofrontalis m., frontal belly

Temporoparietal m.

Orbicularis oculi m., palpebral part

Orbicularis oculi m., orbital part

Levator labii superioris alaeque nasi m.

Zygomaticus minor m.

Levator labii superioris m.

Zygomaticus major m.

Levator anguli oris m.

Orbicularis oris m., marginal part

Risorius m.

Platysma

Depressor supercilii m.

Procerus m.

Nasal bone

Corrugator supercilii m.

Med. palpebral lig.

Levator labii superioris alaeque nasi m.

Nasal m.

Orbicularis oculi m., orbital part

Levator labii superioris m.

Zygomaticus minor m.

Zygomaticus major m.

Depressor septi m.

Levator anguli oris m.

Parotid duct*; Buccal fat pad**

Parotid gland

Buccinator m.

Masseter m., superf. part

Orbicularis oris m., labial part

Platysma

Mental foramen

Depressor anguli oris m.

Depressor labii inferioris m.

Sternocleidomastoid m.

Platysma

Superf. layer of cervical fascia

Mentalis m.

Depressor labii inferioris m.

Depressor anguli oris m.

Fig. 131 Facial muscles and muscles of mastication, anterior view (80%). The more superficial layer is shown on the right side of the face, while the deeper muscles are on the left.

* Clinical: STENSEN's duct
** Clinical: BICHAT's fat pad

Facial Muscles: Muscles of the Mouth

Name *Innervation**	Origin	Insertion	Function
1. **Levator labii superioris alaeque nasi muscle** *Facial n. (VII)*	Frontal process of maxilla	Greater alar cartilage and skin of nose, upper lips	Facial expression: Move lips, nasal alae, cheeks, skin of chin
2. **Levator labii superioris muscle** *Facial n. (VII)*	Infraorbital margin, maxilla, zygomatic bone	Upper lip	
3. **Zygomaticus minor muscle** *Facial n. (VII)*	Molar surface of zygomatic bone	Angle of mouth	
4. **Zygomaticus major muscle** *Facial n. (VII)*	Lateral surface of zygomatic bone	Angle of mouth	
5. **Risorius muscle** (part of Platsyma or No. 6) *Facial n. (VII)*	Masseteric fascia	Angle of mouth	
6. **Depressor anguli oris muscle** Facial n. (VII)	Oblique line of mandible	Angle of mouth and lower lip	
7. **Levator anguli oris muscle** *Facial n. (VII)*	Canine fossa of maxilla	Upper lip musculature and angle of mouth	
8. **Depressor labii inferioris muscle** *Facial n. (VII)*	Oblique line of mandible	Lower lip	
9. **Orbicularis oris muscle** *Facial n. (VII)*	Consists of marginal part (from other facial muscles) and labial part (from skin of lip)	Upper and lower lips, philtrum of upper lip	
10. **Mentalis muscle** *Facial n. (VII)*	Incisive fossa of mandible	Skin of chin	
11. **Transverse menti muscle** *Facial n. (VII)*	Mandible	Angle of mouth	
12. **Buccinator muscle** *Facial n. (VII)*	Outer surface of alveolar processes of maxilla and mandible, pterygomandibular raphe	Angle of mouth and lips	Compresses the cheek, forces the air out as in blowing a trumpet (buccinator in Latin), aids in chewing

* All facial muscles are innervated by the facial n. (VII)

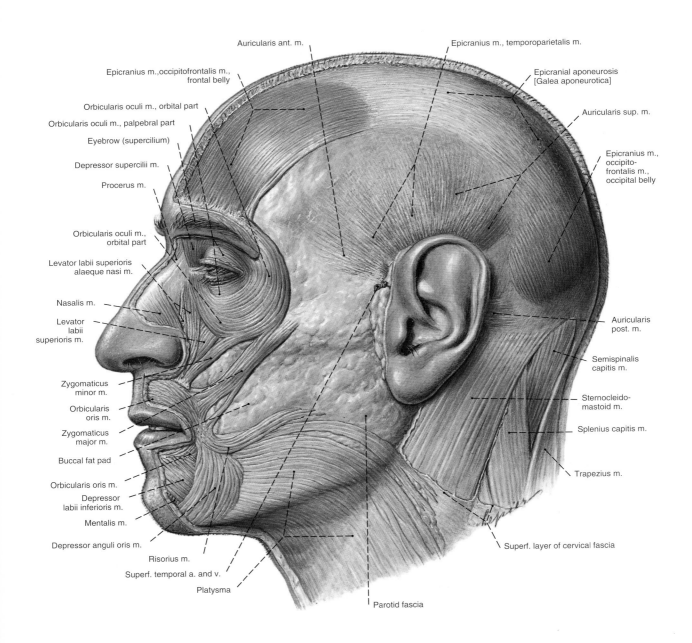

Auricularis ant. m.

Epicranius m., temporoparietalis m.

Epicranius m.,occipitofrontalis m., frontal belly

Epicranial aponeurosis [Galea aponeurotica]

Orbicularis oculi m., orbital part

Auricularis sup. m.

Orbicularis oculi m., palpebral part

Eyebrow (supercilium)

Epicranius m., occipito-frontalis m., occipital belly

Depressor supercilii m.

Procerus m.

Orbicularis oculi m., orbital part

Levator labii superioris alaeque nasi m.

Nasalis m.

Levator labii superioris m.

Auricularis post. m.

Semispinalis capitis m.

Zygomaticus minor m.

Sternocleido-mastoid m.

Orbicularis oris m.

Splenius capitis m.

Zygomaticus major m.

Buccal fat pad

Trapezius m.

Orbicularis oris m.

Depressor labii inferioris m.

Mentalis m.

Depressor anguli oris m.

Superf. layer of cervical fascia

Risorius m.

Superf. temporal a. and v.

Platysma

Parotid fascia

Fig. 132 The facial muscles, lateral view (60%).

Muscles of the Scalp: The Epicranius Muscle

Name *Innervation*	Origin	Insertion	Function
1. **Occipitofrontalis, muscle, frontal belly** *Facial n. (VII)*	Supraorbital margin	Galea aponeurotica	Moves scalp
2. **Occipitofrontalis, muscle, occipital belly** *Facial n. (VII)*	Supreme nuchal line	Galea aponeurotica	
3. **Temporoparietalis muscle** *Facial n. (VII)*	Temporal fascia near ear, superior lamina	Skin or temporal fascia above and in front of ear	

Muscles of the Nose

Name *Innervation*	Origin	Insertion	Function
1. **Nasalis muscle** *Facial n. (VII)*			
Transverse part	Maxilla above canine teeth	Aponeurosis over bridge of nose	Dilates and contracts nostrils
Alar part	Maxilla above lateral incisors	Alar cartilage of nose	
2. **Depressor septi muscle** *Facial n. (VII)*	Maxilla above medial incisors	Nasal septum, cartilaginous part	

Muscles of the Eyelids

Name *Innervation*	Origin	Insertion	Function
1. **Orbicularis oculi muscle** *Facial n. (VII)*			
Orbital part	Frontal process of maxilla, medial angle of eye, medial palpebral ligament	Surrounds orbital opening as a sphincter, some fibers go to eyebrow	Closes eyelids, compresses lacrimal sac, moves eyebrows
Palpebral part	Medial palpebral ligament	Lateral palpebral raphe	
Lacrimal part	Posterior lacrimal crest	Superior and inferior tarsi medial to puncta lacrimalia	
2. **Depressor supercilii muscle** *Facial n. (VII)*	Nasal part of frontal bone bone	Skin of eyebrow	
3. **Corrugator supercilii muscle** *Facial n. (VII)*	Nasal part of frontal bone	Skin of eyebrow	
4. **Procerus muscle** *Facial n. (VII)*	Bridge of nose and lateral nasal cartilage	Skin of forehead between eyebrows	Acts upon skin of forehead and eyebrows

Extrinsic Muscles of the Ear

Name *Innervation*	Origin	Insertion	Function
1. **Auricularis anterior muscle** *Facial n. (VII)*	Temporal fascia, superficial lamina	Spine of the helix	Moves the auricula
2. **Auricularis superior muscle** *Facial n. (VII)*	Galea aponeurotica	Root of auricula	
3. **Auricularis posterior muscle** *Facial n. (VII)*	Mastoid process of temporal bone, tendon of sternoclei-domastoid muscle	Auricula at convexity of concha	

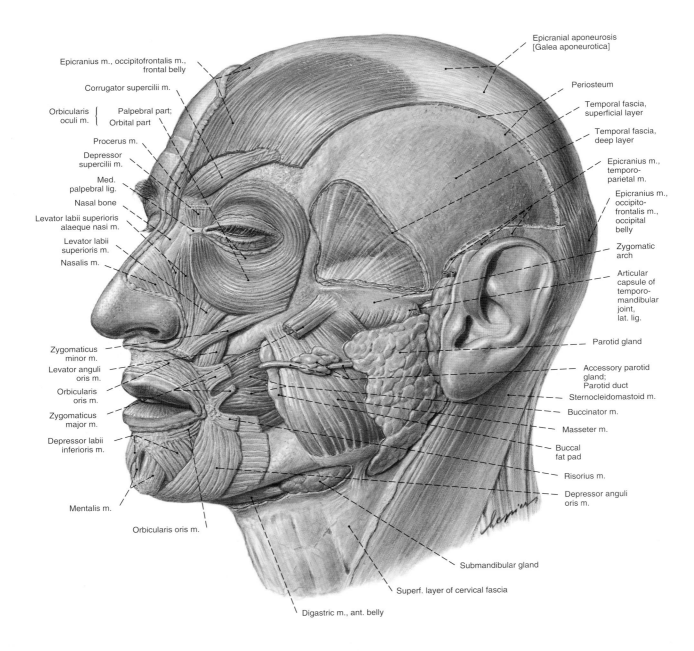

Epicranius m., occipitofrontalis m., frontal belly

Corrugator supercilii m.

Orbicularis oculi m. { Palpebral part; Orbital part

Procerus m.

Depressor supercilii m.

Med. palpebral lig.

Nasal bone

Levator labii superioris alaeque nasi m.

Levator labii superioris m.

Nasalis m.

Zygomaticus minor m.

Levator anguli oris m.

Orbicularis oris m.

Zygomaticus major m.

Depressor labii inferioris m.

Mentalis m.

Orbicularis oris m.

Digastric m., ant. belly

Superf. layer of cervical fascia

Submandibular gland

Epicranial aponeurosis [Galea aponeurotica]

Periosteum

Temporal fascia, superficial layer

Temporal fascia, deep layer

Epicranius m., temporo-parietal m.

Epicranius m., occipito-frontalis m., occipital belly

Zygomatic arch

Articular capsule of temporo-mandibular joint, lat. lig.

Parotid gland

Accessory parotid gland; Parotid duct

Sternocleidomastoid m.

Buccinator m.

Masseter m.

Buccal fat pad

Risorius m.

Depressor anguli oris m.

Fig. 133 Facial muscles and muscles of mastication, lateral view (60%). The temporal and the superficial fasciae have been partially removed, and the masseteric and parotid fasciae have been completely removed.

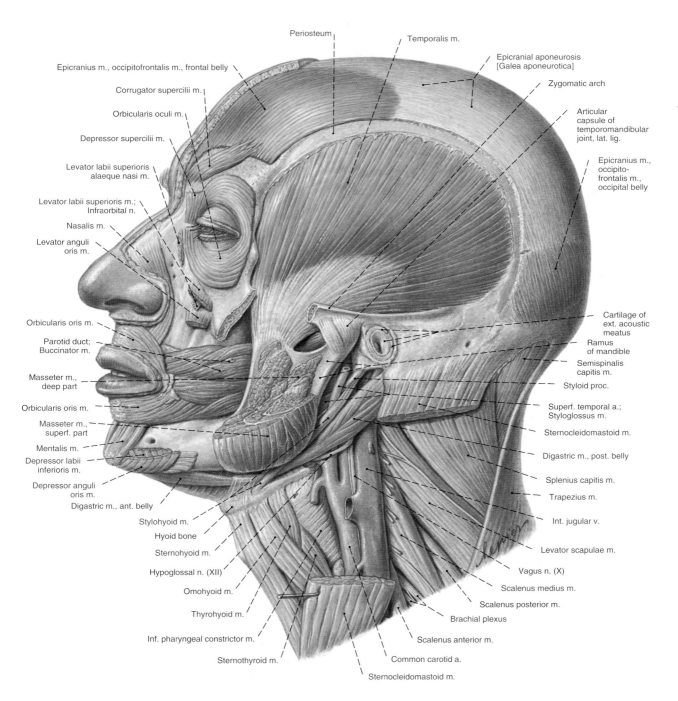

Periosteum

Temporalis m.

Epicranial aponeurosis [Galea aponeurotica]

Zygomatic arch

Epicranius m., occipitofrontalis m., frontal belly

Corrugator supercilii m.

Orbicularis oculi m.

Depressor supercilii m.

Levator labii superioris alaeque nasi m.

Levator labii superioris m.; Infraorbital n.

Nasalis m.

Levator anguli oris m.

Orbicularis oris m.

Parotid duct; Buccinator m.

Masseter m., deep part

Orbicularis oris m.

Masseter m., superf. part

Mentalis m.

Depressor labii inferioris m.

Depressor anguli oris m.

Digastric m., ant. belly

Stylohyoid m.

Hyoid bone

Sternohyoid m.

Hypoglossal n. (XII)

Omohyoid m.

Thyrohyoid m.

Inf. pharyngeal constrictor m.

Sternothyroid m.

Articular capsule of temporomandibular joint, lat. lig.

Epicranius m., occipito-frontalis m., occipital belly

Cartilage of ext. acoustic meatus

Ramus of mandible

Semispinalis capitis m.

Styloid proc.

Superf. temporal a.; Styloglossus m.

Sternocleidomastoid m.

Digastric m., post. belly

Splenius capitis m.

Trapezius m.

Int. jugular v.

Levator scapulae m.

Vagus n. (X)

Scalenus medius m.

Scalenus posterior m.

Brachial plexus

Scalenus anterior m.

Common carotid a.

Sternocleidomastoid m.

Fig. 134   Facial muscles, muscles of mastication, and supra- and infrahyoid muscles, lateral view (60%). The external ear, the zygomatic arch, the masseter muscle and several muscles of facial expression have been partially removed.

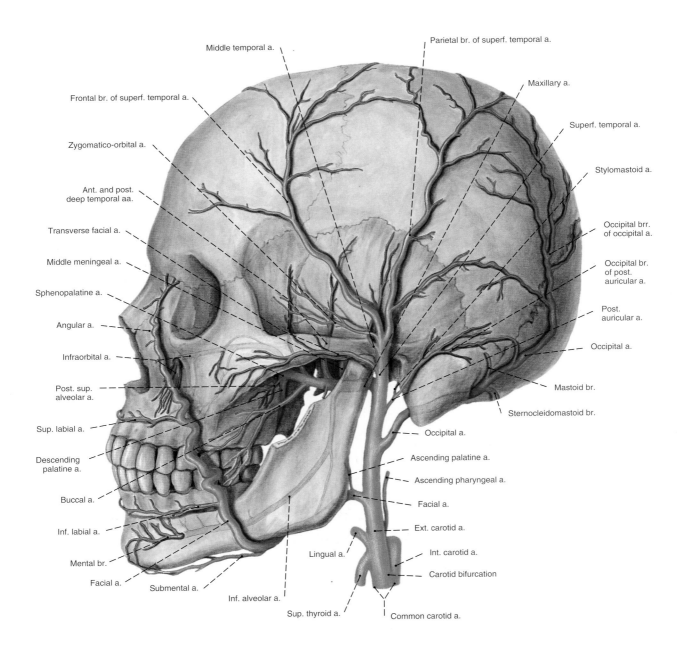

Middle temporal a.

Parietal br. of superf. temporal a.

Frontal br. of superf. temporal a.

Maxillary a.

Zygomatico-orbital a.

Superf. temporal a.

Ant. and post.
deep temporal aa.

Stylomastoid a.

Transverse facial a.

Occipital brr.
of occipital a.

Middle meningeal a.

Occipital br.
of post.
auricular a.

Sphenopalatine a.

Post.
auricular a.

Angular a.

Occipital a.

Infraorbital a.

Post. sup.
alveolar a.

Mastoid br.

Sternocleidomastoid br.

Sup. labial a.

Occipital a.

Descending
palatine a.

Ascending palatine a.

Ascending pharyngeal a.

Buccal a.

Facial a.

Inf. labial a.

Ext. carotid a.

Mental br.

Lingual a.

Int. carotid a.

Carotid bifurcation

Facial a.

Submental a.

Inf. alveolar a.

Sup. thyroid a.

Common carotid a.

Fig. 135 The external carotid artery and its branches, lateral aspect (60%).

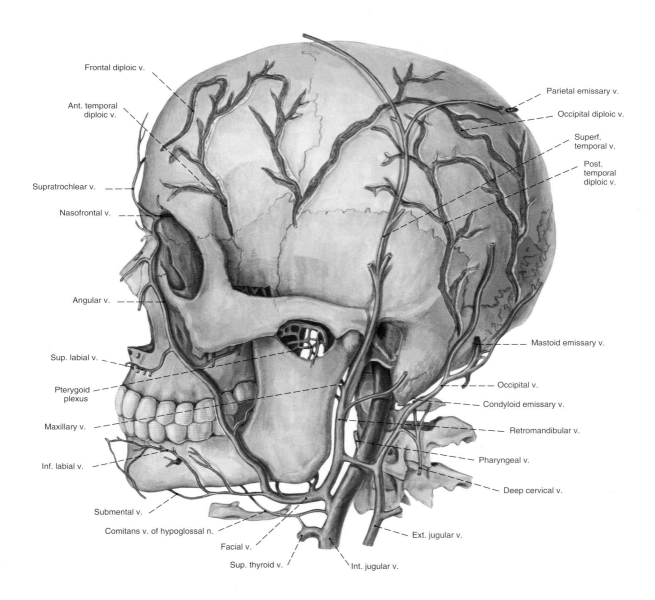

Frontal diploic v.

Ant. temporal diploic v.

Supratrochlear v.

Nasofrontal v.

Angular v.

Sup. labial v.

Pterygoid plexus

Maxillary v.

Inf. labial v.

Submental v.

Comitans v. of hypoglossal n.

Facial v.

Sup. thyroid v.

Parietal emissary v.

Occipital diploic v.

Superf. temporal v.

Post. temporal diploic v.

Mastoid emissary v.

Occipital v.

Condyloid emissary v.

Retromandibular v.

Pharyngeal v.

Deep cervical v.

Ext. jugular v.

Int. jugular v.

Fig. 136 The internal jugular vein and its extracranial tributaries, lateral aspect (60%).

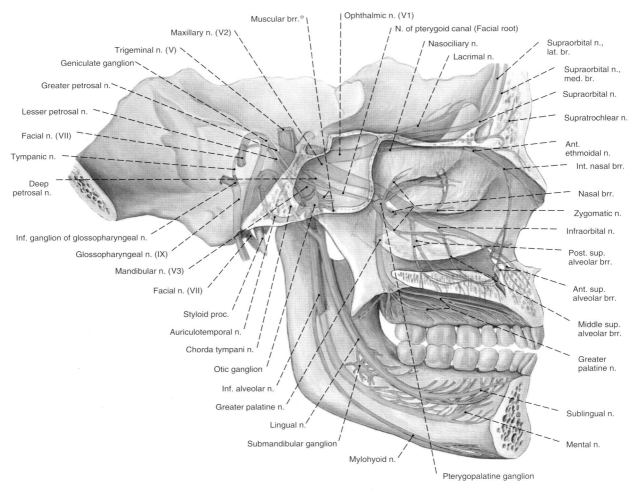

Muscular brr.*
Ophthalmic n. (V1)
Maxillary n. (V2)
N. of pterygoid canal (Facial root)
Trigeminal n. (V)
Nasociliary n.
Geniculate ganglion
Lacrimal n.
Greater petrosal n.
Supraorbital n., lat. br.
Lesser petrosal n.
Supraorbital n., med. br.
Facial n. (VII)
Supraorbital n.
Tympanic n.
Supratrochlear n.
Deep petrosal n.
Ant. ethmoidal n.
Int. nasal brr.
Inf. ganglion of glossopharyngeal n.
Nasal brr.
Glossopharyngeal n. (IX)
Zygomatic n.
Mandibular n. (V3)
Infraorbital n.
Facial n. (VII)
Post. sup. alveolar brr.
Styloid proc.
Ant. sup. alveolar brr.
Auriculotemporal n.
Middle sup. alveolar brr.
Chorda tympani n.
Greater palatine n.
Otic ganglion
Inf. alveolar n.
Greater palatine n.
Sublingual n.
Lingual n.
Mental n.
Submandibular ganglion
Mylohyoid n.
Pterygopalatine ganglion

Fig. 137 The nerves of the face, the trigeminal (V), facial (VII), glossopharyngeal (IX) nerves and their branches. A paramedian section of the skull with exposed nerves in yellow and nerves covered by bone, light yellow; medial view (60%).
* Branches to muscles of mastication

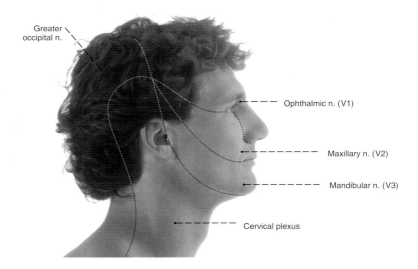

Greater occipital n.
Ophthalmic n. (V1)
Maxillary n. (V2)
Mandibular n. (V3)
Cervical plexus

Fig. 138 Sensory innervation of the face and neck, lateral aspect (30%).

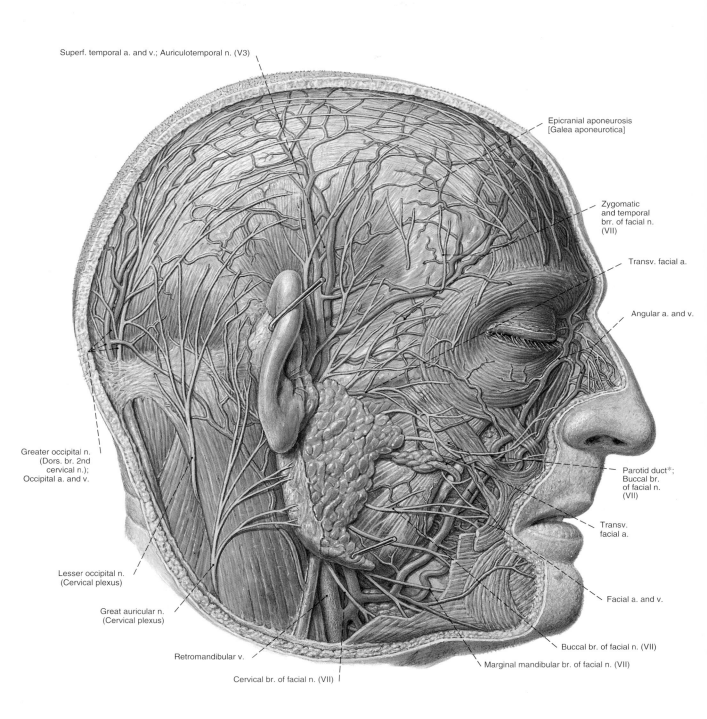

Superf. temporal a. and v.; Auriculotemporal n. (V3)

Epicranial aponeurosis
[Galea aponeurotica]

Zygomatic
and temporal
brr. of facial n.
(VII)

Transv. facial a.

Angular a. and v.

Parotid duct*;
Buccal br.
of facial n.
(VII)

Transv.
facial a.

Greater occipital n.
(Dors. br. 2nd
cervical n.);
Occipital a. and v.

Facial a. and v.

Lesser occipital n.
(Cervical plexus)

Great auricular n.
(Cervical plexus)

Buccal br. of facial n. (VII)

Retromandibular v.

Marginal mandibular br. of facial n. (VII)

Cervical br. of facial n. (VII)

Fig. 139 Vessels and nerves of the
head, superficial layer, lateral view (90%).

* Clinical: STENSEN's duct

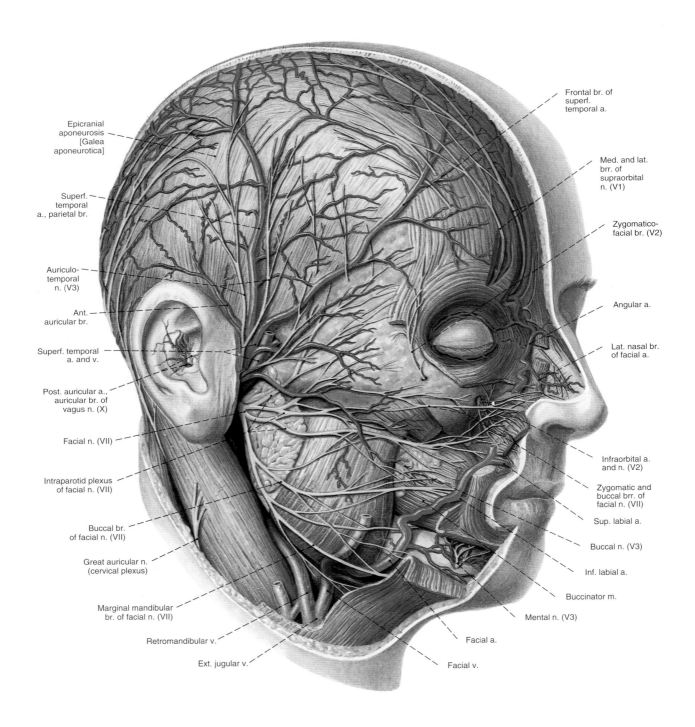

Epicranial aponeurosis [Galea aponeurotica]

Superf. temporal a., parietal br.

Auriculo-temporal n. (V3)

Ant. auricular br.

Superf. temporal a. and v.

Post. auricular a., auricular br. of vagus n. (X)

Facial n. (VII)

Intraparotid plexus of facial n. (VII)

Buccal br. of facial n. (VII)

Great auricular n. (cervical plexus)

Marginal mandibular br. of facial n. (VII)

Retromandibular v.

Ext. jugular v.

Frontal br. of superf. temporal a.

Med. and lat. brr. of supraorbital n. (V1)

Zygomatico-facial br. (V2)

Angular a.

Lat. nasal br. of facial a.

Infraorbital a. and n. (V2)

Zygomatic and buccal brr. of facial n. (VII)

Sup. labial a.

Buccal n. (V3)

Inf. labial a.

Buccinator m.

Mental n. (V3)

Facial a.

Facial v.

Fig. 140 Vessels and nerves of the head, lateral aspect (90%).The middle layer after removal of the superfical part of the parotid gland to expose the intraparotid plexus (VII).

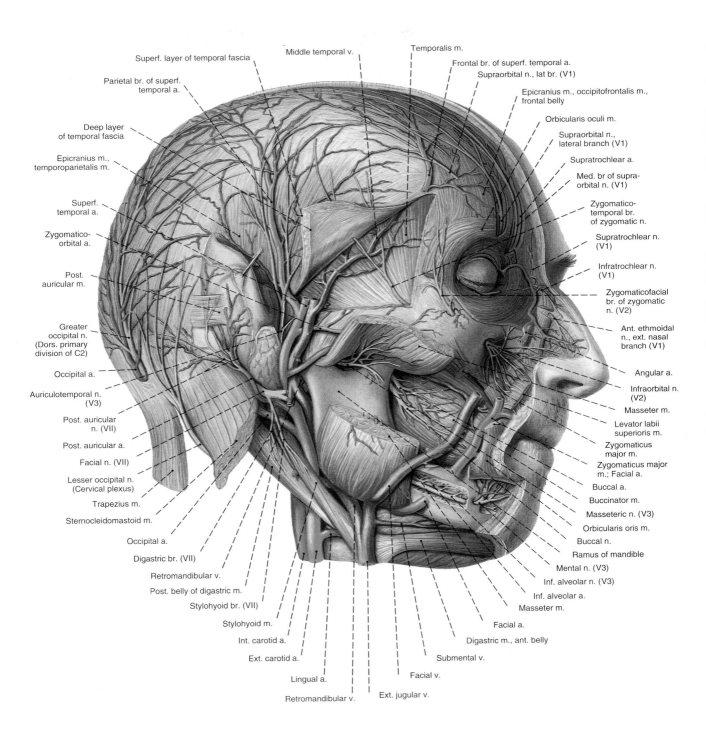

Fig. 141 Vessels and nerves of the head, lateral aspect (90%). The facial muscles, the parotid gland and branches of the facial nerve have been extensively removed; the masseter muscle and the temporal fascia are sectioned and reflected; and the mandibular canal is exposed.

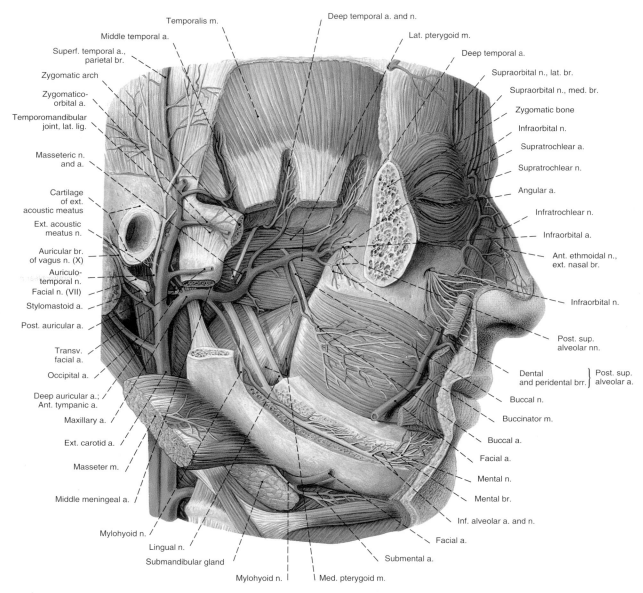

Temporalis m.

Deep temporal a. and n.

Middle temporal a.

Lat. pterygoid m.

Superf. temporal a., parietal br.

Deep temporal a.

Zygomatic arch

Supraorbital n., lat. br.

Zygomatico-orbital a.

Supraorbital n., med. br.

Temporomandibular joint, lat. lig.

Zygomatic bone

Masseteric n. and a.

Infraorbital n.

Cartilage of ext. acoustic meatus

Supratrochlear a.

Ext. acoustic meatus n.

Supratrochlear n.

Auricular br. of vagus n. (X)

Angular a.

Auriculo-temporal n.

Infratrochlear n.

Facial n. (VII)

Infraorbital a.

Stylomastoid a.

Ant. ethmoidal n., ext. nasal br.

Post. auricular a.

Infraorbital n.

Transv. facial a.

Post. sup. alveolar nn.

Occipital a.

Dental and peridental brr. | Post. sup. alveolar a.

Deep auricular a.; Ant. tympanic a.

Buccal n.

Maxillary a.

Buccinator m.

Ext. carotid a.

Buccal a.

Masseter m.

Facial a.

Middle meningeal a.

Mental n.

Mylohyoid n.

Mental br.

Lingual n.

Inf. alveolar a. and n.

Submandibular gland

Facial a.

Mylohyoid n.

Submental a.

Med. pterygoid m.

Fig. 142 Vessels and nerves of the face, lateral view. The deep layer after partial removal of the zygomatic arch and the ramus of the mandible with the masseter and temporalis muscles. The mandibular canal has been opened.

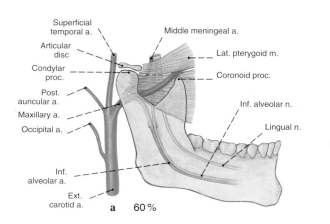

Superficial temporal a.

Middle meningeal a.

Articular disc

Lat. pterygoid m.

Condylar proc.

Coronoid proc.

Post. auricular a.

Inf. alveolar n.

Maxillary a.

Lingual n.

Occipital a.

Inf. alveolar a.

Ext. carotid a.

a 60 %

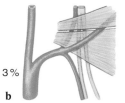

3 %

b

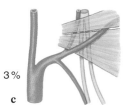

3 %

c

Fig. 143 a–c Variations of the maxillary artery. Percentages indicate the frequency of occurrence.

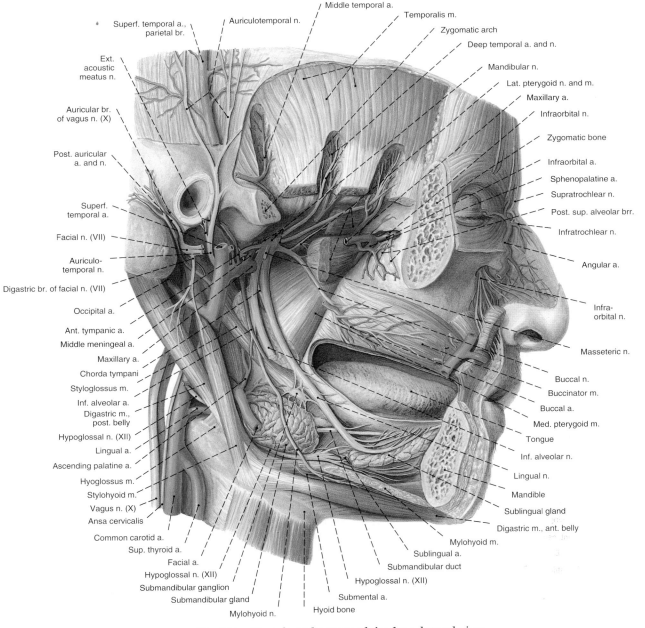

Superf. temporal a., parietal br.
Auriculotemporal n.
Middle temporal a.
Temporalis m.
Zygomatic arch
Deep temporal a. and n.
Ext. acoustic meatus n.
Mandibular n.
Lat. pterygoid n. and m.
Maxillary a.
Auricular br. of vagus n. (X)
Infraorbital n.
Zygomatic bone
Post. auricular a. and n.
Infraorbital a.
Sphenopalatine a.
Supratrochlear n.
Superf. temporal a.
Post. sup. alveolar brr.
Facial n. (VII)
Infratrochlear n.
Auriculo-temporal n.
Angular a.
Digastric br. of facial n. (VII)
Occipital a.
Infra-orbital n.
Ant. tympanic a.
Middle meningeal a.
Maxillary a.
Masseteric n.
Chorda tympani
Styloglossus m.
Buccal n.
Inf. alveolar a.
Buccinator m.
Digastric m., post. belly
Buccal a.
Hypoglossal n. (XII)
Med. pterygoid m.
Lingual a.
Tongue
Ascending palatine a.
Inf. alveolar n.
Hyoglossus m.
Lingual n.
Stylohyoid m.
Mandible
Vagus n. (X)
Sublingual gland
Ansa cervicalis
Digastric m., ant. belly
Common carotid a.
Mylohyoid m.
Sup. thyroid a.
Sublingual a.
Facial a.
Submandibular duct
Hypoglossal n. (XII)
Hypoglossal n. (XII)
Submandibular ganglion
Submental a.
Submandibular gland
Mylohyoid n.
Hyoid bone

Fig. 144 Vessels and nerves of the face, lateral view. The deep layer after removal of the zygomatic arch and a large part of the right mandible. Portions of the buccinator muscle and underlying oral mucous membrane have been removed.

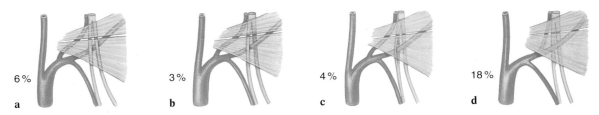

6 % a   3 % b   4 % c   18 % d

Fig. 145 a–d Variations of the maxillary artery. Percentages indicate frequency of occurrence.

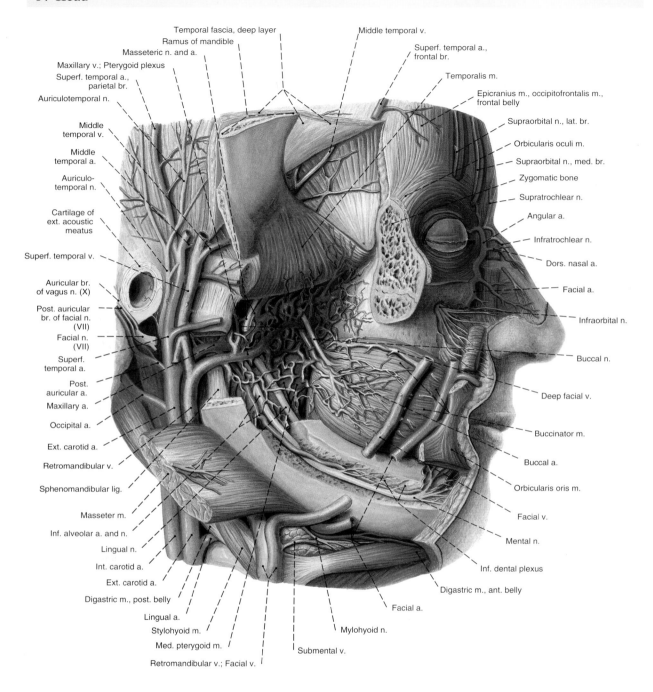

Temporal fascia, deep layer
Ramus of mandible
Masseteric n. and a.
Maxillary v.; Pterygoid plexus
Superf. temporal a., parietal br.
Auriculotemporal n.
Middle temporal v.
Middle temporal a.
Auriculo-temporal n.
Cartilage of ext. acoustic meatus
Superf. temporal v.
Auricular br. of vagus n. (X)
Post. auricular br. of facial n. (VII)
Facial n. (VII)
Superf. temporal a.
Post. auricular a.
Maxillary a.
Occipital a.
Ext. carotid a.
Retromandibular v.
Sphenomandibular lig.
Masseter m.
Inf. alveolar a. and n.
Lingual n.
Int. carotid a.
Ext. carotid a.
Digastric m., post. belly
Lingual a.
Stylohyoid m.
Med. pterygoid m.
Retromandibular v.; Facial v.
Submental v.
Mylohyoid n.
Facial a.
Digastric m., ant. belly
Inf. dental plexus
Mental n.
Facial v.
Orbicularis oris m.
Buccal a.
Buccinator m.
Deep facial v.
Buccal n.
Infraorbital n.
Facial a.
Dors. nasal a.
Infratrochlear n.
Angular a.
Supratrochlear n.
Zygomatic bone
Supraorbital n., med. br.
Orbicularis oculi m.
Supraorbital n., lat. br.
Epicranius m., occipitofrontalis m., frontal belly
Temporalis m.
Superf. temporal a., frontal br.
Middle temporal v.

Fig. 146 Vessels and nerves of the face, deep layer, lateral view. The specimen is similar to Figure 142.

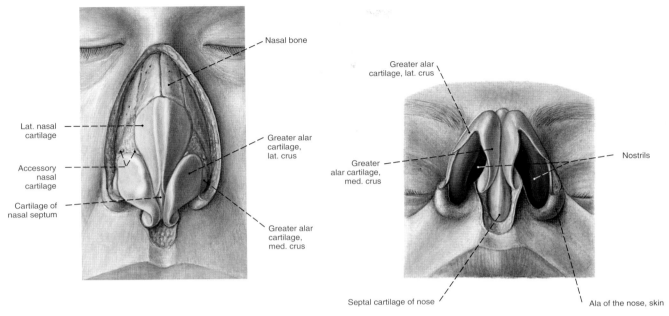

Nasal bone

Lat. nasal
cartilage

Accessory
nasal
cartilage

Cartilage of
nasal septum

Greater alar
cartilage,
lat. crus

Greater alar
cartilage,
med. crus

Fig. 147 The nasal skeleton,
anterior view (90%).

Greater alar
cartilage, lat. crus

Greater
alar cartilage,
med. crus

Nostrils

Septal cartilage of nose

Ala of the nose, skin

Fig. 148 Cartilages of the nose, viewed
from below (90%).

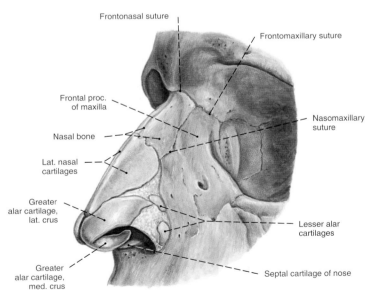

Frontonasal suture

Frontomaxillary suture

Frontal proc.
of maxilla

Nasal bone

Lat. nasal
cartilages

Greater
alar cartilage,
lat. crus

Greater
alar cartilage,
med. crus

Nasomaxillary
suture

Lesser alar
cartilages

Septal cartilage of nose

Fig. 149 The nasal
skeleton, lateral view (90%).

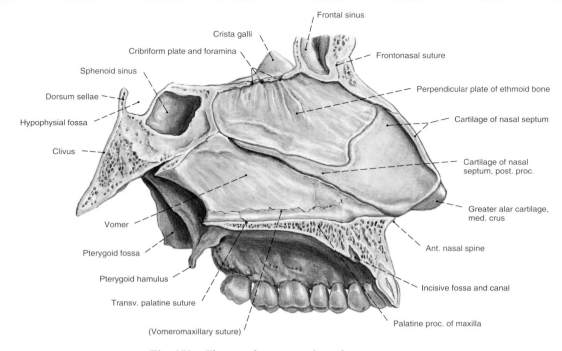

Crista galli

Frontal sinus

Cribriform plate and foramina

Frontonasal suture

Sphenoid sinus

Dorsum sellae

Perpendicular plate of ethmoid bone

Hypophysial fossa

Cartilage of nasal septum

Clivus

Cartilage of nasal septum, post. proc.

Greater alar cartilage, med. crus

Vomer

Pterygoid fossa

Ant. nasal spine

Pterygoid hamulus

Incisive fossa and canal

Transv. palatine suture

(Vomeromaxillary suture)

Palatine proc. of maxilla

Fig. 150 The nasal septum, viewed laterally from the right.

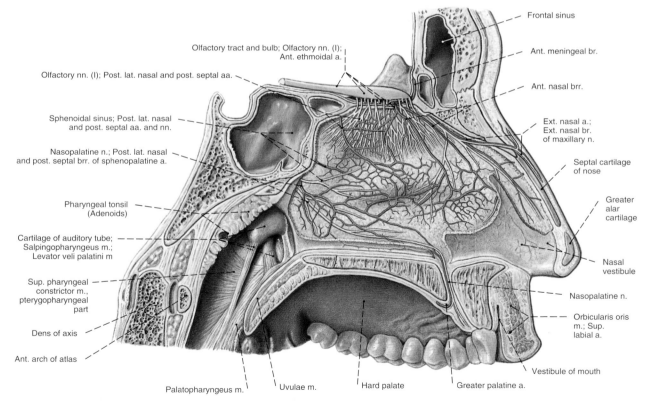

Frontal sinus

Olfactory tract and bulb; Olfactory nn. (I);
Ant. ethmoidal a.

Ant. meningeal br.

Olfactory nn. (I); Post. lat. nasal and post. septal aa.

Ant. nasal brr.

Sphenoidal sinus; Post. lat. nasal and post. septal aa. and nn.

Ext. nasal a.;
Ext. nasal br.
of maxillary n.

Nasopalatine n.; Post. lat. nasal and post. septal brr. of sphenopalatine a.

Septal cartilage of nose

Pharyngeal tonsil (Adenoids)

Greater alar cartilage

Cartilage of auditory tube;
Salpingopharyngeus m.;
Levator veli palatini m

Nasal vestibule

Sup. pharyngeal constrictor m., pterygopharyngeal part

Nasopalatine n.

Dens of axis

Orbicularis oris m.; Sup. labial a.

Ant. arch of atlas

Vestibule of mouth

Palatopharyngeus m.

Uvulae m.

Hard palate

Greater palatine a.

Fig. 151 Arteries and nerves of the nasal septum, viewed laterally from the right. A paramedian section after extensive removal of the nasal mucous membrane. Note: The pharyngeal tonsil becomes smaller with age and is often barely identifiable.

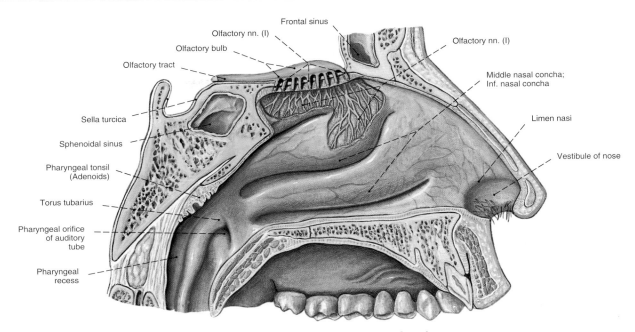

Fig. 152 The lateral wall of the left nasal cavity, medial view. A paramedian section with the nasal mucous membrane partially removed.

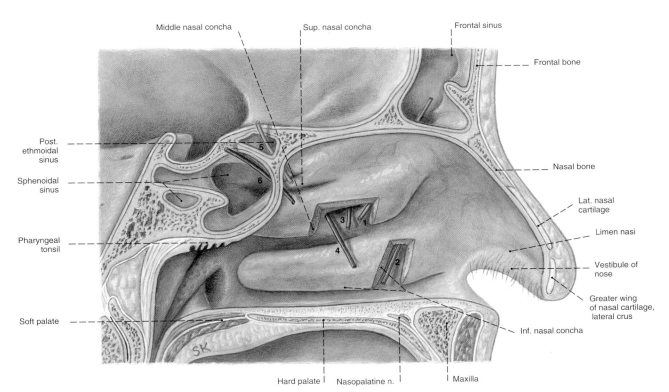

1 Frontal sinus
2 Nasolacrimal duct
3 Ant. ethmoidal sinus
4 Maxillary sinus
5 Post. ethmoidal sinus
6 Sphenoidal sinus

Fig. 153 The left nasal cavity and openings of the paranasal sinuses, and the nasolacrimal duct, medial view. A paramedian section after partial removal of the middle and lower conchae. Colored probes are located in the openings of the paranasal sinuses and nasolacrimal duct.

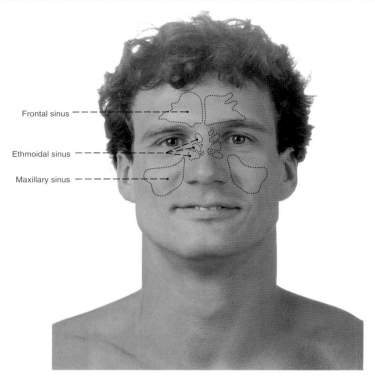

Frontal sinus

Ethmoidal sinus

Maxillary sinus

Fig. 154 The paranasal sinuses projected onto the face, anterior view. The sphenoidal sinuses are not shown.

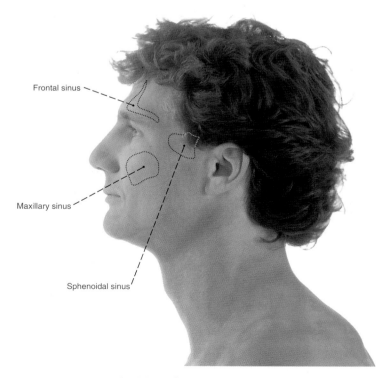

Frontal sinus

Maxillary sinus

Sphenoidal sinus

Fig. 155 The paranasal sinuses projected onto the face, lateral view. The ethmoidal sinuses are not shown.

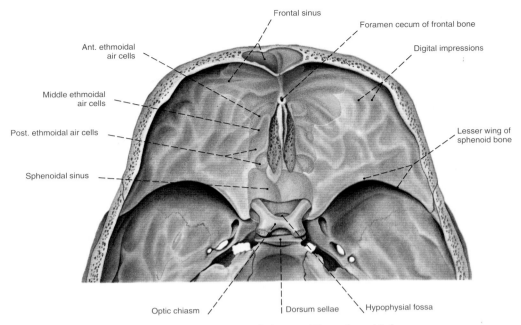

Fig. 156 The paranasal sinuses. The sphenoidal, ethmoidal, and frontal sinuses are projected onto the anterior cranial fossa, viewed from above (80%).

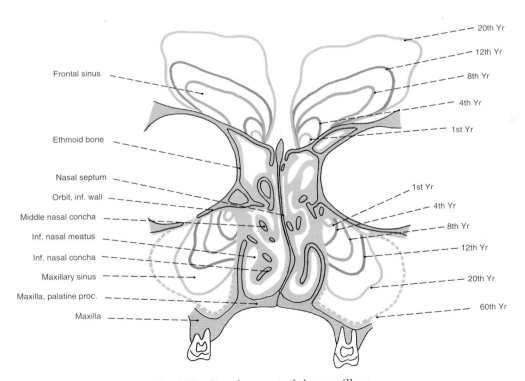

Fig. 157 Development of the maxillary and frontal sinuses. Yr = age in years.

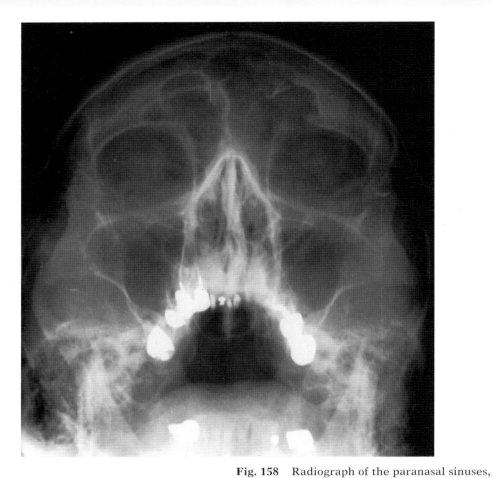

Fig. 158 Radiograph of the paranasal sinuses, PA projection, antero-inferior view (80%). The beam is oriented in the occipito-oral direction with the mouth open.

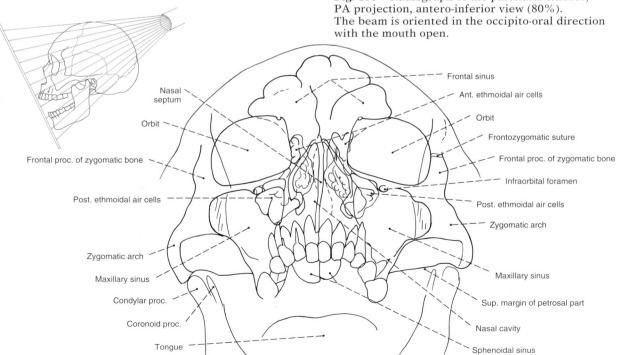

Frontal sinus

Ant. ethmoidal air cells

Nasal septum

Orbit

Orbit

Frontozygomatic suture

Frontal proc. of zygomatic bone

Frontal proc. of zygomatic bone

Infraorbital foramen

Post. ethmoidal air cells

Post. ethmoidal air cells

Zygomatic arch

Zygomatic arch

Maxillary sinus

Maxillary sinus

Condylar proc.

Sup. margin of petrosal part

Coronoid proc.

Nasal cavity

Tongue

Sphenoidal sinus

Fig. 159 The paranasal sinuses: line drawing of Figure 158.

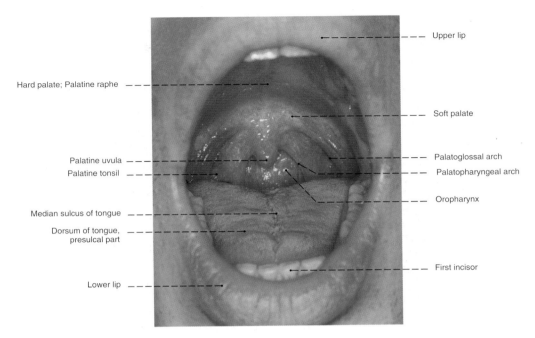

Upper lip

Hard palate; Palatine raphe

Soft palate

Palatine uvula

Palatine tonsil

Palatoglossal arch

Palatopharyngeal arch

Oropharynx

Median sulcus of tongue

Dorsum of tongue,
presulcal part

First incisor

Lower lip

Fig. 160 The oral cavity,
anterior view.

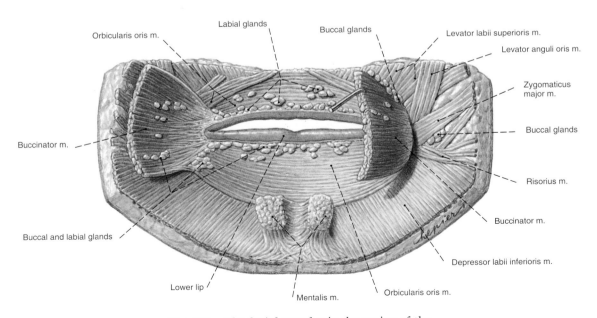

Orbicularis oris m.

Labial glands

Buccal glands

Levator labii superioris m.

Levator anguli oris m.

Zygomaticus
major m.

Buccal glands

Buccinator m.

Risorius m.

Buccinator m.

Depressor labii inferioris m.

Buccal and labial glands

Lower lip

Mentalis m.

Orbicularis oris m.

Fig. 161 The facial muscles in the region of the
mouth, internal aspect (80%). The oral mucous
membrane has been removed, and some small
salivary glands remain.

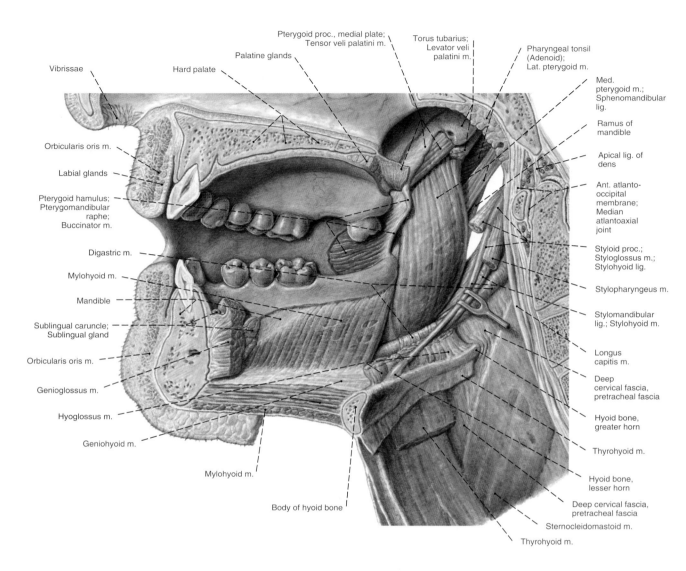

Vibrissae

Orbicularis oris m.

Labial glands

Pterygoid hamulus;
Pterygomandibular
raphe;
Buccinator m.

Digastric m.

Mylohyoid m.

Mandible

Sublingual caruncle;
Sublingual gland

Orbicularis oris m.

Genioglossus m.

Hyoglossus m.

Geniohyoid m.

Mylohyoid m.

Body of hyoid bone

Hard palate

Palatine glands

Pterygoid proc., medial plate;
Tensor veli palatini m.

Torus tubarius;
Levator veli
palatini m.

Pharyngeal tonsil
(Adenoid);
Lat. pterygoid m.

Med.
pterygoid m.;
Sphenomandibular
lig.

Ramus of
mandible

Apical lig. of
dens

Ant. atlanto-
occipital
membrane;
Median
atlantoaxial
joint

Styloid proc.;
Styloglossus m.;
Stylohyoid lig.

Stylopharyngeus m.

Stylomandibular
lig.; Stylohyoid m.

Longus
capitis m.

Deep
cervical fascia,
pretracheal fascia

Hyoid bone,
greater horn

Thyrohyoid m.

Hyoid bone,
lesser horn

Deep cervical fascia,
pretracheal fascia

Sternocleidomastoid m.

Thyrohyoid m.

Fig. 162   The oral cavity, medial view.
A paramedian section after removal
of the pharynx and larynx.

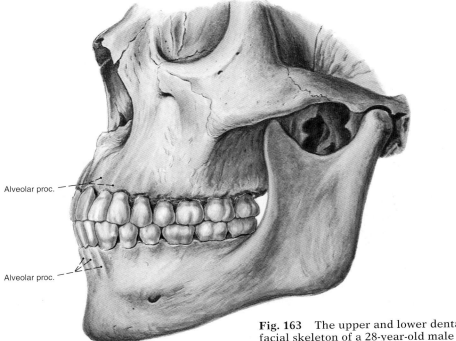

Alveolar proc.

Alveolar proc.

Fig. 163 The upper and lower dental arches in the facial skeleton of a 28-year-old male in centric occlusion, lateral view.

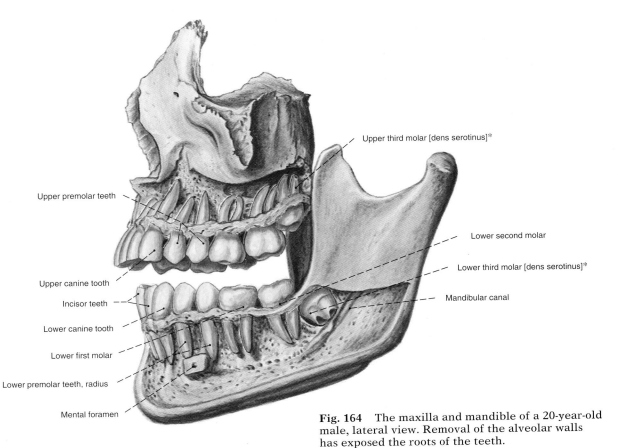

Upper third molar [dens serotinus]*

Upper premolar teeth

Lower second molar

Lower third molar [dens serotinus]*

Upper canine tooth

Incisor teeth

Mandibular canal

Lower canine tooth

Lower first molar

Lower premolar teeth, radius

Mental foramen

Fig. 164 The maxilla and mandible of a 20-year-old male, lateral view. Removal of the alveolar walls has exposed the roots of the teeth.

* The lower third molar has not yet erupted.

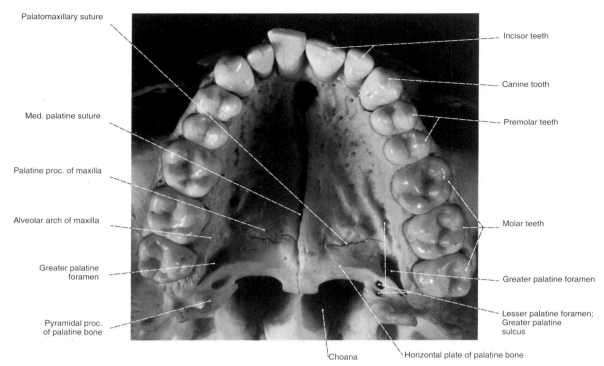

Palatomaxillary suture

Med. palatine suture

Palatine proc. of maxilla

Alveolar arch of maxilla

Greater palatine foramen

Pyramidal proc. of palatine bone

Incisor teeth

Canine tooth

Premolar teeth

Molar teeth

Greater palatine foramen

Lesser palatine foramen; Greater palatine sulcus

Choana

Horizontal plate of palatine bone

Fig. 165 The hard palate and dental arch of the maxilla, inferior aspect (150%). Photograph of an adult specimen.

Note the displacement of the four incisors from their normal position (Fig. 184).

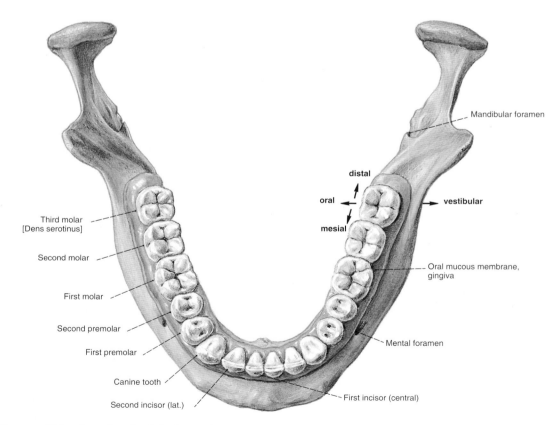

Third molar [Dens serotinus]

Second molar

First molar

Second premolar

First premolar

Canine tooth

Second incisor (lat.)

distal

oral — vestibular

mesial

Mandibular foramen

Oral mucous membrane, gingiva

Mental foramen

First incisor (central)

Fig. 166 The mandible, dental arch of the lower jaw, and gingiva, superior aspect (110%). Oral is synonymous with lingual in the mandible and with palatal in the maxilla.

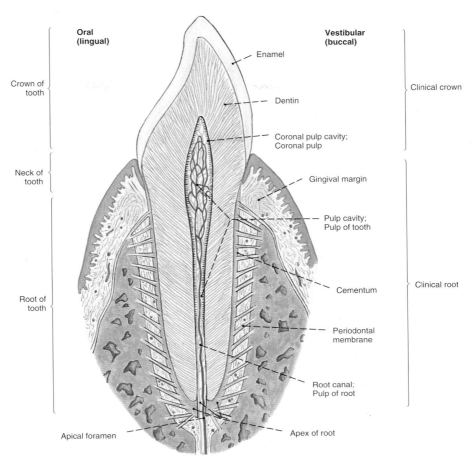

Oral
(lingual)

Vestibular
(buccal)

Enamel

Crown of
tooth

Clinical crown

Dentin

Coronal pulp cavity;
Coronal pulp

Gingival margin

Neck of
tooth

Pulp cavity;
Pulp of tooth

Cementum

Clinical root

Root of
tooth

Periodontal
membrane

Root canal;
Pulp of root

Apical foramen

Apex of root

Fig. 167 Schematic longitudinal section through an
incisor tooth in its alveolar bony socket.

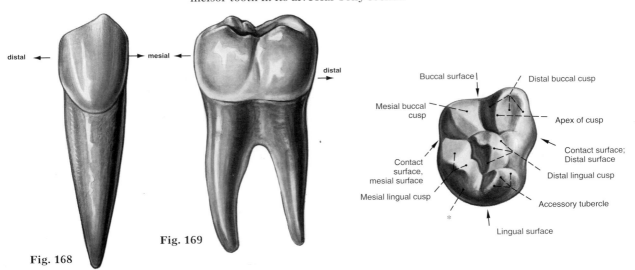

distal ←

mesial ←

distal →

Fig. 169

Fig. 168

Buccal surface

Distal buccal cusp

Mesial buccal
cusp

Apex of cusp

Contact
surface,
mesial surface

Contact surface;
Distal surface

Distal lingual cusp

Mesial lingual cusp

Accessory tubercle

*

Lingual surface

Fig. 168 The right lower permanent canine tooth,
buccal surface (400%).

Fig. 169 The left lower deciduous second molar
tooth, buccal surface (400%). The two sturdy roots of
this molar are bent somewhat distally (a typical
feature of these roots).

Fig. 170 The right lower permanent first molar,
occlusal surface (250%). The occlusal surface
usually has two buccal (vestibular) and two
lingual (oral) cusps.

* Occasionally a fifth cusp may appear on the mesiolingual
surface of the crown, the tubercle of CARABELLI.

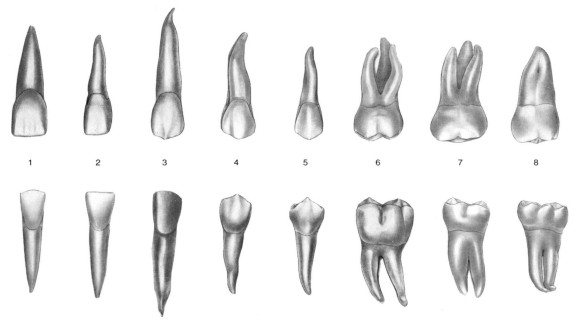

Fig. 171 The left upper and lower permanent teeth, viewed from the buccal surface (120%).

1 First incisor
2 Second incisor
3 Canine tooth
4 First premolar

5 Second premolar
6 First molar
7 Second molar
8 Third molar [Dens serotinus]

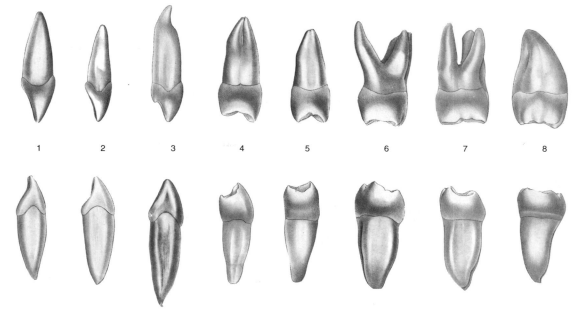

Fig. 172 The left upper and lower permanent teeth, viewed from the mesial surface (120%).

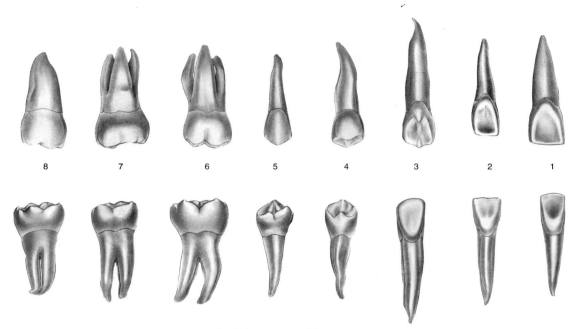

Fig. 173 The left upper and lower permanent
teeth, lingual surface (120%).
(See page 96 for identification of numbers)

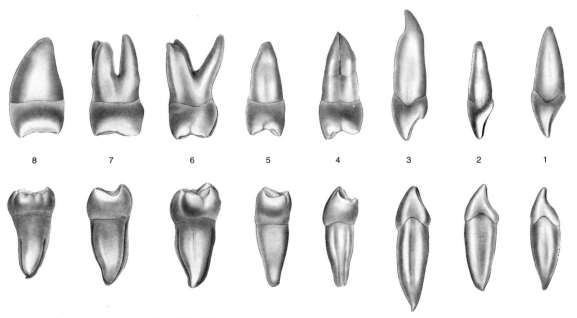

Fig. 174 The left upper and lower permanent
teeth, distal surface (120%).
(See page 96 for identification of numbers)

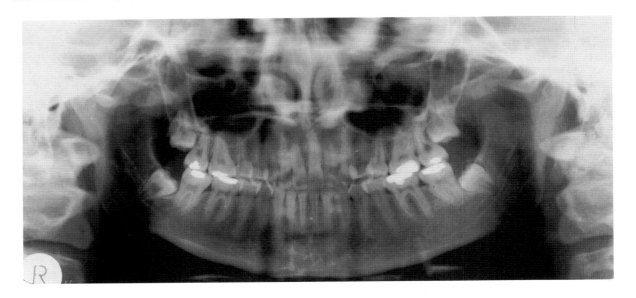

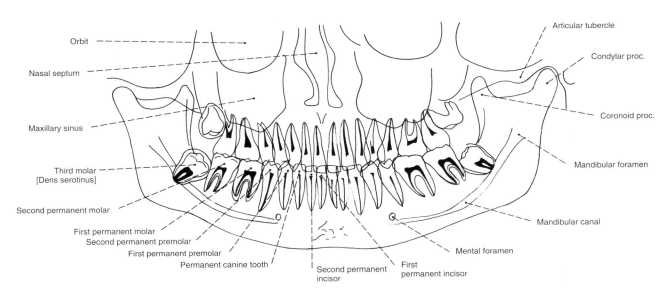

Fig. 175 Panoramic radiograph of the maxilla and mandible of an 18-year-old female. Complete dentition with impacted wisdom teeth (third molars) and some molars with amalgam restorations.

	Maxilla		
Right	18 17 16 15 14 13 12 11	21 22 23 24 25 26 27 28	Left
	48 47 46 45 44 43 42 41	31 32 33 34 35 36 37 38	
	Mandible		

Adult dentition

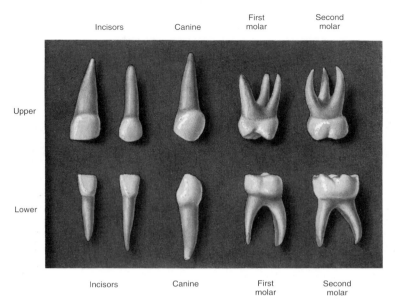

Fig. 176   The left deciduous teeth of a 3-year-old child, buccal surface (130%).

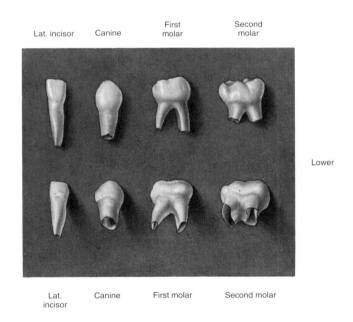

Fig. 177   The left deciduous teeth of a 2-year-old child. The top row shows the buccal surface; the bottom row views the teeth obliquely from below (130%). The dental roots are not yet completely calcified.

		Maxilla								
Right	55 54 53 52 51					61 62 63 64 65					Left
	85 84 83 82 81					71 72 73 74 75					

Mandible

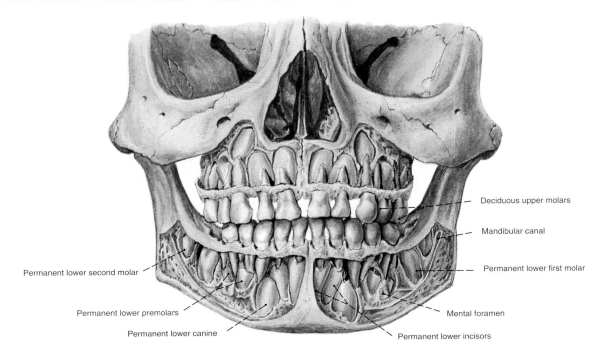

Deciduous upper molars

Mandibular canal

Permanent lower first molar

Permanent lower second molar

Permanent lower premolars

Permanent lower canine

Mental foramen

Permanent lower incisors

Fig. 178 Facial skeleton and deciduous teeth of a 5-year-old child, anterior view. The rudiments of the permanent teeth are shown in light blue.

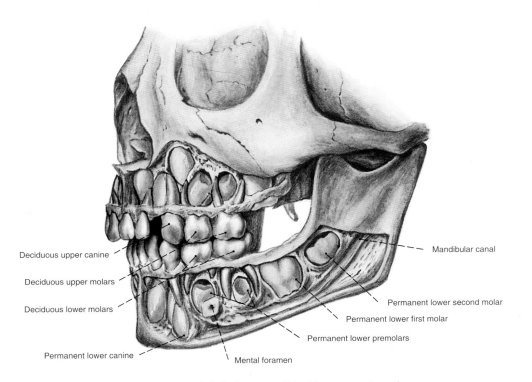

Deciduous upper canine

Deciduous upper molars

Deciduous lower molars

Permanent lower canine

Mental foramen

Mandibular canal

Permanent lower second molar

Permanent lower first molar

Permanent lower premolars

Fig. 179 Facial skeleton and deciduous teeth, as in the specimen of Fig. 178, lateral aspect.

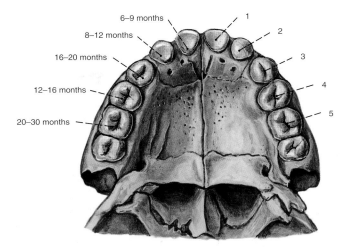

6–9 months
8–12 months
16–20 months
12–16 months
20–30 months

1
2
3
4
5

Fig. 180 Maxilla with deciduous teeth, inferior aspect. Numbers on the left side of the figure indicate the age of eruption of each tooth in months, and those on the right indicate the sequential order of appearance for the erupted deciduous teeth. Eruption times vary considerably and may differ between males and females and between the maxilla and mandible.

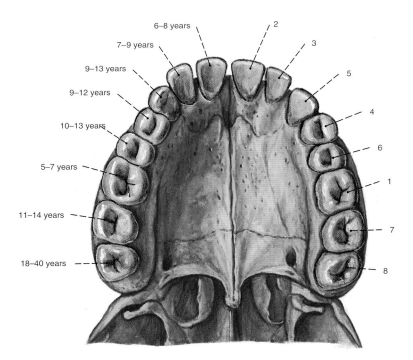

6–8 years
7–9 years
9–13 years
9–12 years
10–13 years
5–7 years
11–14 years
18–40 years

2
3
5
4
6
1
7
8

Fig. 181 Maxilla with permanent teeth, inferior aspect. Numbers on the left side of the figure indicate the age of eruption of each tooth in years, and those on the right indicate the sequential order of appearance for the erupted permanent teeth. Eruption times vary considerably.

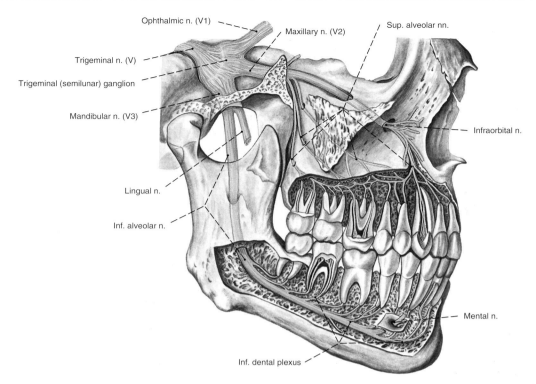

Ophthalmic n. (V1)

Maxillary n. (V2)

Sup. alveolar nn.

Trigeminal n. (V)

Trigeminal (semilunar) ganglion

Mandibular n. (V3)

Infraorbital n.

Lingual n.

Inf. alveolar n.

Mental n.

Inf. dental plexus

Fig. 182 Maxillary nerve (V2) and mandibular nerve (V3), lateral aspect. Parts of the maxilla and mandible have been removed and the mandibular canal has been exposed.

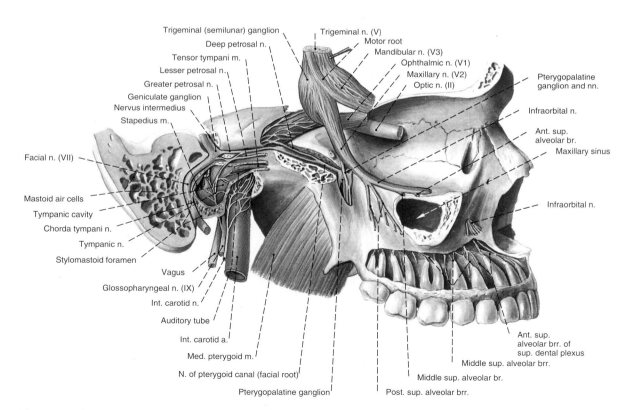

Trigeminal (semilunar) ganglion

Deep petrosal n.

Tensor tympani m.

Lesser petrosal n.

Greater petrosal n.

Geniculate ganglion

Nervus intermedius

Stapedius m.

Facial n. (VII)

Mastoid air cells

Tympanic cavity

Chorda tympani n.

Tympanic n.

Stylomastoid foramen

Vagus

Glossopharyngeal n. (IX)

Int. carotid n.

Auditory tube

Int. carotid a.

Med. pterygoid m.

N. of pterygoid canal (facial root)

Pterygopalatine ganglion

Trigeminal n. (V)

Motor root

Mandibular n. (V3)

Ophthalmic n. (V1)

Maxillary n. (V2)

Optic n. (II)

Pterygopalatine ganglion and nn.

Infraorbital n.

Ant. sup. alveolar br.

Maxillary sinus

Infraorbital n.

Ant. sup. alveolar brr. of sup. dental plexus

Middle sup. alveolar brr.

Middle sup. alveolar br.

Post. sup. alveolar brr.

Fig. 183 The roots of the pterygopalatine ganglion, lateral aspect. A sagittal section with the facial canal, the tympanic cavity, and the pterygoid canal exposed and the trigeminal ganglion retracted laterally.

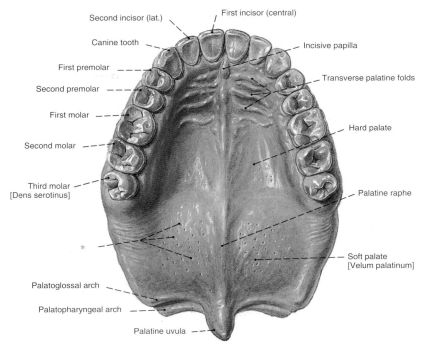

Second incisor (lat.)

First incisor (central)

Canine tooth

Incisive papilla

First premolar

Second premolar

Transverse palatine folds

First molar

Hard palate

Second molar

Third molar
[Dens serotinus]

Palatine raphe

*

Soft palate
[Velum palatinum]

Palatoglossal arch

Palatopharyngeal arch

Palatine uvula

Fig. 184 The hard and soft palates and the upper dental arch, viewed from below.

* Openings of the palatine glands

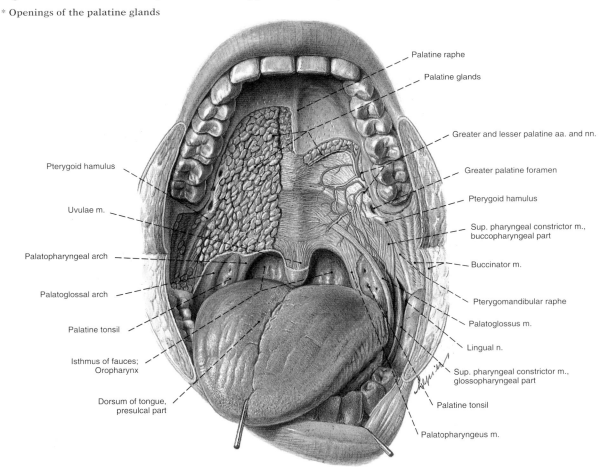

Palatine raphe

Palatine glands

Pterygoid hamulus

Greater and lesser palatine aa. and nn.

Greater palatine foramen

Uvulae m.

Pterygoid hamulus

Sup. pharyngeal constrictor m.,
buccopharyngeal part

Palatopharyngeal arch

Buccinator m.

Palatoglossal arch

Pterygomandibular raphe

Palatine tonsil

Palatoglossus m.

Lingual n.

Isthmus of fauces;
Oropharynx

Sup. pharyngeal constrictor m.,
glossopharyngeal part

Dorsum of tongue,
presulcal part

Palatine tonsil

Palatopharyngeus m.

Fig. 185 The oral cavity and palatine muscles, anterior view. The tongue has been protracted and the palatine mucosa extensively removed to show the palatine glands and the directions of the muscle fibers of the soft palate.

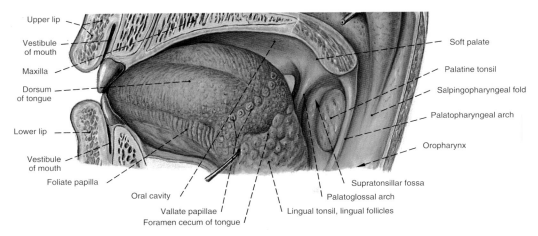

Upper lip

Vestibule of mouth

Maxilla

Dorsum of tongue

Lower lip

Vestibule of mouth

Foliate papilla

Oral cavity

Vallate papillae

Foramen cecum of tongue

Soft palate

Palatine tonsil

Salpingopharyngeal fold

Palatopharyngeal arch

Oropharynx

Supratonsillar fossa

Palatoglossal arch

Lingual tonsil, lingual follicles

Fig. 186 The oral cavity and pharynx, medial view of a paramedian section. The tongue has been protracted across the plane of the section, making it fully visible.

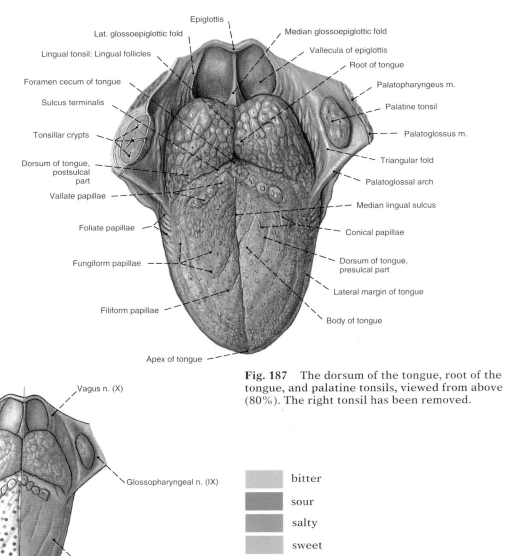

Epiglottis

Lat. glossoepiglottic fold

Lingual tonsil; Lingual follicles

Foramen cecum of tongue

Sulcus terminalis

Tonsillar crypts

Dorsum of tongue, postsulcal part

Vallate papillae

Foliate papillae

Fungiform papillae

Filiform papillae

Apex of tongue

Median glossoepiglottic fold

Vallecula of epiglottis

Root of tongue

Palatopharyngeus m.

Palatine tonsil

Palatoglossus m.

Triangular fold

Palatoglossal arch

Median lingual sulcus

Conical papillae

Dorsum of tongue, presulcal part

Lateral margin of tongue

Body of tongue

Fig. 187 The dorsum of the tongue, root of the tongue, and palatine tonsils, viewed from above (80%). The right tonsil has been removed.

Vagus n. (X)

Glossopharyngeal n. (IX)

Lingual n. (Mandibular n., V₃)

bitter

sour

salty

sweet

Fig. 188 Innervation and taste modalities of the dorsum of the tongue.

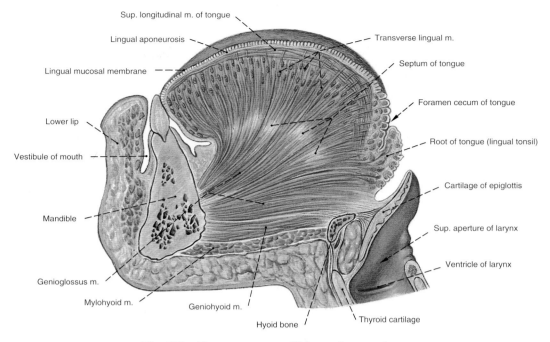

Sup. longitudinal m. of tongue

Lingual aponeurosis

Lingual mucosal membrane

Transverse lingual m.

Septum of tongue

Foramen cecum of tongue

Lower lip

Vestibule of mouth

Root of tongue (lingual tonsil)

Cartilage of epiglottis

Mandible

Sup. aperture of larynx

Ventricle of larynx

Genioglossus m.

Mylohyoid m.

Geniohyoid m.

Thyroid cartilage

Hyoid bone

Fig. 189 The tongue, mandible, and parts of the larynx, median section, lateral aspect.

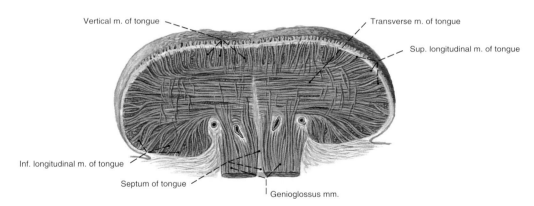

Vertical m. of tongue

Transverse m. of tongue

Sup. longitudinal m. of tongue

Inf. longitudinal m. of tongue

Septum of tongue

Genioglossus mm.

Fig. 190 The tongue. Cross section at the level of the middle segment, anterior view.

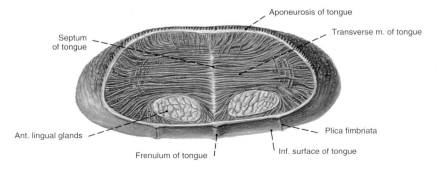

Aponeurosis of tongue

Septum of tongue

Transverse m. of tongue

Ant. lingual glands

Plica fimbriata

Frenulum of tongue

Inf. surface of tongue

Fig. 191 The tongue, anterior view. Cross section through the apex (tip), anterior view.

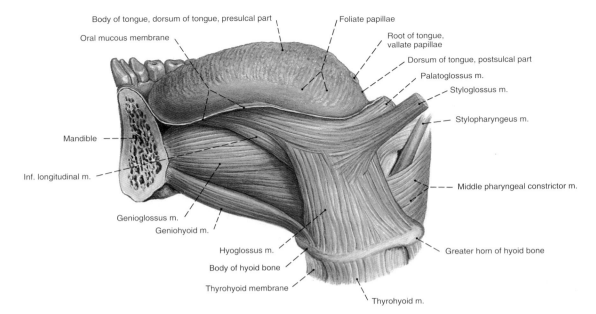

Body of tongue, dorsum of tongue, presulcal part

Oral mucous membrane

Foliate papillae

Root of tongue, vallate papillae

Dorsum of tongue, postsulcal part

Palatoglossus m.

Styloglossus m.

Stylopharyngeus m.

Mandible

Inf. longitudinal m.

Middle pharyngeal constrictor m.

Genioglossus m.

Geniohyoid m.

Hyoglossus m.

Body of hyoid bone

Thyrohyoid membrane

Greater horn of hyoid bone

Thyrohyoid m.

Fig. 192 Muscles of the tongue, lateral view (80%). The mandible has been resected.

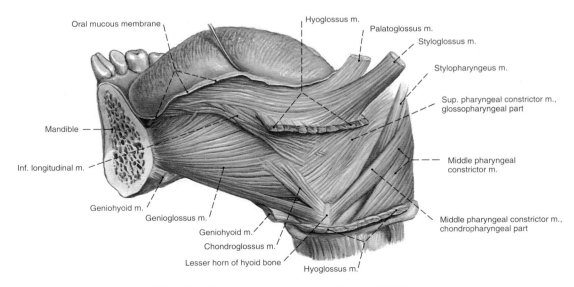

Oral mucous membrane

Hyoglossus m.

Palatoglossus m.

Styloglossus m.

Stylopharyngeus m.

Sup. pharyngeal constrictor m., glossopharyngeal part

Mandible

Inf. longitudinal m.

Middle pharyngeal constrictor m.

Geniohyoid m.

Genioglossus m.

Geniohyoid m.

Chondroglossus m.

Lesser horn of hyoid bone

Hyoglossus m.

Middle pharyngeal constrictor m., chondropharyngeal part

Fig. 193 Muscles of the tongue, lateral view (80%). The mandible has been resected and the hyoglossus muscle partially removed.

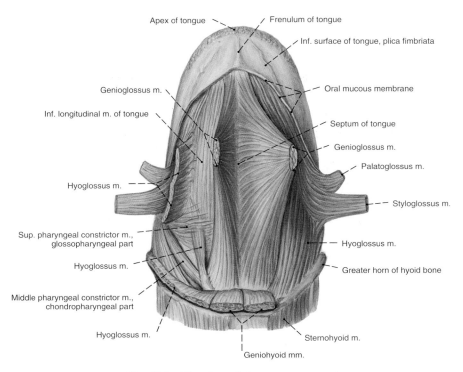

Apex of tongue — Frenulum of tongue

Inf. surface of tongue, plica fimbriata

Genioglossus m.

Inf. longitudinal m. of tongue

Oral mucous membrane

Septum of tongue

Genioglossus m.

Palatoglossus m.

Hyoglossus m.

Styloglossus m.

Sup. pharyngeal constrictor m., glossopharyngeal part

Hyoglossus m.

Hyoglossus m.

Greater horn of hyoid bone

Middle pharyngeal constrictor m., chondropharyngeal part

Hyoglossus m.

Sternohyoid m.

Geniohyoid mm.

Fig. 194 Muscles of the tongue, anterior view from below (80%). The genioglossus muscles have been resected from the mandible.

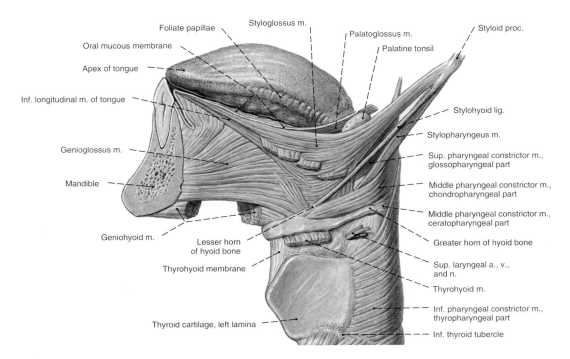

Foliate papillae

Styloglossus m.

Palatoglossus m.

Styloid proc.

Oral mucous membrane

Palatine tonsil

Apex of tongue

Inf. longitudinal m. of tongue

Stylohyoid lig.

Stylopharyngeus m.

Genioglossus m.

Sup. pharyngeal constrictor m., glossopharyngeal part

Mandible

Middle pharyngeal constrictor m., chondropharyngeal part

Middle pharyngeal constrictor m., ceratopharyngeal part

Geniohyoid m.

Greater horn of hyoid bone

Lesser horn of hyoid bone

Sup. laryngeal a., v., and n.

Thyrohyoid membrane

Thyrohyoid m.

Inf. pharyngeal constrictor m., thyropharyngeal part

Thyroid cartilage, left lamina

Inf. thyroid tubercle

Fig. 195 Muscles of the tongue, pharyngeal muscles, and larynx, lateral view (60%). The hyoglossus, genioglossus and thyrohyoid muscles have been sectioned.

Muscles of the Tongue

Name *Innervation*	Origin	Insertion	Function
1. **Genioglossus muscle** *Hypoglossal n. (XII)*	Mental spine of mandible	Fans out to body of tongue and lingual aponeurosis	Protrudes and depresses the tongue
2. **Hyoglossus muscle** *Hypoglossal n. (XII)*	Body and greater horn of hyoid bone	Lateral parts of tongue, lingual aponeurosis	Depresses and retracts the tongue
3. **Chondroglossus muscle** *Hypoglossal n. (XII)*	Lesser horn of hyoid bone	Lateral parts of tongue, lingual aponeurosis	Depresses and retracts the tongue
4. **Styloglossus muscle** *Hypoglossal n. (XII)*	Styloid process of temporal bone	Enters lateral parts of tongue from above and behind	Retracts and elevates the tongue (in sucking and swallowing)
5. **Palatoglossus muscle** *Accessory n. (XI)* *via Vagus n. (X)* *(pharyngeal plexus)*	Palatal aponeurosis	Upper, posterior parts of tongue	Constricts isthmus of the fauces
6. **Superior longitudinal muscle** *Hypoglossal n. (XII)*	Close to epiglottis and lingual septum	Apex of tongue	
7. **Inferior longitudinal muscle** *Hypoglossal n. (XII)*	Inferior surface of tongue at root	Apex of tongue	Muscles 6–9 alter shape of the tongue
8. **Transverse lingual muscle** *Hypoglossal n. (XII)*	Lingual septum	Lateral margins of tongue	
9. **Vertical lingual muscle** *Hypoglossal n. (XII)*	Upper surface anterior part of tongue	Inferior surface anterior part of tongue	

Muscles of the Palate

Name *Innervation*	Origin	Insertion	Function
1. **Uvulae muscle** *Accessory n. (XI)* *via vagus n. (X)* *(pharyngeal plexus)*	Palatine aponeurosis, post. nasal spine of palatine bone	Stroma of the uvula	Raises uvula
2. **Levator veli palatini muscle** *Accessory n. (XI)* *via vagus n. (X)* *(pharyngeal plexus)*	Temporal bone, inf. surface of petrous part, auditory tube cartilage	Muscles of both sides interdigitate in palatine velum without a tendon	Elevates the soft palate against dorsal pharyngeal wall (in deglutition)
3. **Tensor veli palatini muscle** *(Mandibular n., V3)*	Scaphoid fossa of med. pterygoid plate, spine of sphenoid, auditory tube cartilage	Runs as flat tendon through sulcus of pterygoid hamulus, forming palatine aponeurosis with tendon of opposite side	Tenses the soft palate, dilates auditory tube (in deglutition)
4. **Palatoglossus muscle** *Accessory n. (XI)* *via vagus n. (X)* *(pharyngeal plexus)*	Ant. surface of soft palate	Side of tongue, dorsum and transverse muscle of tongue	Constricts the fauces (in deglutition), draws root of tongue upward, lowers soft palate
5. **Palatopharyngeus muscle** *Accessory n. (XI)* *via vagus n. (X)* *(pharyngeal plexus)*	Soft palate midline	Post. border of thyroid cartilage, lateral wall of pharynx	Pulls pharynx upward (in deglutition), lowers soft palate

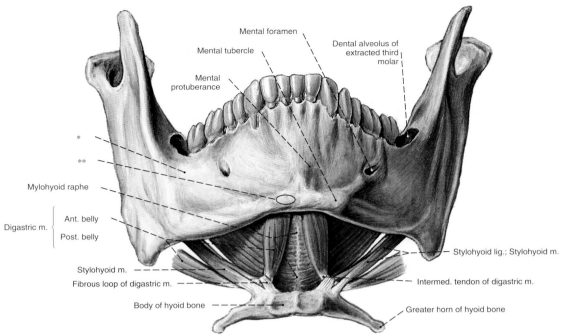

Mental foramen

Mental tubercle

Mental protuberance

Dental alveolus of extracted third molar

*

**

Mylohyoid raphe

Digastric m. { Ant. belly / Post. belly }

Stylohyoid m.

Fibrous loop of digastric m.

Body of hyoid bone

Stylohyoid lig.; Stylohyoid m.

Intermed. tendon of digastric m.

Greater horn of hyoid bone

Fig. 196 Mandible and suprahyoid muscles, antero-inferior view.

* Line of origin of the mylohyoid muscle
** Region of insertion of the anterior belly of the digastric muscle

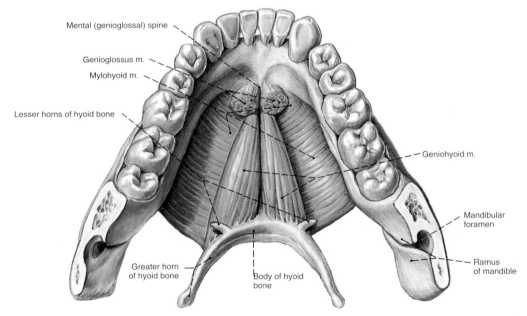

Mental (genioglossal) spine

Genioglossus m.

Mylohyoid m.

Lesser horns of hyoid bone

Geniohyoid m.

Mandibular foramen

Ramus of mandible

Greater horn of hyoid bone

Body of hyoid bone

Fig. 197 Mandible, suprahyoid muscles, and hyoid bone, viewed from above.

The mylohyoid muscles and the mandible have been sectioned.

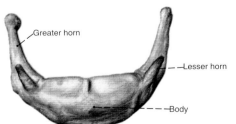

Greater horn

Lesser horn

Body

Fig. 198 Hyoid bone, anterosuperior view.

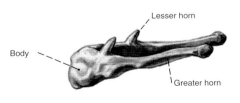

Lesser horn

Body

Greater horn

Fig. 199 Hyoid bone, oblique lateral view.

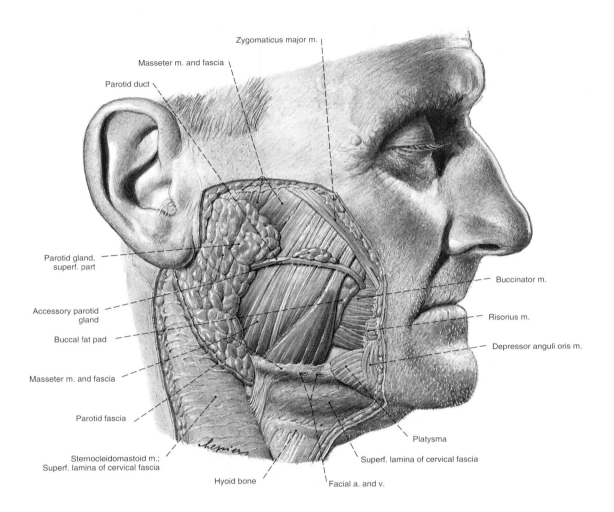

Zygomaticus major m.

Masseter m. and fascia

Parotid duct

Parotid gland, superf. part

Accessory parotid gland

Buccal fat pad

Masseter m. and fascia

Parotid fascia

Sternocleidomastoid m.; Superf. lamina of cervical fascia

Hyoid bone

Buccinator m.

Risorius m.

Depressor anguli oris m.

Platysma

Superf. lamina of cervical fascia

Facial a. and v.

Fig. 200 The parotid gland, lateral view (70%). Note the accessory parotid gland along the parotid duct.

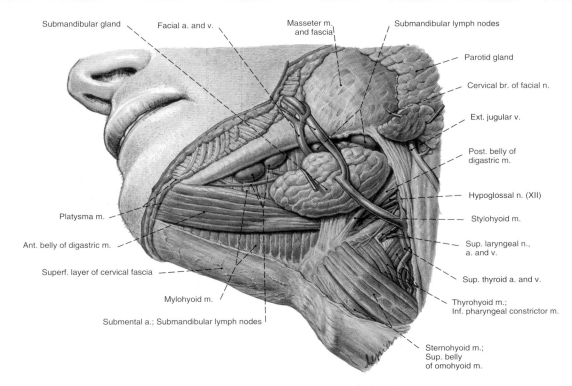

Fig. 201 The submandibular gland, latero-inferior view (80%). The platysma has been removed.

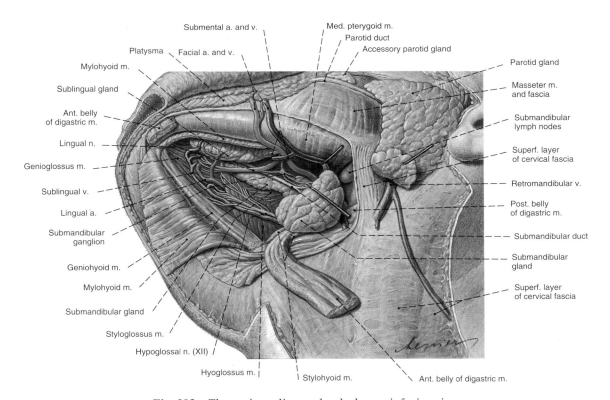

Fig. 202 The major salivary glands, latero-inferior view (80%). The mylohyoid muscle and the anterior belly of the digastric muscle have been sectioned.

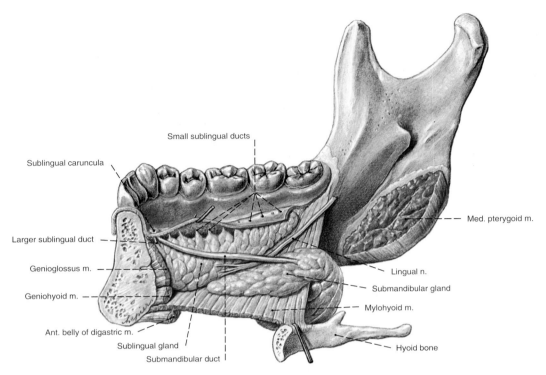

Small sublingual ducts

Sublingual caruncula

Larger sublingual duct

Genioglossus m.

Geniohyoid m.

Ant. belly of digastric m.

Sublingual gland

Submandibular duct

Med. pterygoid m.

Lingual n.

Submandibular gland

Mylohyoid m.

Hyoid bone

Fig. 203 The submandibular and the sublingual glands. A median section through the mandible and the hyoid bone, medial aspect.

Note the position of the lingual nerve in relation to the submandibular duct.

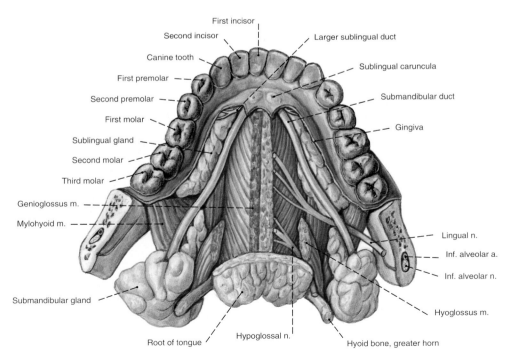

First incisor

Second incisor

Canine tooth

First premolar

Second premolar

First molar

Sublingual gland

Second molar

Third molar

Genioglossus m.

Mylohyoid m.

Submandibular gland

Root of tongue

Hypoglossal n.

Larger sublingual duct

Sublingual caruncula

Submandibular duct

Gingiva

Lingual n.

Inf. alveolar a.

Inf. alveolar n.

Hyoglossus m.

Hyoid bone, greater horn

Fig. 204 The sublingual and the submandibular glands, viewed from above. The genioglossus and the hyoglossus muscles have been sectioned and the tongue has been removed. Note the position of the lingual nerve in relation to the submandibular duct.

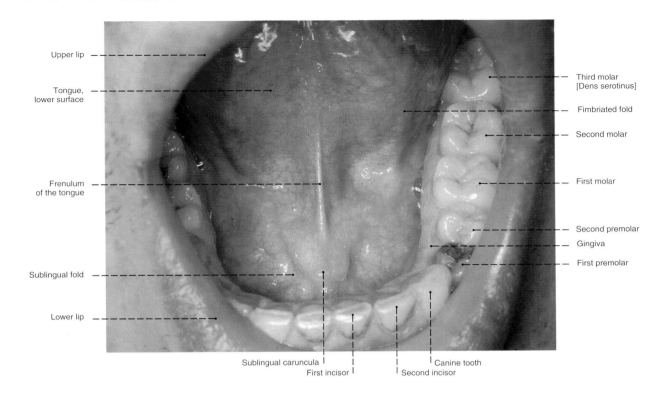

Upper lip

Tongue, lower surface

Frenulum of the tongue

Sublingual fold

Lower lip

Third molar [Dens serotinus]

Fimbriated fold

Second molar

First molar

Second premolar

Gingiva

First premolar

Sublingual caruncula

First incisor

Second incisor

Canine tooth

Fig. 205   The oral cavity and the opening of the submandibular duct, the sublingual caruncula, viewed obliquely from above (170%). Note the filling in the first premolar of the left mandible.

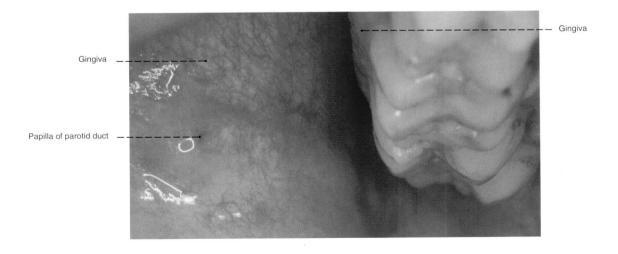

Gingiva

Gingiva

Papilla of parotid duct

Fig. 206   The opening of the parotid duct, the papilla of the parotid duct, anterior view (300%). The papilla is located opposite the second molar of the maxilla.

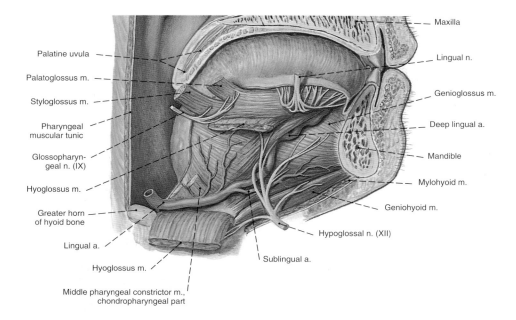

Maxilla

Palatine uvula

Lingual n.

Palatoglossus m.

Genioglossus m.

Styloglossus m.

Pharyngeal
muscular tunic

Deep lingual a.

Glossopharyn-
geal n. (IX)

Mandible

Hyoglossus m.

Mylohyoid m.

Greater horn
of hyoid bone

Geniohyoid m.

Lingual a.

Hypoglossal n. (XII)

Hyoglossus m.

Sublingual a.

Middle pharyngeal constrictor m.,
chondropharyngeal part

Fig. 207 Arteries and nerves of the tongue, medial view
(80%). Paramedian section with the pharynx opened
and the hyoglossus muscle sectioned.

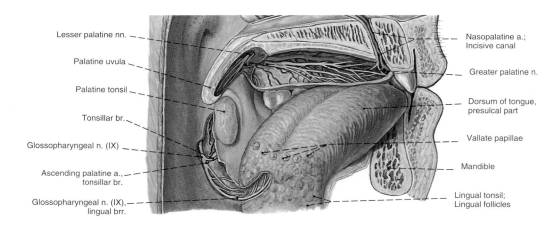

Lesser palatine nn.

Nasopalatine a.;
Incisive canal

Palatine uvula

Greater palatine n.

Palatine tonsil

Tonsillar br.

Dorsum of tongue,
presulcal part

Glossopharyngeal n. (IX)

Vallate papillae

Ascending palatine a.,
tonsillar br.

Mandible

Glossopharyngeal n. (IX),
lingual brr.

Lingual tonsil;
Lingual follicles

Fig. 208 Arteries and nerves of the palate and root
of the tongue, medial view (80%). A median section
with the tongue protracted and the mucous
membrane partially removed.

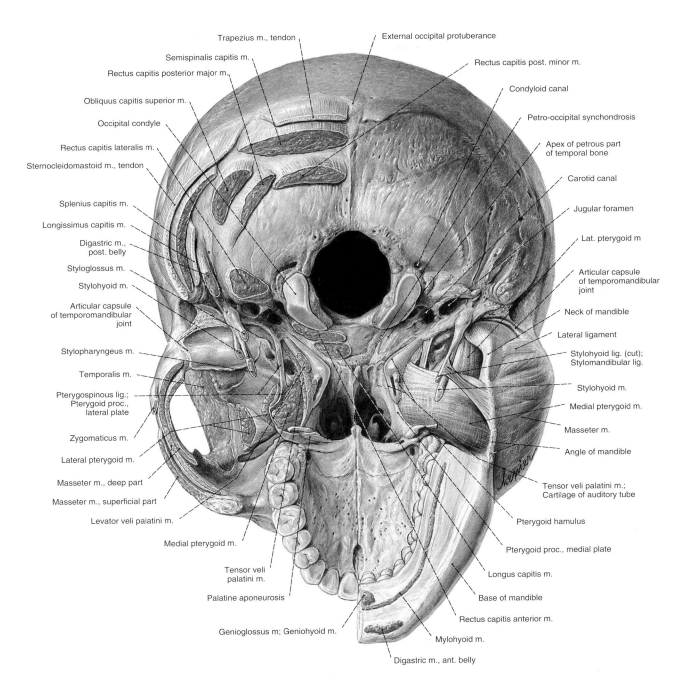

Trapezius m., tendon

External occipital protuberance

Semispinalis capitis m.

Rectus capitis post. minor m.

Rectus capitis posterior major m.

Condyloid canal

Obliquus capitis superior m.

Petro-occipital synchondrosis

Occipital condyle

Apex of petrous part of temporal bone

Rectus capitis lateralis m.

Carotid canal

Sternocleidomastoid m., tendon

Jugular foramen

Splenius capitis m.

Lat. pterygoid m

Longissimus capitis m.

Articular capsule of temporomandibular joint

Digastric m., post. belly

Styloglossus m.

Neck of mandible

Stylohyoid m.

Lateral ligament

Articular capsule of temporomandibular joint

Stylohyoid lig. (cut); Stylomandibular lig.

Stylopharyngeus m.

Stylohyoid m.

Temporalis m.

Medial pterygoid m.

Pterygospinous lig.; Pterygoid proc., lateral plate

Masseter m.

Zygomaticus m.

Angle of mandible

Lateral pterygoid m.

Tensor veli palatini m.; Cartilage of auditory tube

Masseter m., deep part

Masseter m., superficial part

Pterygoid hamulus

Levator veli palatini m.

Pterygoid proc., medial plate

Medial pterygoid m.

Longus capitis m.

Tensor veli palatini m.

Base of mandible

Palatine aponeurosis

Rectus capitis anterior m.

Genioglossus m; Geniohyoid m.

Mylohyoid m.

Digastric m., ant. belly

Fig. 209 The base of the skull with muscle origins and the muscles of mastication, inferior view (80%). The left half of the mandible has been removed.

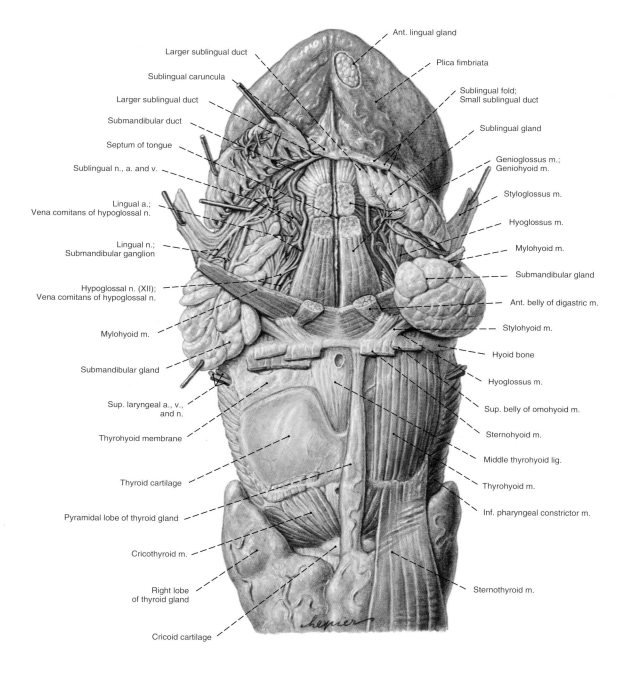

Larger sublingual duct

Sublingual caruncula

Larger sublingual duct

Submandibular duct

Septum of tongue

Sublingual n., a. and v.

Lingual a.;
Vena comitans of hypoglossal n.

Lingual n.;
Submandibular ganglion

Hypoglossal n. (XII);
Vena comitans of hypoglossal n.

Mylohyoid m.

Submandibular gland

Sup. laryngeal a., v.,
and n.

Thyrohyoid membrane

Thyroid cartilage

Pyramidal lobe of thyroid gland

Cricothyroid m.

Right lobe
of thyroid gland

Cricoid cartilage

Ant. lingual gland

Plica fimbriata

Sublingual fold;
Small sublingual duct

Sublingual gland

Genioglossus m.;
Geniohyoid m.

Styloglossus m.

Hyoglossus m.

Mylohyoid m.

Submandibular gland

Ant. belly of digastric m.

Stylohyoid m.

Hyoid bone

Hyoglossus m.

Sup. belly of omohyoid m.

Sternohyoid m.

Middle thyrohyoid lig.

Thyrohyoid m.

Inf. pharyngeal constrictor m.

Sternothyroid m.

Fig. 210 Vessels and nerves of the tongue, major salivary glands, larynx, and thyroid gland, viewed anteriorly from below (140%). The muscles of the floor of the mouth have been sectioned and the infrahyoid muscles partially removed.

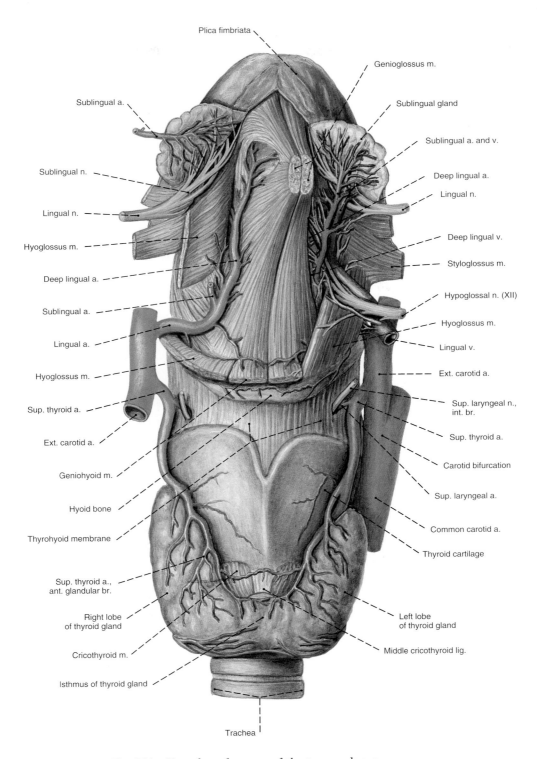

Plica fimbriata

Genioglossus m.

Sublingual a.

Sublingual gland

Sublingual a. and v.

Sublingual n.

Deep lingual a.

Lingual n.

Lingual n.

Hyoglossus m.

Deep lingual v.

Styloglossus m.

Deep lingual a.

Hypoglossal n. (XII)

Sublingual a.

Hyoglossus m.

Lingual a.

Lingual v.

Hyoglossus m.

Ext. carotid a.

Sup. thyroid a.

Sup. laryngeal n., int. br.

Ext. carotid a.

Sup. thyroid a.

Geniohyoid m.

Carotid bifurcation

Hyoid bone

Sup. laryngeal a.

Thyrohyoid membrane

Common carotid a.

Thyroid cartilage

Sup. thyroid a., ant. glandular br.

Right lobe of thyroid gland

Left lobe of thyroid gland

Cricothyroid m.

Middle cricothyroid lig.

Isthmus of thyroid gland

Trachea

Fig. 211 Vessels and nerves of the tongue, larynx, and thyroid gland, viewed anteriorly from below (140%). The muscles of the floor of the mouth have been sectioned and the infrahyoid muscles removed.

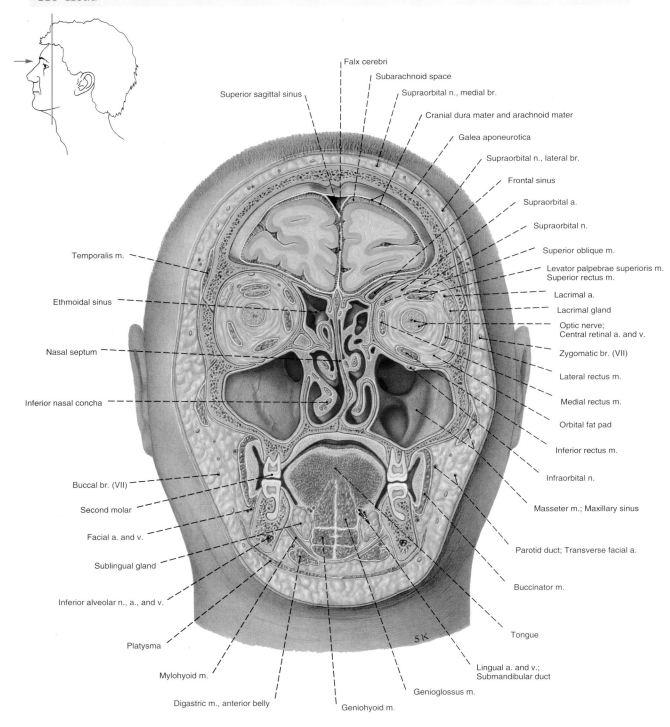

Falx cerebri

Subarachnoid space

Superior sagittal sinus

Supraorbital n., medial br.

Cranial dura mater and arachnoid mater

Galea aponeurotica

Supraorbital n., lateral br.

Frontal sinus

Supraorbital a.

Supraorbital n.

Superior oblique m.

Temporalis m.

Levator palpebrae superioris m.
Superior rectus m.

Lacrimal a.

Ethmoidal sinus

Lacrimal gland

Optic nerve;
Central retinal a. and v.

Nasal septum

Zygomatic br. (VII)

Lateral rectus m.

Medial rectus m.

Inferior nasal concha

Orbital fat pad

Inferior rectus m.

Infraorbital n.

Buccal br. (VII)

Masseter m.; Maxillary sinus

Second molar

Facial a. and v.

Parotid duct; Transverse facial a.

Sublingual gland

Buccinator m.

Inferior alveolar n., a., and v.

Tongue

Platysma

Lingual a. and v.;
Submandibular duct

Mylohyoid m.

Genioglossus m.

Digastric m., anterior belly

Geniohyoid m.

SK

Fig. 212   The oral cavity, maxillary sinus, orbit, and
cranial cavity, anterior view. Frontal section through
the head of a 48-year-old male at the level of the second
upper molar, with the oral cavity, maxillary sinus, and
cranial cavity opened. Note the size of the maxillary sinus.

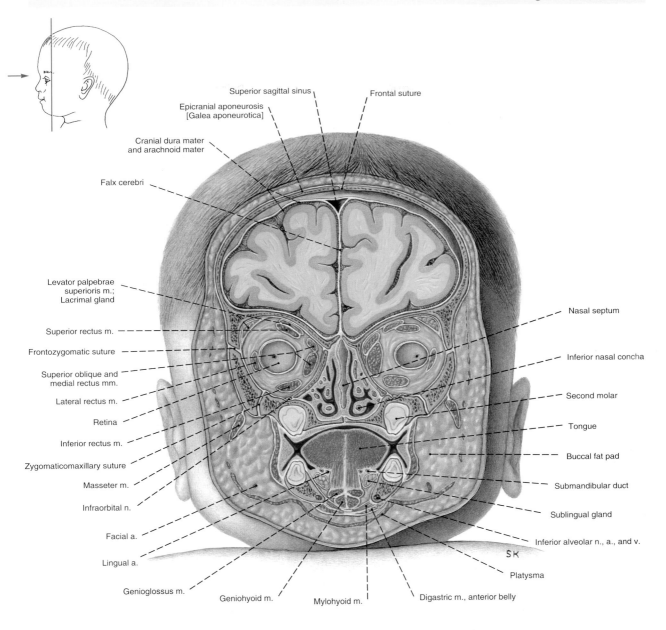

Superior sagittal sinus

Frontal suture

Epicranial aponeurosis
[Galea aponeurotica]

Cranial dura mater
and arachnoid mater

Falx cerebri

Levator palpebrae
superioris m.;
Lacrimal gland

Superior rectus m.

Frontozygomatic suture

Superior oblique and
medial rectus mm.

Lateral rectus m.

Retina

Inferior rectus m.

Zygomaticomaxillary suture

Masseter m.

Infraorbital n.

Facial a.

Lingual a.

Genioglossus m.

Geniohyoid m.

Mylohyoid m.

Digastric m., anterior belly

Nasal septum

Inferior nasal concha

Second molar

Tongue

Buccal fat pad

Submandibular duct

Sublingual gland

Inferior alveolar n., a., and v.

Platysma

S K

Fig. 213 The oral cavity, orbit, and cranial cavity, anterior view. Frontal section through the head of a newborn at the level of the second upper molar, with the oral cavity and cranial cavity opened. Note the absence of the maxillary sinus and the proximity of the teeth to the orbits. Compare with Figure 212.

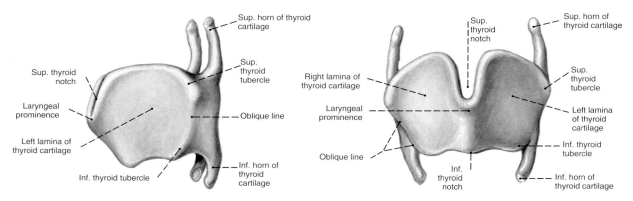

Fig. 214 Thyroid cartilage, lateral view.

Fig. 215 Thyroid cartilage, anterior view.

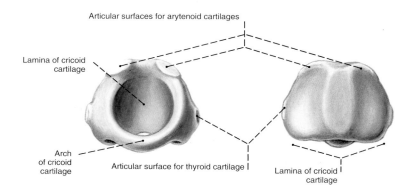

Fig. 216 Cricoid cartilage, viewed from anterior and above.

Fig. 217 Cricoid cartilage, posterior view.

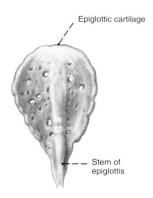

Fig. 218 Epiglottis, posterior view.

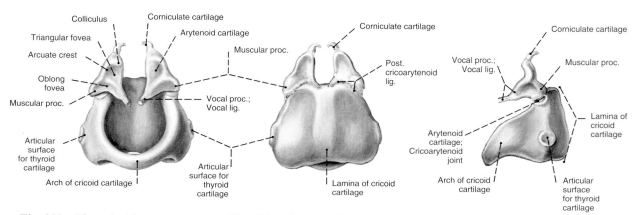

Fig. 219 The cricoid, arytenoid, and corniculate cartilages, viewed from anterior and above.

Fig. 220 The cricoid, arytenoid, and corniculate cartilages, posterior view.

Fig. 221 The cricoid, arytenoid, and corniculate cartilages, lateral view.

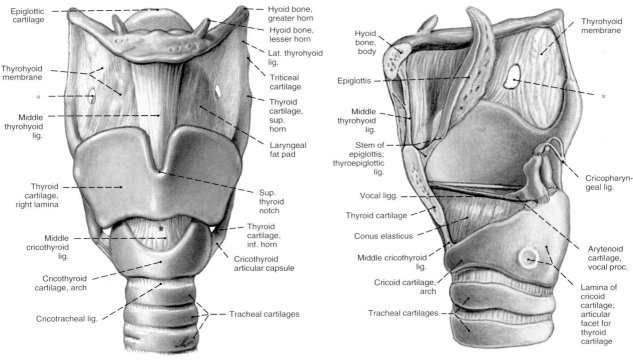

Fig. 222   Larynx, hyoid bone, and trachea, anterior view. The laryngeal fat pad fills the space between the thyrohyoid membrane and the epiglottis.

* Foramen for the superior laryngeal artery and vein and for the internal branch of the superior laryngeal nerve

Fig. 223   Larynx and hyoid bone, lateral view. The upper part of the larynx and the hyoid bone have been sectioned in the median plane. Both arytenoid cartilages, the cricoid cartilage, and the upper tracheal cartilages are intact.

* Foramen for the superior laryngeal artery and vein and for the internal branch of the superior laryngeal nerve

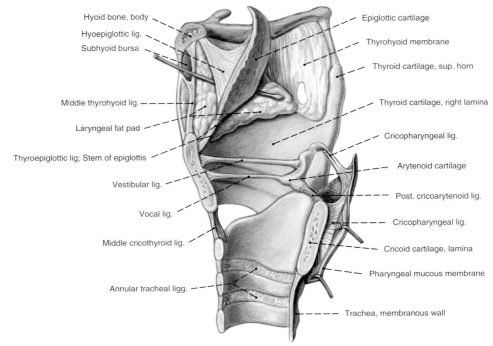

Fig. 224   Larynx and hyoid bone. Right half of a median section, lateral view. The probe lies between the epiglottis and the laryngeal fat pad.

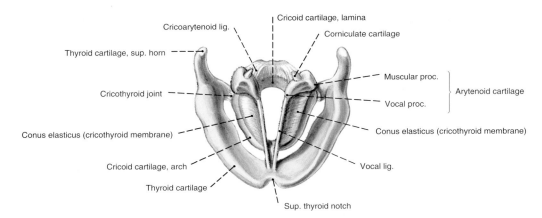

Fig. 225 Laryngeal cartilages, vocal ligament, and conus elasticus, viewed from anterior and above.

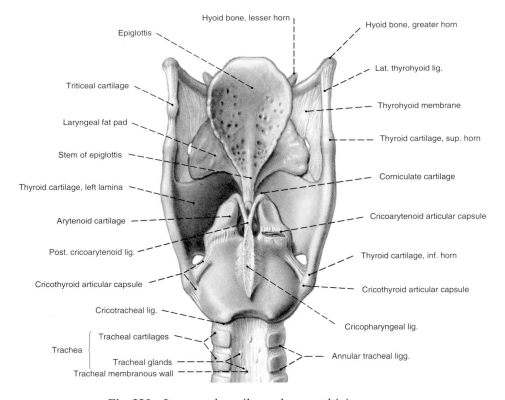

Fig. 226 Laryngeal cartilages, laryngeal joints, hyoid bone, trachea, and larynx of a juvenile, posterior view. In the adult, the laryngeal cartilages are calcified and ossified.

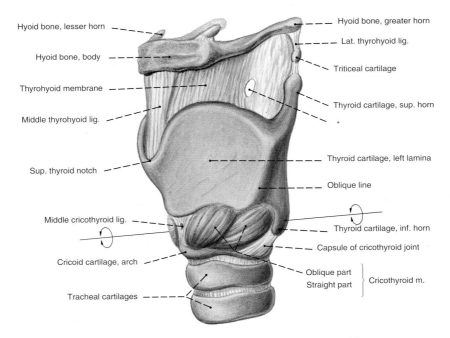

Hyoid bone, lesser horn

Hyoid bone, body

Thyrohyoid membrane

Middle thyrohyoid lig.

Sup. thyroid notch

Middle cricothyroid lig.

Cricoid cartilage, arch

Tracheal cartilages

Hyoid bone, greater horn

Lat. thyrohyoid lig.

Triticeal cartilage

Thyroid cartilage, sup. horn

Thyroid cartilage, left lamina

Oblique line

Thyroid cartilage, inf. horn

Capsule of cricothyroid joint

Oblique part
Straight part } Cricothyroid m.

Fig. 227 Larynx, hyoid bone, and the cricothyroid muscle, anterolateral view.

* Foramen for the internal branch of the superior laryngeal nerve and the superior laryngeal artery

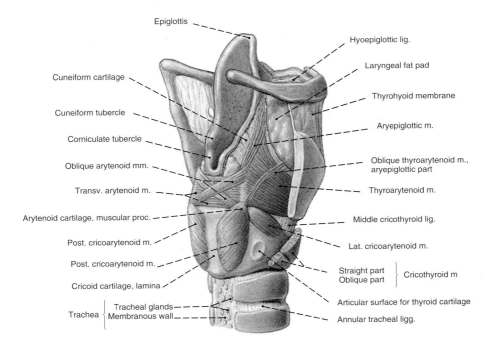

Epiglottis

Cuneiform cartilage

Cuneiform tubercle

Corniculate tubercle

Oblique arytenoid mm.

Transv. arytenoid m.

Arytenoid cartilage, muscular proc.

Post. cricoarytenoid m.

Post. cricoarytenoid m.

Cricoid cartilage, lamina

Trachea { Tracheal glands
Membranous wall

Hyoepiglottic lig.

Laryngeal fat pad

Thyrohyoid membrane

Aryepiglottic m.

Oblique thyroarytenoid m., aryepiglottic part

Thyroarytenoid m.

Middle cricothyroid lig.

Lat. cricoarytenoid m.

Straight part
Oblique part } Cricothyroid m

Articular surface for thyroid cartilage

Annular tracheal ligg.

Fig. 228 The laryngeal muscles, posterolateral view.

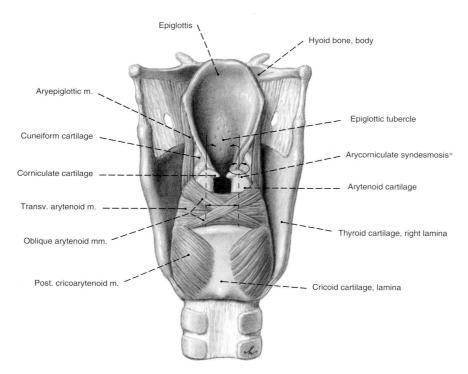

Epiglottis

Hyoid bone, body

Aryepiglottic m.

Epiglottic tubercle

Cuneiform cartilage

Arycorniculate syndesmosis*

Corniculate cartilage

Arytenoid cartilage

Transv. arytenoid m.

Oblique arytenoid mm.

Thyroid cartilage, right lamina

Post. cricoarytenoid m.

Cricoid cartilage, lamina

Fig. 229   The laryngeal muscles, posterior view.

* The arytenoid and corniculate cartilages may be either fused or articulated with each other.

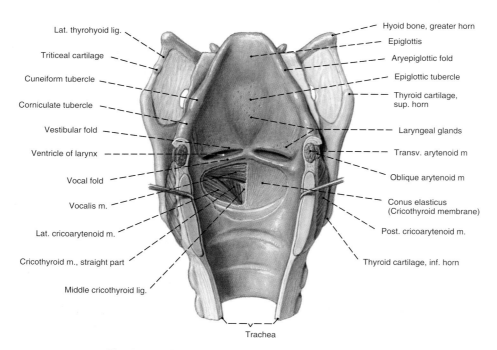

Lat. thyrohyoid lig.

Hyoid bone, greater horn

Triticeal cartilage

Epiglottis

Cuneiform tubercle

Aryepiglottic fold

Corniculate tubercle

Epiglottic tubercle

Vestibular fold

Thyroid cartilage, sup. horn

Ventricle of larynx

Laryngeal glands

Vocal fold

Transv. arytenoid m

Vocalis m.

Oblique arytenoid m

Lat. cricoarytenoid m.

Conus elasticus (Cricothyroid membrane)

Cricothyroid m., straight part

Post. cricoarytenoid m.

Middle cricothyroid lig.

Thyroid cartilage, inf. horn

Trachea

Fig. 230   The larynx, posterior view. The posterior wall of the larynx has been split in the median plane with the two halves retracted laterally. On the left, the mucous membrane has been removed from beneath the vocal fold to the superior border of the arch of the cricoid cartilage.

Muscles of the Larynx

Name *Innervation**	Origin	Insertion	Function
1. **Cricothyroid muscle** (superficial straight part and a deeper oblique part) *Superior laryngeal n., External branch*	Outer surface of cricoid cartilage	Caudal margin and inferior horn of thyroid cartilage	Tenses the vocal folds (true vocal cords)
2. **Posterior cricoarytenoid muscle** *Inferior laryngeal n., from recurrent laryngeal n.*	Dorsal surface of cricoid cartilage	Muscular process on the posterior surface of arytenoid cartilage	Opens the rima glottidis
3. **Lateral cricoarytenoid muscle** *Inferior laryngeal n., from recurrent laryngeal n.,*	Cranial margin of lateral part of cricoid cartilage		Closes the rima glottidis (intermembranous part)
4. **Transverse arytenoid muscle** *Inferior laryngeal n., from recurrent laryngeal n.*	Lateral edge and dorsal surface of arytenoid cartilage	To the same part on the opposite side (crosses transversely between the 2 cartilages)	Closes the rima glottidis (intercartilaginous part)
5. **Oblique arytenoid muscle** *Inferior laryngeal n., from recurrent laryngeal n.*	Muscular process on the posterior surface of one arytenoid cartilage	Apex of muscular process of opposite arytenoid cartilage	
6. **Vocalis muscle** *Inferior laryngeal n., from recurrent laryngeal n.*	From medial fibers of thyroarytenoid muscle adherent to the vocal ligament	Along vocal ligament extending to the vocal process of arytenoid cartilage	Tenses the vocal folds (forming their edge)
7. **Aryepiglottic muscle** *Inferior laryngeal n., from recurrent laryngeal n.*	Variable fibers of the oblique arytenoid muscle in the aryepiglottic folds	Lateral border of epiglottis	Narrows the laryngeal entrance
8. **Thyroarytenoid muscle** *Inferior laryngeal n., from recurrent laryngeal n.*	Inner surface of angle of the thyroid cartilage	Muscular process and lateral surface of arytenoid cartilage	Narrows the rima glottidis
9. **Thyroepiglottic muscle** *Inferior laryngeal n., from recurrent laryngeal n.*	Continuation of thyroarytenoid muscle in the aryepiglottic fold	Margin of epiglottis	Narrows the laryngeal entrance

* With the exception of the cricothyroid muscle, all laryngeal muscles are innervated by the inferior laryngeal n. from the recurrent laryngeal n.

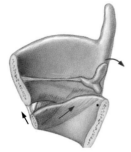

a Cricothyroid m.

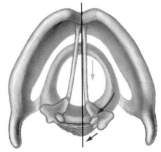

b Arytenoid m.

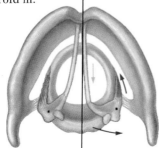

c Lateral cricoarytenoid m.

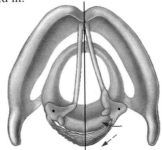

d Posterior cricoarytenoid m.

Fig. 231 a–d Diagrams showing the functioning of the laryngeal muscles, viewed from above. The arrows indicate the direction of movement, those in yellow indicating tension. The muscles on the left are relaxed, those on the right are contracted.

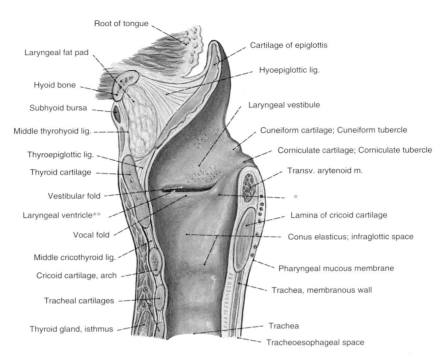

Root of tongue

Laryngeal fat pad

Hyoid bone

Subhyoid bursa

Middle thyrohyoid lig.

Thyroepiglottic lig.

Thyroid cartilage

Vestibular fold

Laryngeal ventricle**

Vocal fold

Middle cricothyroid lig.

Cricoid cartilage, arch

Tracheal cartilages

Thyroid gland, isthmus

Cartilage of epiglottis

Hyoepiglottic lig.

Laryngeal vestibule

Cuneiform cartilage; Cuneiform tubercle

Corniculate cartilage; Corniculate tubercle

Transv. arytenoid m.

*

Lamina of cricoid cartilage

Conus elasticus; infraglottic space

Pharyngeal mucous membrane

Trachea, membranous wall

Trachea

Tracheoesophageal space

Fig. 232   Larynx. Medial view of the right half of a median section (90%).

*   Clinically known as the macula flava, where the elastic tissue shines yellowish through the mucous membrane.
** Clinical: MORGAGNI's ventricle

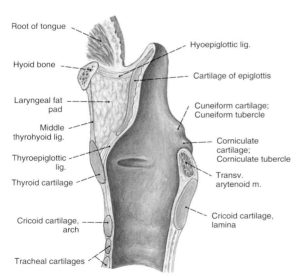

Root of tongue

Hyoid bone

Laryngeal fat pad

Middle thyrohyoid lig.

Thyroepiglottic lig.

Thyroid cartilage

Cricoid cartilage, arch

Tracheal cartilages

Hyoepiglottic lig.

Cartilage of epiglottis

Cuneiform cartilage; Cuneiform tubercle

Corniculate cartilage; Corniculate tubercle

Transv. arytenoid m.

Cricoid cartilage, lamina

Fig. 233   Larynx. Medial view of the right half of a median section with the epiglottis positioned for respiration (80%).

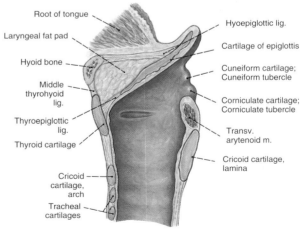

Root of tongue

Laryngeal fat pad

Hyoid bone

Middle thyrohyoid lig.

Thyroepiglottic lig.

Thyroid cartilage

Cricoid cartilage, arch

Tracheal cartilages

Hyoepiglottic lig.

Cartilage of epiglottis

Cuneiform cartilage; Cuneiform tubercle

Corniculate cartilage; Corniculate tubercle

Transv. arytenoid m.

Cricoid cartilage, lamina

Fig. 234   Larynx. Medial view of the right half of a median section with the epiglottis positioned for swallowing (80%). In swallowing, as the larynx is elevated, the laryngeal fat pad passively pushes the epiglottis posteriorly.

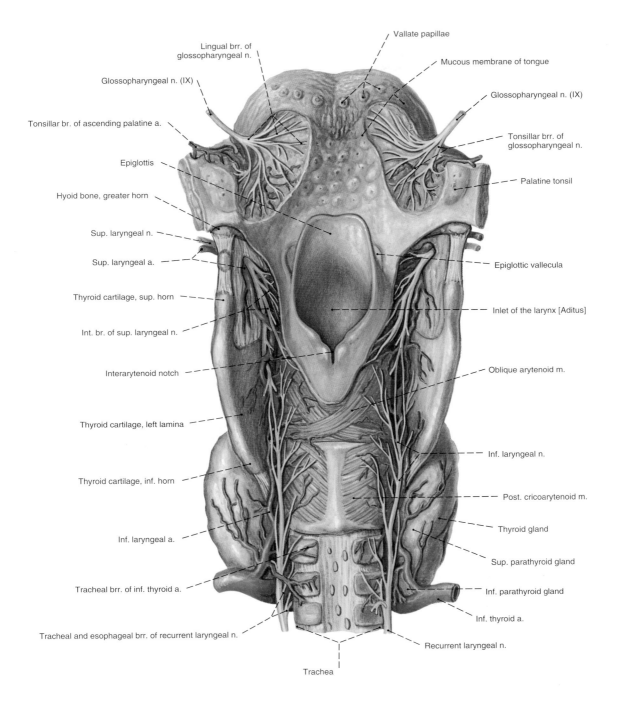

Lingual brr. of glossopharyngeal n.

Vallate papillae

Mucous membrane of tongue

Glossopharyngeal n. (IX)

Glossopharyngeal n. (IX)

Tonsillar br. of ascending palatine a.

Tonsillar brr. of glossopharyngeal n.

Epiglottis

Palatine tonsil

Hyoid bone, greater horn

Sup. laryngeal n.

Epiglottic vallecula

Sup. laryngeal a.

Thyroid cartilage, sup. horn

Inlet of the larynx [Aditus]

Int. br. of sup. laryngeal n.

Interarytenoid notch

Oblique arytenoid m.

Thyroid cartilage, left lamina

Inf. laryngeal n.

Thyroid cartilage, inf. horn

Post. cricoarytenoid m.

Thyroid gland

Inf. laryngeal a.

Sup. parathyroid gland

Tracheal brr. of inf. thyroid a.

Inf. parathyroid gland

Inf. thyroid a.

Tracheal and esophageal brr. of recurrent laryngeal n.

Recurrent laryngeal n.

Trachea

Fig. 235 Arteries and nerves of the larynx and the root of the tongue, posterior view (140%). The mucous membrane of the root of the tongue has been partially removed.

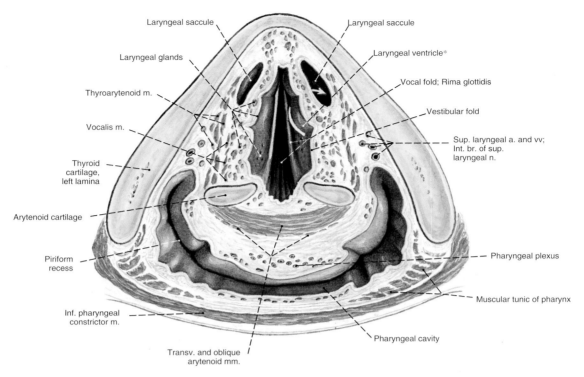

Laryngeal saccule

Laryngeal glands

Thyroarytenoid m.

Vocalis m.

Thyroid cartilage, left lamina

Arytenoid cartilage

Piriform recess

Inf. pharyngeal constrictor m.

Transv. and oblique arytenoid mm.

Laryngeal saccule

Laryngeal ventricle*

Vocal fold; Rima glottidis

Vestibular fold

Sup. laryngeal a. and vv; Int. br. of sup. laryngeal n.

Pharyngeal plexus

Muscular tunic of pharynx

Pharyngeal cavity

Fig. 236 Larynx. Cross section at the level of the vestibular folds, viewed from above (200%).

The white arrow indicates the connection between the ventricle and the saccule of the larynx.

* Clinical: MORGAGNI's ventricle

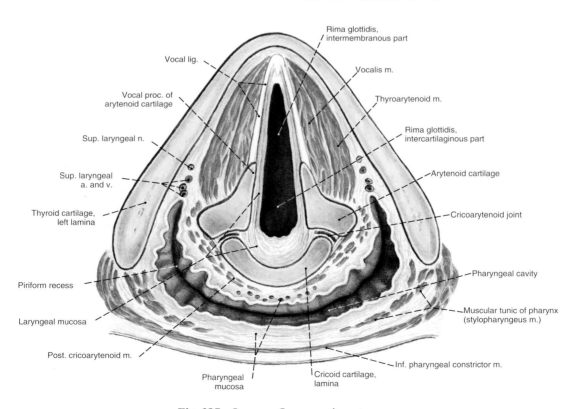

Vocal lig.

Vocal proc. of arytenoid cartilage

Sup. laryngeal n.

Sup. laryngeal a. and v.

Thyroid cartilage, left lamina

Piriform recess

Laryngeal mucosa

Post. cricoarytenoid m.

Pharyngeal mucosa

Rima glottidis, intermembranous part

Vocalis m.

Thyroarytenoid m.

Rima glottidis, intercartilaginous part

Arytenoid cartilage

Cricoarytenoid joint

Pharyngeal cavity

Muscular tunic of pharynx (stylopharyngeus m.)

Inf. pharyngeal constrictor m.

Cricoid cartilage, lamina

Fig. 237 Larynx. Cross section at the level of the vocal folds, viewed from above (200%).

Fig. 238 a,b Laryngoscopy.

a Indirect laryngoscopy.
Pulling the tongue forward
allows access for the
laryngoscope, enabling the
vocal folds to be visualized.

b Direct endoscopic
laryngoscopy.

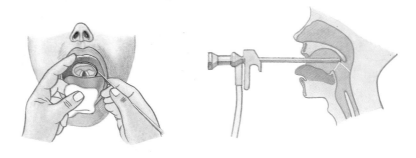

a   b

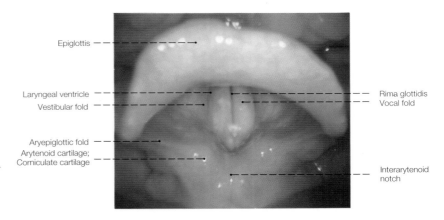

Epiglottis

Vocal fold — — — Rima glottidis

Vestibular fold

Arytenoid cartilage;
Corniculate cartilage

Piriform recess — — — Interarytenoid notch

Fig. 239 Direct laryngoscopy.
Respiratory position, with
vocal folds open for deep
inspiration.

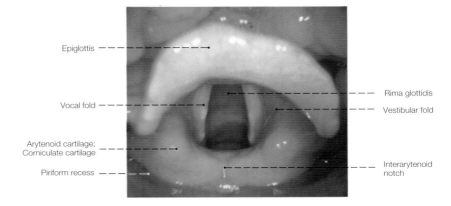

Epiglottis

Laryngeal ventricle — — — Rima glottidis

Vestibular fold — — — Vocal fold

Aryepiglottic fold — — —

Arytenoid cartilage;
Corniculate cartilage

Interarytenoid notch

Fig. 240 Direct laryngoscopy.
Phonation position, with
vocal folds closed.

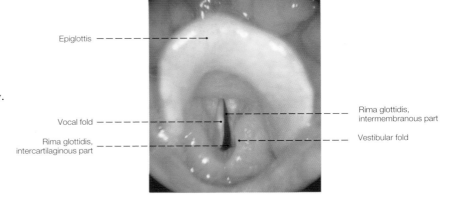

Epiglottis — — —

Vocal fold — — — Rima glottidis,
intermembranous part

Rima glottidis,
intercartilaginous part

Vestibular fold

Fig. 241 Direct laryngoscopy.
The intercartilaginous part
of the rima glottidis
is open, as during whispering.
Note the bulge in the
vestibular fold.

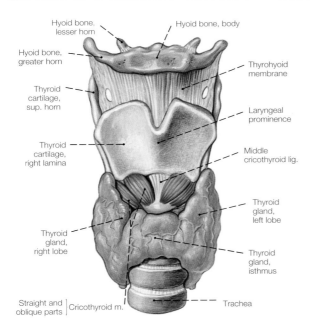

Fig. 242 Hyoid bone, larynx, thyroid gland, and trachea, anterior view (80%)

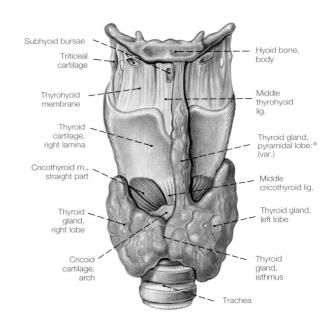

Fig. 243 Hyoid bone, larynx, thyroid gland, and trachea, anterior view (80%).

* The pyramidal lobe frequently extends to the middle thyrohyoid lig. as a developmental variant.

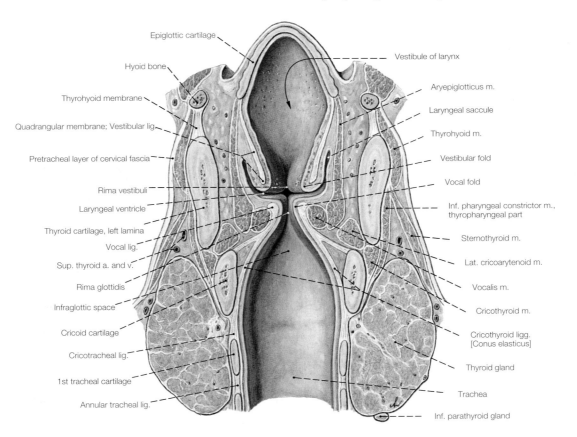

Fig. 244 Larynx and thyroid gland. Frontal section through the middle of the larynx, posterior view (120%).

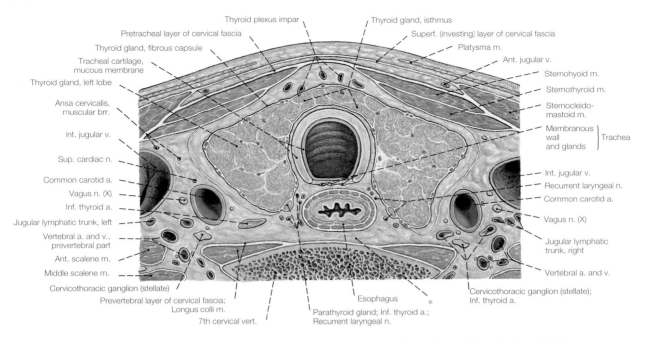

Thyroid plexus impar
Pretracheal layer of cervical fascia
Thyroid gland, fibrous capsule
Tracheal cartilage, mucous membrane
Thyroid gland, left lobe
Ansa cervicalis, muscular brr.
Int. jugular v.
Sup. cardiac n.
Common carotid a.
Vagus n. (X)
Inf. thyroid a.
Jugular lymphatic trunk, left
Vertebral a. and v., prevertebral part
Ant. scalene m.
Middle scalene m.
Cervicothoracic ganglion (stellate)
Prevertebral layer of cervical fascia; Longus colli m.
7th cervical vert.

Thyroid gland, isthmus
Superf. (investing) layer of cervical fascia
Platysma m.
Ant. jugular v.
Sternohyoid m.
Sternothyroid m.
Sternocleido-mastoid m.
Membranous wall and glands } Trachea
Int. jugular v.
Recurrent laryngeal n.
Common carotid a.
Vagus n. (X)
Jugular lymphatic trunk, right
Vertebral a. and v.
Cervicothoracic ganglion (stellate); Inf. thyroid a.
Esophagus
Parathyroid gland; Inf. thyroid a.; Recurrent laryngeal n.

Fig. 245 Thyroid gland. Horizontal section through the cervical viscera at the level of the second tracheal cartilage, viewed from below (90%).
* Clinical: Retroesophageal space

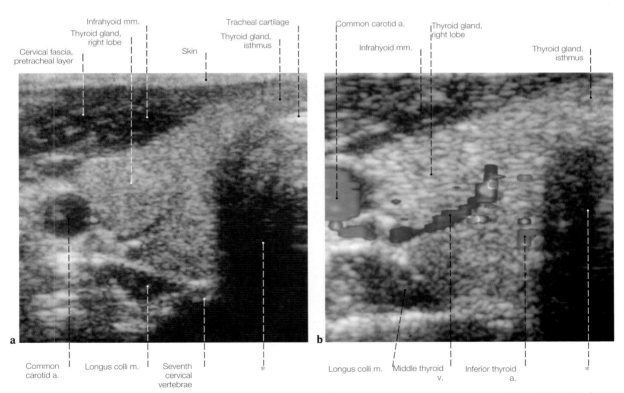

Infrahyoid mm.
Thyroid gland, right lobe
Cervical fascia, pretracheal layer
Skin
Tracheal cartilage
Thyroid gland, isthmus

Common carotid a.
Longus colli m.
Seventh cervical vertebrae
*

Common carotid a.
Infrahyoid mm.
Thyroid gland, right lobe
Thyroid gland, isthmus

Longus colli m.
Middle thyroid v.
Inferior thyroid a.
*

Fig. 246 a,b Thyroid gland.
a Ultrasonogram. A cross section of the right gland, ventrodorsal beam direction, viewed from below (200%).

* Shadow of the trachea

b Ultrasonogram. A cross section of the right gland, ventrodorsal beam direction, viewed from below (200%). The colors indicate the direction of blood flow (red: toward the probe, artery; blue, away from the probe, vein; color-coded Doppler sonography).

* Shadow of the trachea

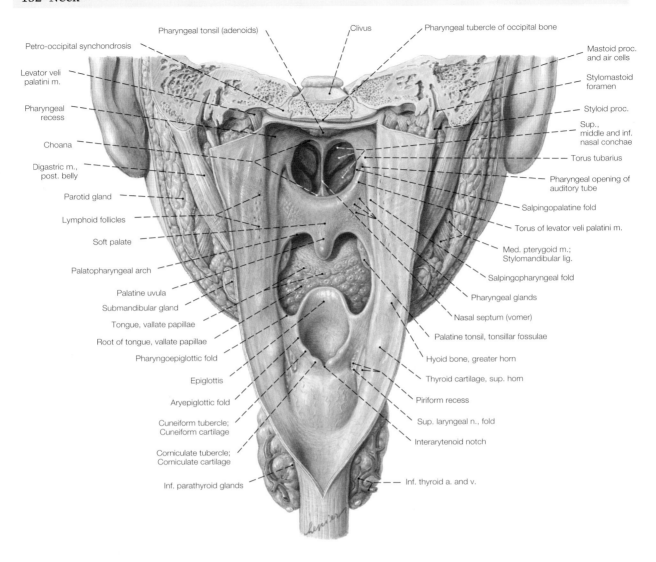

Pharyngeal tonsil (adenoids)
Clivus
Pharyngeal tubercle of occipital bone
Petro-occipital synchondrosis
Levator veli palatini m.
Pharyngeal recess
Choana
Digastric m., post. belly
Parotid gland
Lymphoid follicles
Soft palate
Palatopharyngeal arch
Palatine uvula
Submandibular gland
Tongue, vallate papillae
Root of tongue, vallate papillae
Pharyngoepiglottic fold
Epiglottis
Aryepiglottic fold
Cuneiform tubercle; Cuneiform cartilage
Corniculate tubercle; Corniculate cartilage
Inf. parathyroid glands

Mastoid proc. and air cells
Stylomastoid foramen
Styloid proc.
Sup., middle and inf. nasal conchae
Torus tubarius
Pharyngeal opening of auditory tube
Salpingopalatine fold
Torus of levator veli palatini m.
Med. pterygoid m.; Stylomandibular lig.
Salpingopharyngeal fold
Pharyngeal glands
Nasal septum (vomer)
Palatine tonsil, tonsillar fossulae
Hyoid bone, greater horn
Thyroid cartilage, sup. horn
Piriform recess
Sup. laryngeal n., fold
Interarytenoid notch
Inf. thyroid a. and v.

Fig. 247 Pharynx. Frontal section at the level of the mastoid process with the pharynx opened by a longitudinal midline incision, posterior view (80%).

Constrictor Muscles of the Pharynx

Name *Innervation*	Origin	Insertion	Function
1. Superior pharyngeal constrictor muscle *Pharyngeal plexus (Glossopharyngeal n., IX, Vagus n., X)*		Pharyngobasilar fascia, median raphe	Constricts the pharynx; In swallowing, arches the mucosa forward, closing the nasopharynx with the soft palate
Pterygopharyngeal part	Pterygoid hamulus of sphenoid bone		
Buccopharyngeal part	Pterygomandibular raphe, buccinator muscle		
Mylopharyngeal part	Mylohyoid line of mandible		
Glossopharyngeal part	Transverse muscle of the tongue		

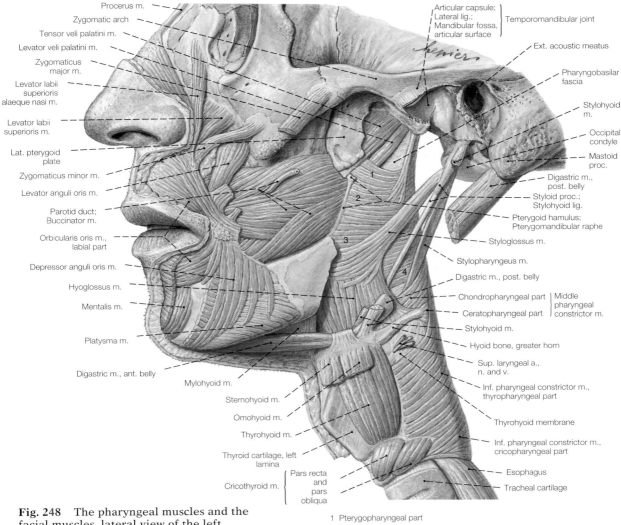

Procerus m.
Zygomatic arch
Tensor veli palatini m.
Levator veli palatini m.
Zygomaticus major m.
Levator labii superioris alaeque nasi m.
Levator labii superioris m.
Lat. pterygoid plate
Zygomaticus minor m.
Levator anguli oris m.
Parotid duct; Buccinator m.
Orbicularis oris m., labial part
Depressor anguli oris m.
Hyoglossus m.
Mentalis m.
Platysma m.
Digastric m., ant. belly
Mylohyoid m.
Sternohyoid m.
Omohyoid m.
Thyrohyoid m.
Thyroid cartilage, left lamina
Cricothyroid m.
Pars recta and pars obliqua

Articular capsule; Lateral lig.; Mandibular fossa, articular surface | Temporomandibular joint
Ext. acoustic meatus
Pharyngobasilar fascia
Stylohyoid m.
Occipital condyle
Mastoid proc.
Digastric m., post. belly
Styloid proc.; Stylohyoid lig.
Pterygoid hamulus; Pterygomandibular raphe
Styloglossus m.
Stylopharyngeus m.
Digastric m., post. belly
Chondropharyngeal part | Middle pharyngeal constrictor m.
Ceratopharyngeal part
Stylohyoid m.
Hyoid bone, greater horn
Sup. laryngeal a., n. and v.
Inf. pharyngeal constrictor m., thyropharyngeal part
Thyrohyoid membrane
Inf. pharyngeal constrictor m., cricopharyngeal part
Esophagus
Tracheal cartilage

Fig. 248 The pharyngeal muscles and the facial muscles, lateral view of the left side. The mandible has been partially removed.

1 Pterygopharyngeal part
2 Buccopharyngeal part
3 Mylopharyngeal part
4 Glossopharyngeal part of the superior pharyngeal constrictor m.

Constrictor Muscles of the Pharynx (continued)

Name *Innervation*	Origin	Insertion	Function
2. Middle pharyngeal constrictor muscle *Pharyngeal plexus (Glossopharyngeal n., IX, Vagus n., X)*			All constrict the pharynx during swallowing
Chondropharyngeal part	Lesser horn of hyoid bone		
Ceratopharyngeal part	Greater horn of hyoid bone		
3. Inferior pharyngeal constrictor muscle *Pharyngeal plexus (Glossopharyngeal n., IX, Vagus n., X)*			
Thyropharyngeal part	Oblique line of thyroid cartilage		
Cricopharyngeal part	Lateral margin of cricoid cartilage		

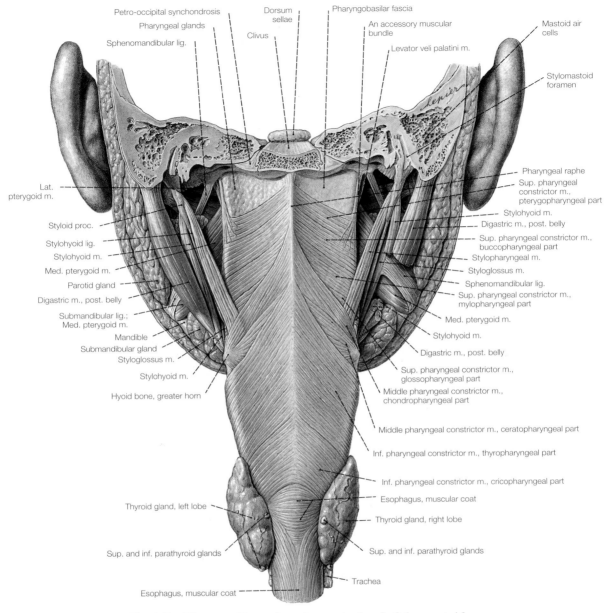

Petro-occipital synchondrosis
Pharyngeal glands
Sphenomandibular lig.
Dorsum sellae
Clivus
Pharyngobasilar fascia
An accessory muscular bundle
Levator veli palatini m.
Mastoid air cells
Stylomastoid foramen
Lat. pterygoid m.
Styloid proc.
Stylohyoid lig.
Stylohyoid m.
Med. pterygoid m.
Parotid gland
Digastric m., post. belly
Submandibular lig.; Med. pterygoid m.
Mandible
Submandibular gland
Styloglossus m.
Stylohyoid m.
Hyoid bone, greater horn
Pharyngeal raphe
Sup. pharyngeal constrictor m., pterygopharyngeal part
Stylohyoid m.
Digastric m., post. belly
Sup. pharyngeal constrictor m., buccopharyngeal part
Stylopharyngeal m.
Styloglossus m.
Sphenomandibular lig.
Sup. pharyngeal constrictor m., mylopharyngeal part
Med. pterygoid m.
Stylohyoid m.
Digastric m., post. belly
Sup. pharyngeal constrictor m., glossopharyngeal part
Middle pharyngeal constrictor m., chondropharyngeal part
Middle pharyngeal constrictor m., ceratopharyngeal part
Inf. pharyngeal constrictor m., thyropharyngeal part
Thyroid gland, left lobe
Inf. pharyngeal constrictor m., cricopharyngeal part
Esophagus, muscular coat
Thyroid gland, right lobe
Sup. and inf. parathyroid glands
Sup. and inf. parathyroid glands
Esophagus, muscular coat
Trachea

Fig. 249   Pharynx. Frontal section at the level of the mastoid processes with the fascia removed, posterior view (80%).

Levator Muscles of the Pharynx

Name *Innervation*	Origin	Insertion	Function
1. Stylopharyngeus muscle *Br. to stylopharyngeus m.* *(Glossopharyngeal n., IX)*	Styloideus proc. (temporal bone)	Lateral pharyngeal wall	Elevates the pharynx toward the base of the skull
2. Salpingopharyngeus muscle *Pharyngeal plexus* *(Glossopharyngeal n., IX, Vagus n., X)*	Cartilage of auditory tube	Lateral pharyngeal wall	Opens auditory tube (during swallowing, yawning)
3. Palatopharyngeus muscle (described with muscles of the palate, p. 108)			

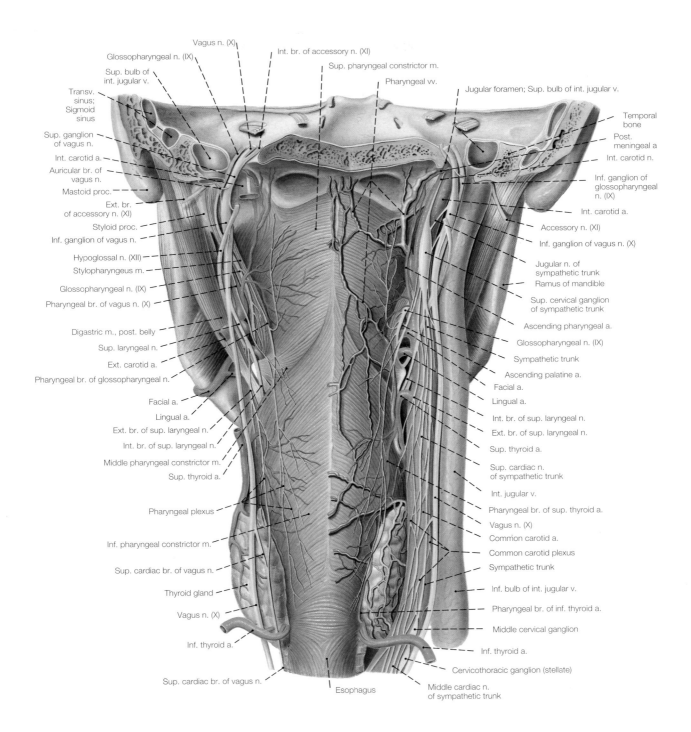

Vagus n. (X)

Glossopharyngeal n. (IX)

Int. br. of accessory n. (XI)

Sup. pharyngeal constrictor m.

Sup. bulb of int. jugular v.

Pharyngeal vv.

Transv. sinus; Sigmoid sinus

Jugular foramen; Sup. bulb of int. jugular v.

Temporal bone

Sup. ganglion of vagus n.

Post. meningeal a

Int. carotid a.

Int. carotid n.

Auricular br. of vagus n.

Inf. ganglion of glossopharyngeal n. (IX)

Mastoid proc.

Ext. br. of accessory n. (XI)

Int. carotid a.

Styloid proc.

Accessory n. (XI)

Inf. ganglion of vagus n.

Inf. ganglion of vagus n. (X)

Hypoglossal n. (XII)

Jugular n. of sympathetic trunk

Stylopharyngeus m.

Ramus of mandible

Glossopharyngeal n. (IX)

Sup. cervical ganglion of sympathetic trunk

Pharyngeal br. of vagus n. (X)

Ascending pharyngeal a.

Digastric m., post. belly

Glossopharyngeal n. (IX)

Sup. laryngeal n.

Sympathetic trunk

Ext. carotid a.

Ascending palatine a.

Pharyngeal br. of glossopharyngeal n.

Facial a.

Lingual a.

Facial a.

Int. br. of sup. laryngeal n.

Lingual a.

Ext. br. of sup. laryngeal n.

Ext. br. of sup. laryngeal n.

Sup. thyroid a.

Int. br. of sup. laryngeal n.

Sup. cardiac n. of sympathetic trunk

Middle pharyngeal constrictor m.

Sup. thyroid a.

Int. jugular v.

Pharyngeal plexus

Pharyngeal br. of sup. thyroid a.

Vagus n. (X)

Common carotid a.

Inf. pharyngeal constrictor m.

Common carotid plexus

Sympathetic trunk

Sup. cardiac br. of vagus n.

Thyroid gland

Inf. bulb of int. jugular v.

Vagus n. (X)

Pharyngeal br. of inf. thyroid a.

Middle cervical ganglion

Inf. thyroid a.

Inf. thyroid a.

Cervicothoracic ganglion (stellate)

Sup. cardiac br. of vagus n.

Esophagus

Middle cardiac n. of sympathetic trunk

Fig. 250 Blood vessels and nerves of the pharynx. Frontal section at the level of the jugular foramina, posterior view (80%). The left carotid artery and internal jugular vein have been removed. The weak point at the transition of the inferior pharyngeal constrictor muscle to the muscular coat of the esophagus is known clinically as the Laimer triangle.

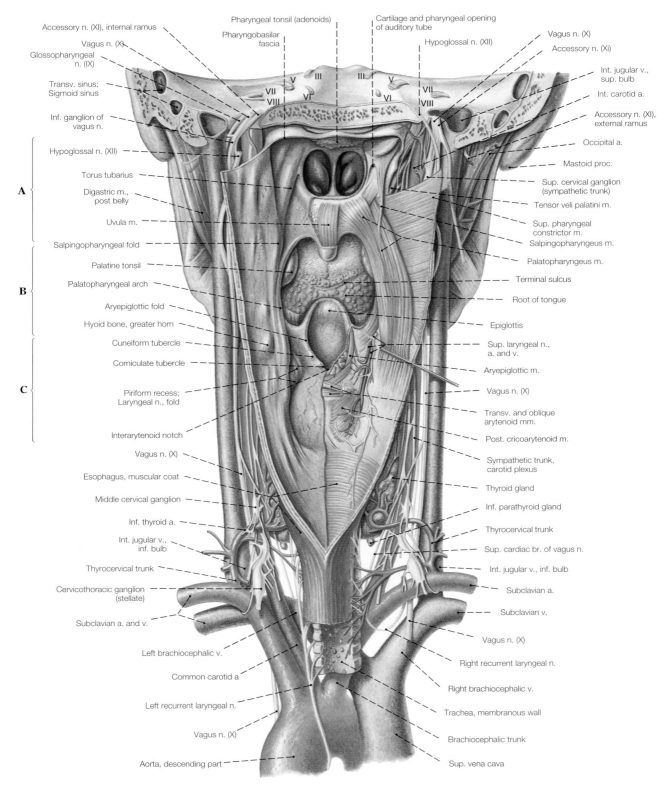

Accessory n. (XI), internal ramus

Vagus n. (X)

Glossopharyngeal n. (IX)

Transv. sinus; Sigmoid sinus

Inf. ganglion of vagus n.

Pharyngeal tonsil (adenoids)

Pharyngobasilar fascia

Cartilage and pharyngeal opening of auditory tube

Hypoglossal n. (XII)

Vagus n. (X)

Accessory n. (Xi)

Int. jugular v., sup. bulb

Int. carotid a.

Accessory n. (XI), external ramus

Occipital a.

Mastoid proc.

Sup. cervical ganglion (sympathetic trunk)

Tensor veli palatini m.

Sup. pharyngeal constrictor m.

Salpingopharyngeus m.

Palatopharyngeus m.

Terminal sulcus

Root of tongue

Epiglottis

Sup. laryngeal n., a. and v.

Aryepiglottic m.

Vagus n. (X)

Transv. and oblique arytenoid mm.

Post. cricoarytenoid m.

Sympathetic trunk, carotid plexus

Thyroid gland

Inf. parathyroid gland

Thyrocervical trunk

Sup. cardiac br. of vagus n.

Int. jugular v., inf. bulb

Subclavian a.

Subclavian v.

Vagus n. (X)

Right recurrent laryngeal n.

Right brachiocephalic v.

Trachea, membranous wall

Brachiocephalic trunk

Sup. vena cava

A

Hypoglossal n. (XII)

Torus tubarius

Digastric m., post belly

Uvula m.

B

Salpingopharyngeal fold

Palatine tonsil

Palatopharyngeal arch

Aryepiglottic fold

Hyoid bone, greater horn

C

Cuneiform tubercle

Corniculate tubercle

Piriform recess; Laryngeal n., fold

Interarytenoid notch

Vagus n. (X)

Esophagus, muscular coat

Middle cervical ganglion

Inf. thyroid a.

Int. jugular v., inf. bulb

Thyrocervical trunk

Cervicothoracic ganglion (stellate)

Subclavian a. and v.

Left brachiocephalic v.

Common carotid a

Left recurrent laryngeal n.

Vagus n. (X)

Aorta, descending part

Fig. 251 Pharynx, larynx, and the parapharyngeal space, posterior view. Frontal section at the level of the jugular foramina, with the pharyngeal wall incised at the midline and the mucous membrane removed on the right. Roman numerals III–VIII correspond to cranial nerves III–VIII.

Levels of the Pharynx:

A Nasal part (epipharynx, nasopharynx)

B Oral part (mesopharynx, oropharynx)

C Laryngeal part (hypopharynx, laryngopharynx)

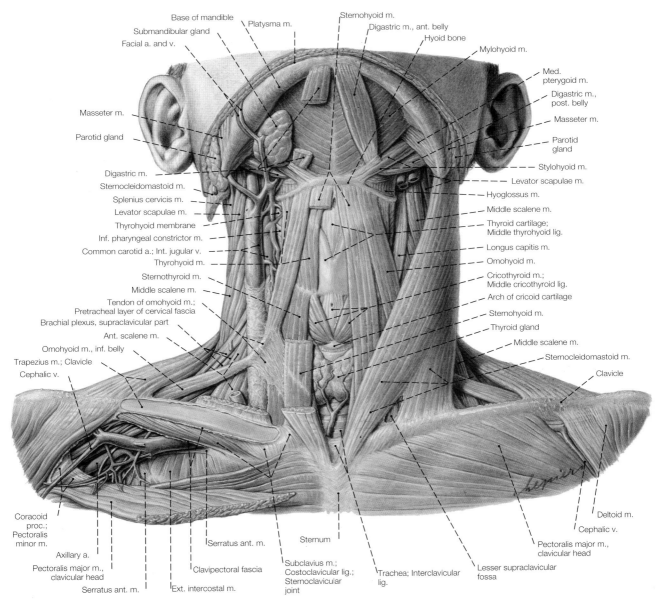

Fig. 252 Muscles of the neck, anterior view (70%). On the left, the contents of the carotid sheath have been removed; on the right, the pectoralis major muscle is reflected.

Sternocleidomastoid Muscle

Name *Innervation*	Origin	Insertion	Function
Sternocleidomastoid muscle *Accessory n. (XI), Cervical plexus*			Both sides together hold the head; ant. fibers flex the head. Post fibers extend the head. One side alone, bends the head laterally, rotates the head toward the opposite side. If the head is fixed, the two sides assist in elevating the thorax during deep inspiration
Sternal head	Ventral surface of the manubrium of the sternum	Lateral surface of mastoid process; lateral half of superior nuchal line of occipital bone	
Clavicular head	Medial third of clavicle		

Suprahyoid Muscles

Name *Innervation*	Origin	Insertion	Function
1. Digastric muscle Anterior belly *Mylohyoid n.* *(Mandibular n., V3)* Posterior belly *Digastric br.* *(Facial n., VII)*	Mastoid notch of temporal bone (posterior belly); divided into two bellies by an intertendon, which is connected to the side of the body and greater horn of the hyoid bone by a fibrous loop	Digastric fossa of mandible (anterior belly)	Opens the mouth by depressing mandible, elevates (fixes) the hyoid bone; assists 3
2. Stylohyoid muscle *Stylohyoid br.* *(Facial n., VII)*	Styloid process of temporal bone	Lateral margin of body of hyoid bone near the greater horn; is perforated by the intertendon of the digastric muscle	Fixes hyoid bone, pulling it backward and upward during deglutition
3. Mylohyoid muscle *Mylohyoid n.* *(Mandibular n., V3)*	Mylohyoid line of the mandible; both together form a plate across the mandibular arch	Mylohyoid raphe and body of hyoid bone	Raises the floor of the mouth in swallowing, depresses the mandible, elevates hyoid bone
4. Geniohyoid muscle *1st cervical n., via* *Hypoglossal n., XII*	Inferior mental spine of the mandible, the muscles of both sides lie close together, with a midline septum between them	Anterior surface of body of hyoid bone	Assists the mylohyoid muscle in elevating the tongue, elevates and fixes the hyoid bone, depresses the mandible

Infrahyoid Muscles

Name *Innervation*	Origin	Insertion	Function
1. Sternohyoid muscle* *Ansa cervicalis* *(Cervical plexus)*	Inner surface of manubrium sterni and sternoclavicular joint	Body of hyoid bone	Depresses the larynx and hyoid after they have been elevated with the pharynx in deglutition (thyrohyoid muscle elevates the larynx); indirectly flexes the head and cervical joints; omohyoid muscle tenses the cervical fascia through the connection of its central tendon to the carotid sheath; assists in respiration (pulls sternum cranially in inspiration)
2. Sternothyroid muscle* *Ansa cervicalis* *(Cervical plexus)*	Inner surface of 1st costal cartilage and manubrium sterni, caudal to 1	Outer surface of thyroid cartilage (opposite the origin of thyrohyoid muscle)	
3. Thyrohyoid muscle *Ansa cervicalis* *(Cervical plexus)*	Outer surface of the thyroid cartilage	Inferior border of greater horn of hyoid bone	
4. Omohyoid muscle** *Ansa cervicalis* *(Cervical plexus)*	Superior margin of scapula between superior angle and scapular notch (inferior belly)	Lower border of body of hyoid bone (superior belly)	

* Often has a transverse tendinous inscription caudally

** Consists of two fleshy bellies united by a central tendon connected to the carotid sheath

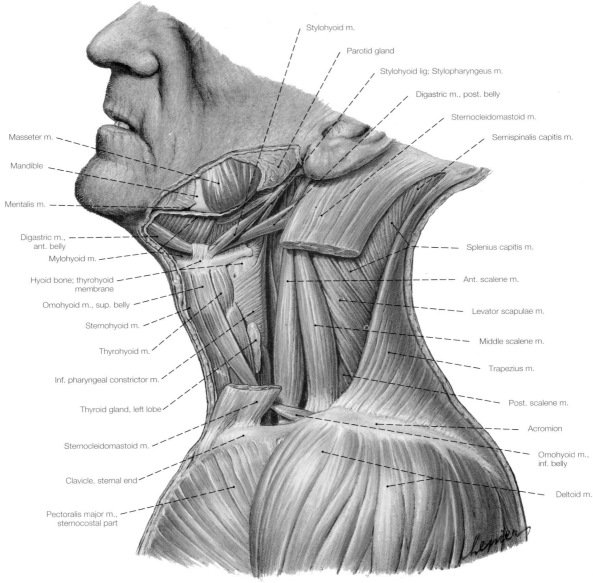

Stylohyoid m.

Parotid gland

Stylohyoid lig; Stylopharyngeus m.

Digastric m., post. belly

Sternocleidomastoid m.

Semispinalis capitis m.

Masseter m.

Mandible

Mentalis m.

Digastric m., ant. belly

Mylohyoid m.

Hyoid bone; thyrohyoid membrane

Omohyoid m., sup. belly

Sternohyoid m.

Thyrohyoid m.

Inf. pharyngeal constrictor m.

Thyroid gland, left lobe

Sternocleidomastoid m.

Clavicle, sternal end

Pectoralis major m., sternocostal part

Splenius capitis m.

Ant. scalene m.

Levator scapulae m.

Middle scalene m.

Trapezius m.

Post. scalene m.

Acromion

Omohyoid m., inf. belly

Deltoid m.

Fig. 253   Muscles of the neck. Lateral view of the left side of the neck after removal of the midportion of the sternocleidomastoid muscle (70%).

Lateral Vertebral Muscles

Name *Innervation*	Origin	Insertion	Function
1. Anterior scalene muscle *Direct branches from cervical plexus and brachial plexus*	Anterior tubercles of transverse processes of 3rd to 6th cervical vertebrae	Scalene tubercle on 1st rib	Elevate 1st and 2nd ribs (muscles of inspiration); flex and laterally rotate vertebral column
2. Middle scalene muscle *Direct branches from cervical plexus and brachial plexus*	Posterior tubercles of transverse processes of last 6 cervical vertebrae	Cranial surface of 1st rib, behind subclavian groove	
3. Posterior scalene muscle *Direct branches from cervical plexus and brachial plexus*	Posterior tubercles of transverse processes of 4th to 6th cervical vertebrae	Outer surface of 2nd rib	

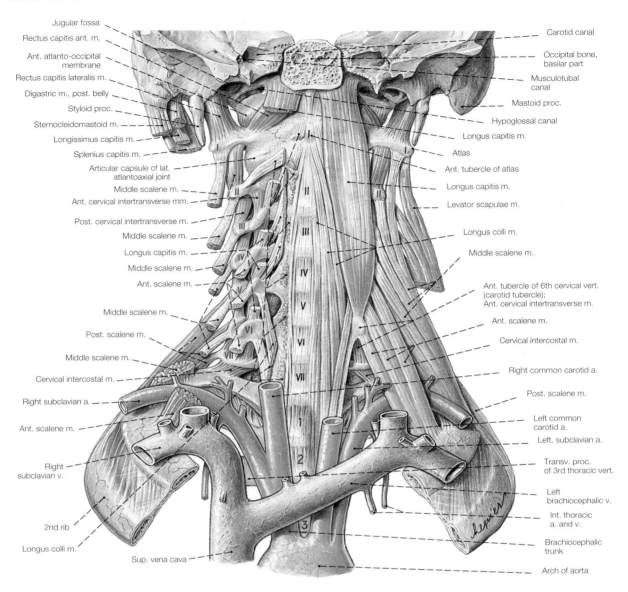

Fig. 254 Muscles of the neck. Frontal section at the level of the apices of the petrous portion of the temporal bone with the cervical viscera removed, anterior view (80%). The left scalene muscles have been removed.

I–VII = 1st to 7th cervical vertebrae
1–3 = 1st to 3rd thoracic vertebrae

Prevertebral Muscles

Name *Innervation*	Origin	Insertion	Function
1. Longus colli muscle *Direct branches from cervical plexus* Vertical part	Bodies of first 3 thoracic and last 3 cervical vertebrae	Bodies of cervical vertebrae C2–C4	Flexes the cervical vertebral column or the head forward; unilaterally inclines and rotates the head toward the same side

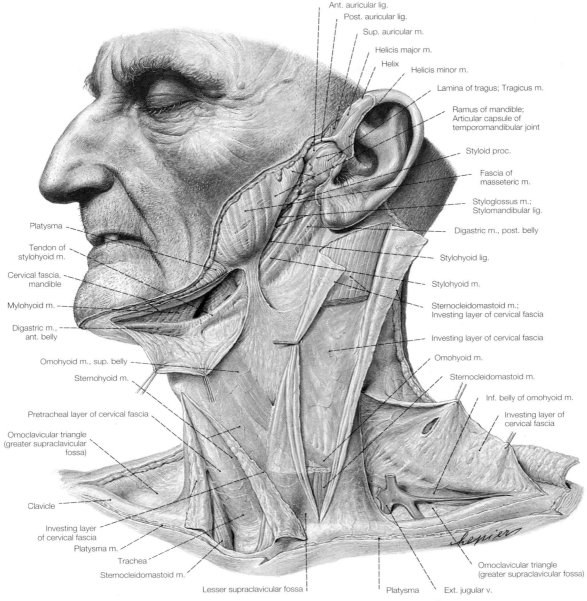

Ant. auricular lig.

Post. auricular lig.

Sup. auricular m.

Helicis major m.

Helix

Helicis minor m.

Lamina of tragus; Tragicus m.

Ramus of mandible;
Articular capsule of
temporomandibular joint

Styloid proc.

Fascia of
masseteric m.

Styloglossus m.;
Stylomandibular lig.

Digastric m., post. belly

Stylohyoid lig.

Stylohyoid m.

Sternocleidomastoid m.;
Investing layer of cervical fascia

Investing layer of cervical fascia

Omohyoid m.

Sternocleidomastoid m.

Inf. belly of omohyoid m.

Investing layer of
cervical fascia

Omoclavicular triangle
(greater supraclavicular fossa)

Ext. jugular v.

Platysma

Platysma

Tendon of
stylohyoid m.

Cervical fascia,
mandible

Mylohyoid m.

Digastric m.,
ant. belly

Omohyoid m., sup. belly

Sternohyoid m.

Pretracheal layer of cervical fascia

Omoclavicular triangle
(greater supraclavicular
fossa)

Clavicle

Investing layer
of cervical fascia

Platysma m.

Trachea

Sternocleidomastoid m.

Lesser supraclavicular fossa

Fig. 255 The fascia of the neck. The head is turned
to the right and portions of the sternocleidomastoid
muscle have been removed, anterolateral view (80%).

Prevertebral Muscles (continued)

Name *Innervation*	Origin	Insertion	Function
Superior oblique part	Anterior tubercles of transverse processes of cervical vertebrae C3–C5	Tubercle on anterior arch of the atlas and body of next cervical vertebrae	Flex the cervical vertebral column or the head forward, unilaterally incline and rotate the head toward the same side
Inferior oblique part	Anterior surface of bodies of first 2 or 3 thoracic vertebrae	Anterior tubercle of the transverse processes of 5th and 6th cervical vertebrae	
2. Longus capitus muscle *Direct branches from cervical plexus*	Anterior tubercles of transverse processes of 3rd–6th cervical vertebrae	Inferior border of basilar part of occipital bone	

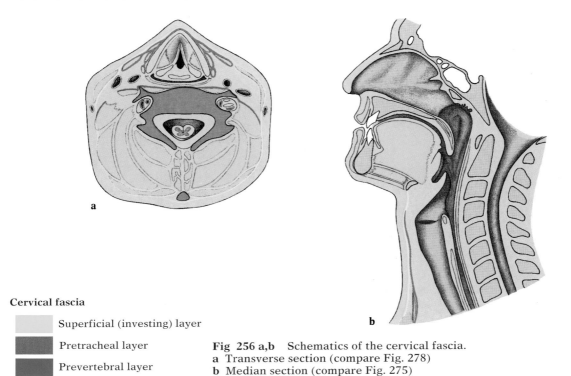

Cervical fascia

- Superficial (investing) layer
- Pretracheal layer
- Prevertebral layer

Fig 256 a,b Schematics of the cervical fascia.
a Transverse section (compare Fig. 278)
b Median section (compare Fig. 275)

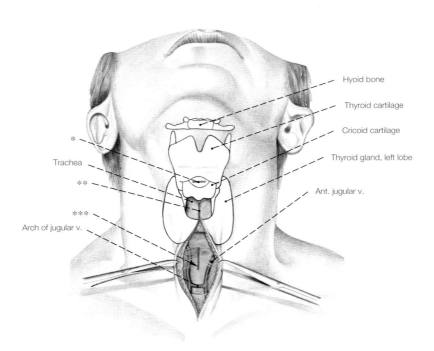

Hyoid bone

Thyroid cartilage

Cricoid cartilage

Thyroid gland, left lobe

*

Trachea

**

Ant. jugular v.

***

Arch of jugular v.

Fig. 257 Projection of the cervical viscera onto the surface and the surgical site of a low tracheotomy, anterior view. The neck is hyperextended posteriorly.

Surgical approaches for opening the trachea are indicated in red:
* Coniotomy
** High tracheotomy (above the isthmus of the thyroid gland)
*** Low tracheotomy (below the isthmus of the thyroid gland)

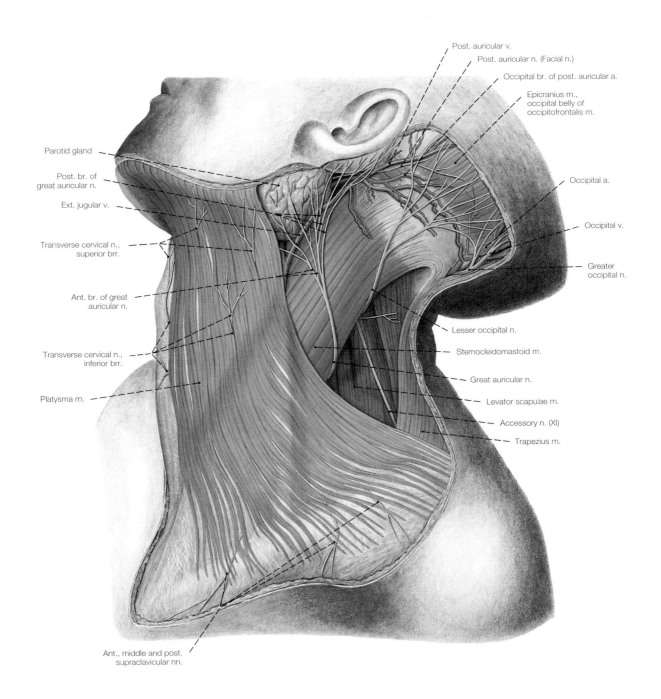

Post. auricular v.

Post. auricular n. (Facial n.)

Occipital br. of post. auricular a.

Epicranius m.,
occipital belly of
occipitofrontalis m.

Parotid gland

Post. br. of
great auricular n.

Ext. jugular v.

Transverse cervical n.,
superior brr.

Ant. br. of great
auricular n.

Transverse cervical n.,
inferior brr.

Platysma m.

Ant., middle and post.
supraclavicular nn.

Occipital a.

Occipital v.

Greater
occipital n.

Lesser occipital n.

Sternocleidomastoid m.

Great auricular n.

Levator scapulae m.

Accessory n. (XI)

Trapezius m.

Fig. 258 Blood vessels and nerves of the anterior
and lateral regions of the neck, superficial layer.
Lateral view of the left side of the neck (70%).

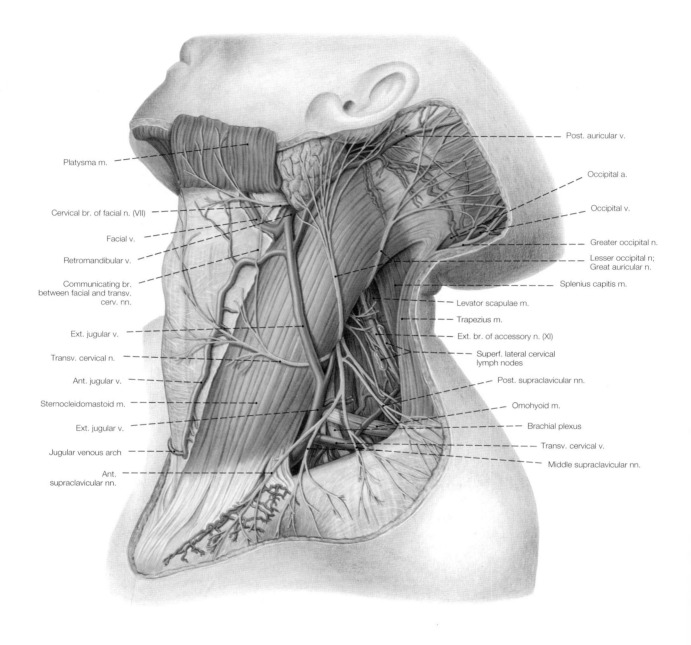

Platysma m.

Cervical br. of facial n. (VII)

Facial v.

Retromandibular v.

Communicating br.
between facial and transv.
cerv. nn.

Ext. jugular v.

Transv. cervical n.

Ant. jugular v.

Sternocleidomastoid m.

Ext. jugular v.

Jugular venous arch

Ant.
supraclavicular nn.

Post. auricular v.

Occipital a.

Occipital v.

Greater occipital n.

Lesser occipital n;
Great auricular n.

Splenius capitis m.

Levator scapulae m.

Trapezius m.

Ext. br. of accessory n. (XI)

Superf. lateral cervical
lymph nodes

Post. supraclavicular nn.

Omohyoid m.

Brachial plexus

Transv. cervical v.

Middle supraclavicular nn.

Fig. 259 Blood vessels and nerves of the lateral region of the neck. Parts of the platysma have been reflected upward and the investing layer of the cervical fascia has been largely removed. Lateral view of the left side of the neck (70%).

The site where the cutaneous branches of the cervical plexus emerge at the posterior border of the sternocleidomastoid muscle is known clinically as ERB's point (punctum nervosum). Due to the danger of damaging the accessory nerve during lymphadenectomy, particular attention should be paid to the positions of the superficial lateral cervical lymph nodes of the neck.

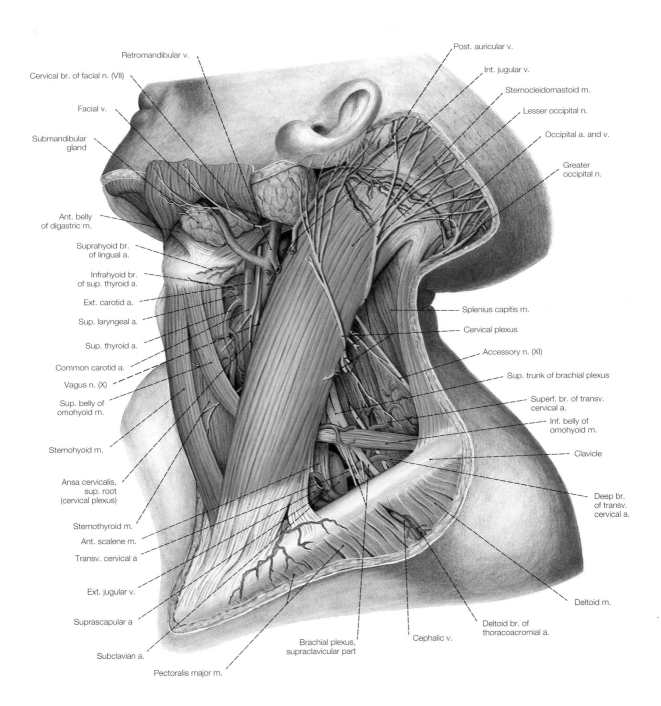

Retromandibular v.

Cervical br. of facial n. (VII)

Facial v.

Submandibular
gland

Ant. belly
of digastric m.

Suprahyoid br.
of lingual a.

Infrahyoid br.
of sup. thyroid a.

Ext. carotid a.

Sup. laryngeal a.

Sup. thyroid a.

Common carotid a.

Vagus n. (X)

Sup. belly of
omohyoid m.

Sternohyoid m.

Ansa cervicalis,
sup. root
(cervical plexus)

Sternothyroid m.

Ant. scalene m.

Transv. cervical a

Ext. jugular v.

Suprascapular a

Subclavian a.

Pectoralis major m.

Brachial plexus,
supraclavicular part

Cephalic v.

Deltoid br. of
thoracoacromial a.

Post. auricular v.

Int. jugular v.

Sternocleidomastoid m.

Lesser occipital n.

Occipital a. and v.

Greater
occipital n.

Splenius capitis m.

Cervical plexus

Accessory n. (XI)

Sup. trunk of brachial plexus

Superf. br. of transv.
cervical a.

Inf. belly of
omohyoid m.

Clavicle

Deep br.
of transv.
cervical a.

Deltoid m.

Fig. 260   Blood vessels and nerves of the anterior
and lateral regions of the neck after removal of the
investing layer of the cervical fascia. Lateral view of
the left side of the neck (70%).

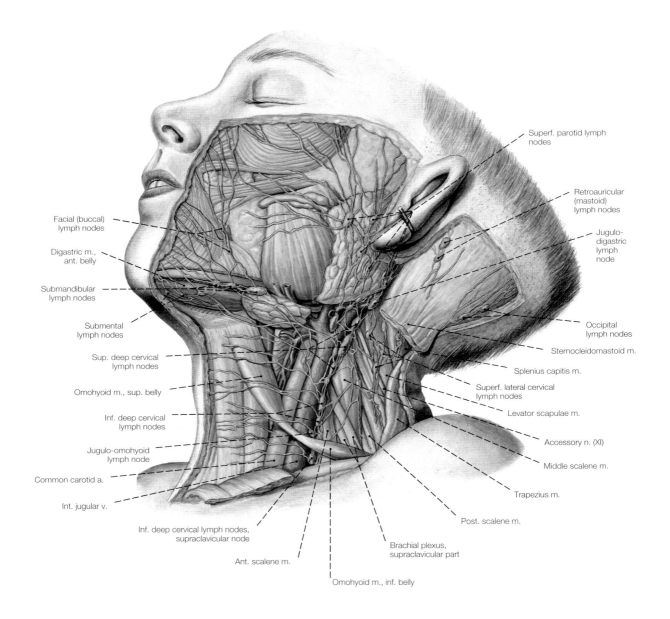

Superf. parotid lymph
nodes

Retroauricular
(mastoid)
lymph nodes

Jugulo-
digastric
lymph
node

Facial (buccal)
lymph nodes

Digastric m.,
ant. belly

Submandibular
lymph nodes

Submental
lymph nodes

Sup. deep cervical
lymph nodes

Omohyoid m., sup. belly

Inf. deep cervical
lymph nodes

Jugulo-omohyoid
lymph node

Common carotid a.

Int. jugular v.

Occipital
lymph nodes

Sternocleidomastoid m.

Splenius capitis m.

Superf. lateral cervical
lymph nodes

Levator scapulae m.

Accessory n. (XI)

Middle scalene m.

Trapezius m.

Post. scalene m.

Inf. deep cervical lymph nodes,
supraclavicular node

Ant. scalene m.

Brachial plexus,
supraclavicular part

Omohyoid m., inf. belly

Fig. 261 The superficial lymphatic vessels and
lymph nodes of the head and neck. The specimen is
from an 8-year-old boy, lateral aspect. The platysma
and superficial cervical fascia have been removed,
as well as the entire cervical plexus and a portion of
the sternocleidomastoid muscle.

The accessory nerve is severely endangered
during surgical removal of the lymph nodes of the
lateral region of the neck.

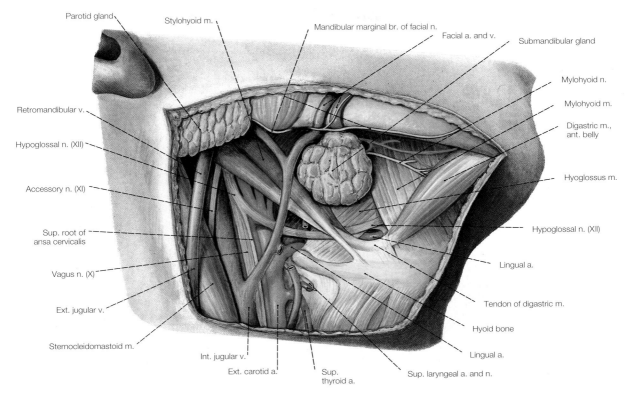

Parotid gland
Stylohyoid m.
Mandibular marginal br. of facial n.
Facial a. and v.
Submandibular gland
Mylohyoid n.
Mylohyoid m.
Retromandibular v.
Digastric m., ant. belly
Hypoglossal n. (XII)
Hyoglossus m.
Accessory n. (XI)
Sup. root of ansa cervicalis
Hypoglossal n. (XII)
Vagus n. (X)
Lingual a.
Ext. jugular v.
Tendon of digastric m.
Sternocleidomastoid m.
Hyoid bone
Int. jugular v.
Lingual a.
Ext. carotid a.
Sup. thyroid a.
Sup. laryngeal a. and n.

Fig. 262   Blood vessels and nerves of the submandibular triangle, viewed laterally from below.

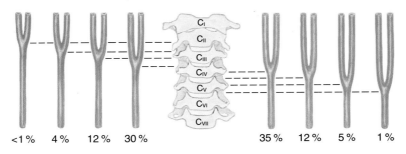

C_I
C_{II}
C_{III}
C_{IV}
C_V
C_{VI}
C_{VII}

<1 %   4 %   12 %   30 %   35 %   12 %   5 %   1 %

Fig. 263   Variations in the levels of bifurcation of the common carotid artery in relation to the cervical vertebrae and their frequency of occurrence.

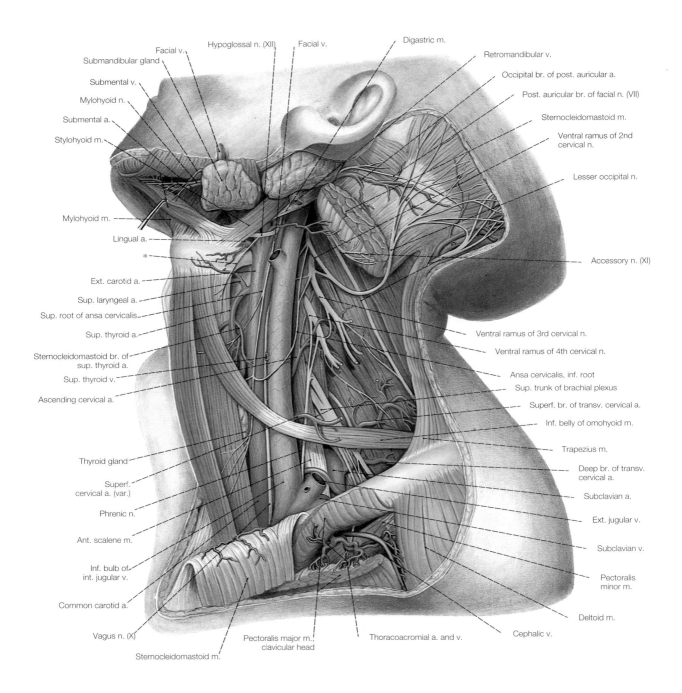

Facial v.
Submandibular gland
Submental v.
Mylohyoid n.
Submental a.
Stylohyoid m.
Hypoglossal n. (XII)
Facial v.
Digastric m.
Retromandibular v.
Occipital br. of post. auricular a.
Post. auricular br. of facial n. (VII)
Sternocleidomastoid m.
Ventral ramus of 2nd cervical n.
Lesser occipital n.
Mylohyoid m.
Lingual a.
*
Ext. carotid a.
Sup. laryngeal a.
Sup. root of ansa cervicalis
Sup. thyroid a.
Sternocleidomastoid br. of sup. thyroid a.
Sup. thyroid v.
Ascending cervical a.
Accessory n. (XI)
Ventral ramus of 3rd cervical n.
Ventral ramus of 4th cervical n.
Ansa cervicalis, inf. root
Sup. trunk of brachial plexus
Superf. br. of transv. cervical a.
Inf. belly of omohyoid m.
Trapezius m.
Thyroid gland
Superf. cervical a. (var.)
Phrenic n.
Ant. scalene m.
Inf. bulb of int. jugular v.
Common carotid a.
Vagus n. (X)
Deep br. of transv. cervical a.
Subclavian a.
Ext. jugular v.
Subclavian v.
Pectoralis minor m.
Deltoid m.
Cephalic v.
Pectoralis major m. clavicular head
Thoracoacromial a. and v.
Sternocleidomastoid m.

Fig. 264 Blood vessels and nerves of the lateral region of the neck. The sternocleidomastoid muscle has been extensively removed; lateral view of the left side of the neck (80%).

* Although derived from the superior root of the ansa cervicalis, the thyrohyoid branch briefly joins the hypoglossal nerve.

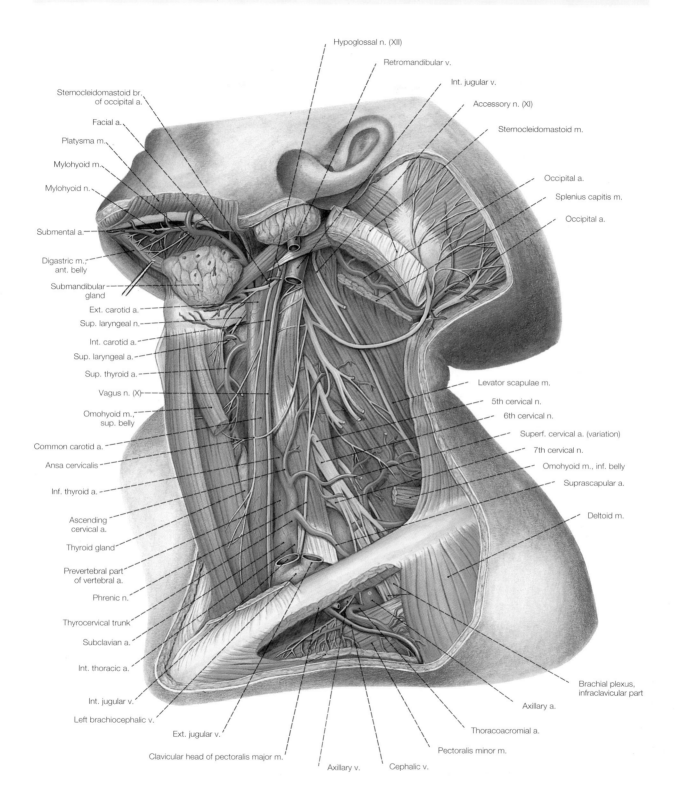

Hypoglossal n. (XII)

Retromandibular v.

Int. jugular v.

Accessory n. (XI)

Sternocleidomastoid m.

Sternocleidomastoid br. of occipital a.

Facial a.

Platysma m.

Mylohyoid m.

Mylohyoid n.

Occipital a.

Splenius capitis m.

Occipital a.

Submental a.

Digastric m., ant. belly

Submandibular gland

Ext. carotid a.

Sup. laryngeal n.

Int. carotid a.

Sup. laryngeal a.

Sup. thyroid a.

Vagus n. (X)

Omohyoid m., sup. belly

Common carotid a.

Ansa cervicalis

Inf. thyroid a.

Ascending cervical a.

Thyroid gland

Prevertebral part of vertebral a.

Phrenic n.

Thyrocervical trunk

Subclavian a.

Int. thoracic a.

Int. jugular v.

Left brachiocephalic v.

Ext. jugular v.

Clavicular head of pectoralis major m.

Axillary v.

Cephalic v.

Pectoralis minor m.

Thoracoacromial a.

Axillary a.

Brachial plexus, infraclavicular part

Deltoid m.

Suprascapular a.

Omohyoid m., inf. belly

7th cervical n.

Superf. cervical a. (variation)

6th cervical n.

5th cervical n.

Levator scapulae m.

Fig. 265 Vessels and nerves of the lateral region of the neck and the deltopectoral triangle. The deep layer after removal of the sternocleidomastoid muscle, the omohyoid muscle and the veins, lateral view of the left side of the neck (80%).

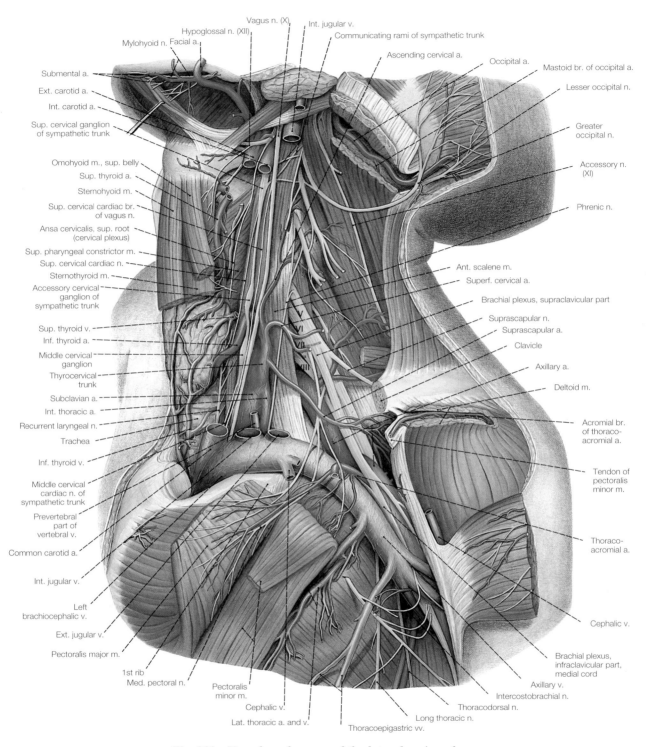

Mylohyoid n. Facial a.
Vagus n. (X)
Hypoglossal n. (XII)
Int. jugular v.
Communicating rami of sympathetic trunk
Ascending cervical a.
Occipital a.
Mastoid br. of occipital a.

Submental a.
Ext. carotid a.
Int. carotid a.
Sup. cervical ganglion of sympathetic trunk
Lesser occipital n.
Greater occipital n.

Omohyoid m., sup. belly
Sup. thyroid a.
Sternohyoid m.
Sup. cervical cardiac br. of vagus n.
Ansa cervicalis, sup. root (cervical plexus)
Sup. pharyngeal constrictor m.
Sup. cervical cardiac n.
Sternothyroid m.
Accessory cervical ganglion of sympathetic trunk
Accessory n. (XI)
Phrenic n.

Sup. thyroid v.
Inf. thyroid a.
Middle cervical ganglion
Thyrocervical trunk
Subclavian a.
Int. thoracic a.
Recurrent laryngeal n.
Trachea
Inf. thyroid v.
Middle cervical cardiac n. of sympathetic trunk
Prevertebral part of vertebral v.
Common carotid a.
Int. jugular v.
Left brachiocephalic v.
Ext. jugular v.
Pectoralis major m.
1st rib
Med. pectoral n.
Pectoralis minor m.
Cephalic v.
Lat. thoracic a. and v.
Thoracoepigastric vv.
Long thoracic n.
Thoracodorsal n.
Intercostobrachial n.
Axillary v.
Brachial plexus, infraclavicular part, medial cord
Cephalic v.
Thoraco-acromial a.
Tendon of pectoralis minor m.
Acromial br. of thoraco-acromial a.
Deltoid m.
Axillary a.
Clavicle
Suprascapular a.
Suprascapular n.
Brachial plexus, supraclavicular part
Superf. cervical a.
Ant. scalene m.

V
VI
VII
VIII

Fig. 266 Vessels and nerves of the lateral region of the neck and the deltopectoral triangle. The deep layer after partial removal of the clavicle, the sternocleidomastoid muscle, trunks of the blood vessels, and caudal parts of the infrahyoid muscles, lateral view of the left side of the neck (80%). Roman numerals V–VIII indicate the roots of the brachial plexus from the ventral primary divisions of the 5th to 8th cervical nerves.

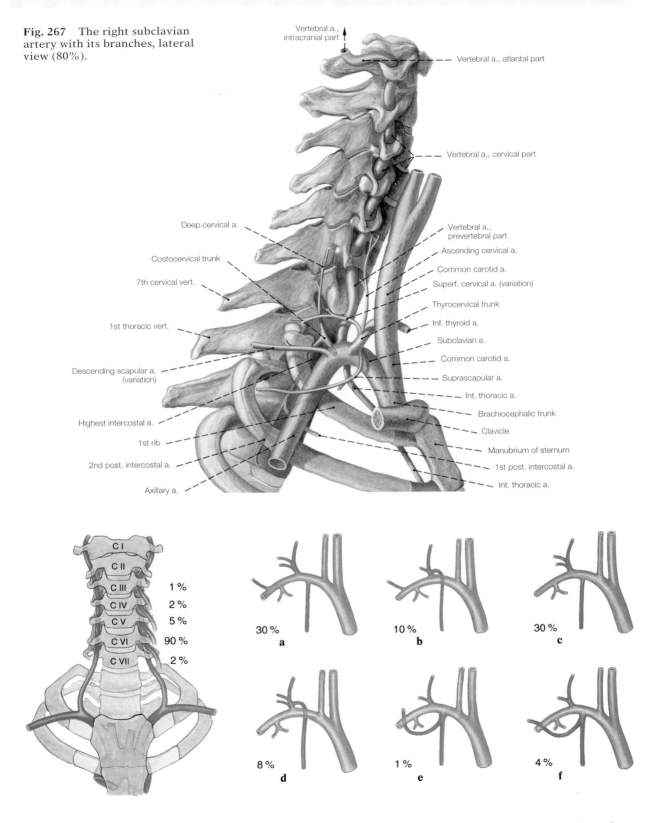

Fig. 267 The right subclavian artery with its branches, lateral view (80%).

Vertebral a., intracranial part

Vertebral a., atlantal part

Vertebral a., cervical part

Deep cervical a.

Costocervical trunk

7th cervical vert.

1st thoracic vert.

Descending scapular a. (variation)

Highest intercostal a.

1st rib

2nd post. intercostal a.

Axillary a.

Vertebral a., prevertebral part

Ascending cervical a.

Common carotid a.

Superf. cervical a. (variation)

Thyrocervical trunk

Inf. thyroid a.

Subclavian a.

Common carotid a.

Suprascapular a.

Int. thoracic a.

Brachiocephalic trunk

Clavicle

Manubrium of sternum

1st post. intercostal a.

Int. thoracic a.

C I
C II
C III   1 %
C IV   2 %
C V   5 %
C VI   90 %
C VII   2 %

30 % **a**

10 % **b**

30 % **c**

8 % **d**

1 % **e**

4 % **f**

Fig. 268 Variations in the levels of entry of the vertebral artery into the transverse foramina. On the right side is shown the classical "textbook case," on the left, variations in entry levels. Percentages indicate the frequency of occurrence.

Fig. 269 a–f Variations in the origin of the branches of the subclavian artery. Percentages indicate the frequency of occurrence.

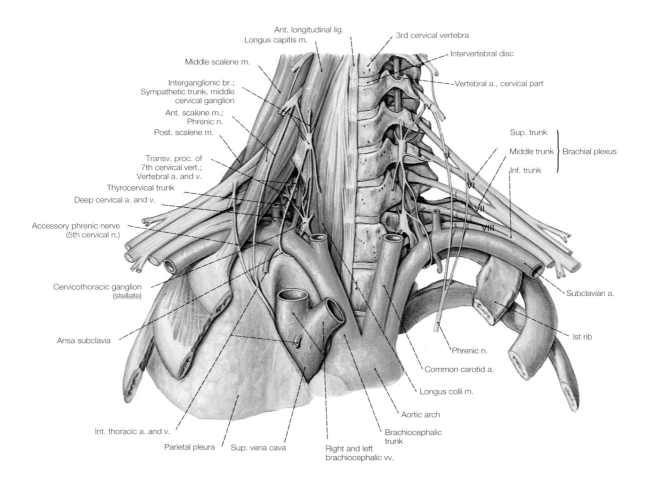

Ant. longitudinal lig.
Longus capitis m.
Middle scalene m.
Interganglionic br.;
Sympathetic trunk, middle
cervical ganglion
Ant. scalene m.;
Phrenic n.
Post. scalene m.
Transv. proc. of
7th cervical vert.;
Vertebral a. and v.
Thyrocervical trunk
Deep cervical a. and v.
Accessory phrenic nerve
(5th cervical n.)
Cervicothoracic ganglion
(stellate)
Ansa subclavia
Int. thoracic a. and v.
Parietal pleura
Sup. vena cava
Right and left
brachiocephalic vv.
3rd cervical vertebra
Intervertebral disc
Vertebral a., cervical part
Sup. trunk
Middle trunk } Brachial plexus
Inf. trunk
Subclavian a.
1st rib
Phrenic n.
Common carotid a.
Longus colli m.
Aortic arch
Brachiocephalic trunk

Fig. 270 Blood vessels and nerves in the cervicothoracic region. Deep layer after removal of the scalene
muscles and the prevertebral muscles on the right side,
anterior view (60%).

Note the close relationship of the sympathetic trunk,
the brachial plexus and the cupola of the lungs.

Roman numerals IV–VIII indicate the roots of the
brachial plexus from the ventral primary divisions of
the 4th to 8th cervical nerves.

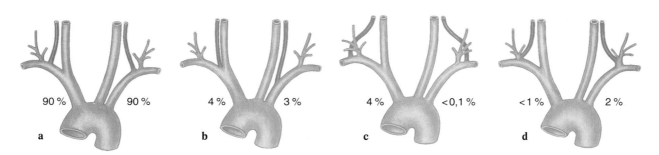

90 %   90 %   4 %   3 %   4 %   <0,1 %   <1 %   2 %
a   b   c   d

Fig. 271 a–d Variations in the origin of the vertebral
artery. Percentages indicate the frequency of occurrence.

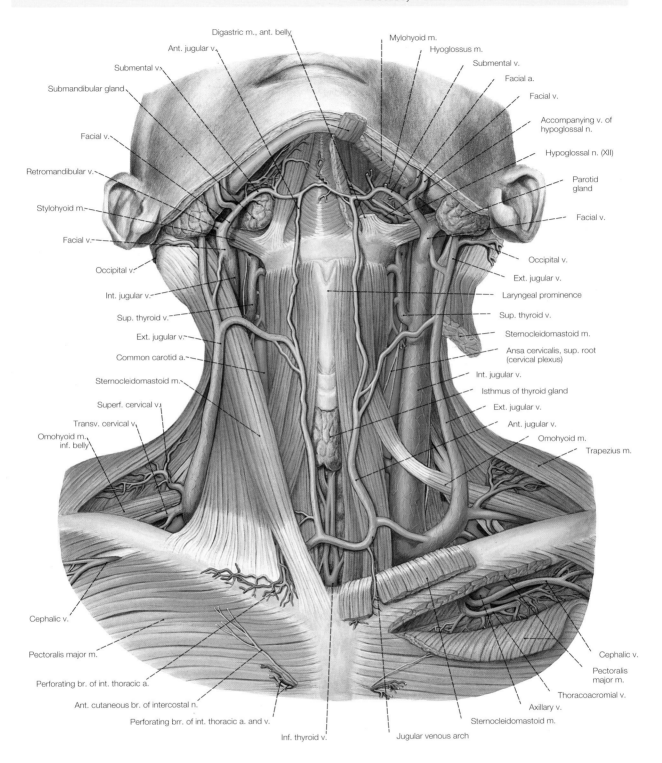

Digastric m., ant. belly

Ant. jugular v.

Submental v.

Submandibular gland

Facial v.

Retromandibular v.

Stylohyoid m.

Facial v.

Occipital v.

Int. jugular v.

Sup. thyroid v.

Ext. jugular v.

Common carotid a.

Sternocleidomastoid m.

Superf. cervical v.

Transv. cervical v.

Omohyoid m., inf. belly

Cephalic v.

Pectoralis major m.

Perforating br. of int. thoracic a.

Ant. cutaneous br. of intercostal n.

Perforating brr. of int. thoracic a. and v.

Inf. thyroid v.

Mylohyoid m.

Hyoglossus m.

Submental v.

Facial a.

Facial v.

Accompanying v. of hypoglossal n.

Hypoglossal n. (XII)

Parotid gland

Facial v.

Occipital v.

Ext. jugular v.

Laryngeal prominence

Sup. thyroid v.

Sternocleidomastoid m.

Ansa cervicalis, sup. root (cervical plexus)

Int. jugular v.

Isthmus of thyroid gland

Ext. jugular v.

Ant. jugular v.

Omohyoid m.

Trapezius m.

Cephalic v.

Pectoralis major m.

Thoracoacromial v.

Axillary v.

Sternocleidomastoid m.

Jugular venous arch

Fig. 272 Veins of the neck, anterior view (80%). The fascial layers of the neck have been removed, and the sternocleidomastoid and pectoralis major muscles on the left side have been partially resected.

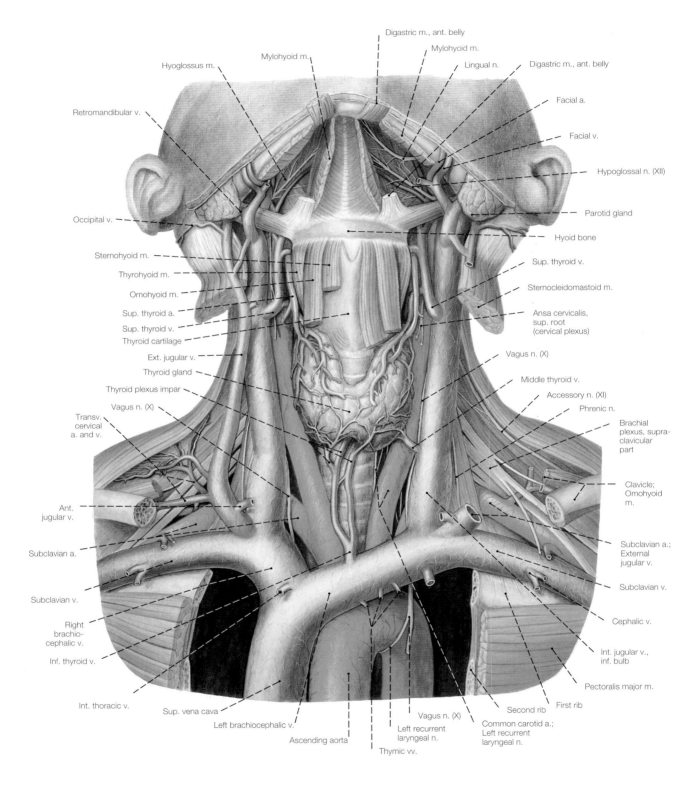

Fig. 273 Vessels and nerves of the neck and the upper thoracic aperture, anterior view (80%). Deep layer after removal of the middle part of the clavicle, the first two ribs and the sternum.

The junction of the internal jugular vein with the subclavian vein is known clinically as the venous angle.

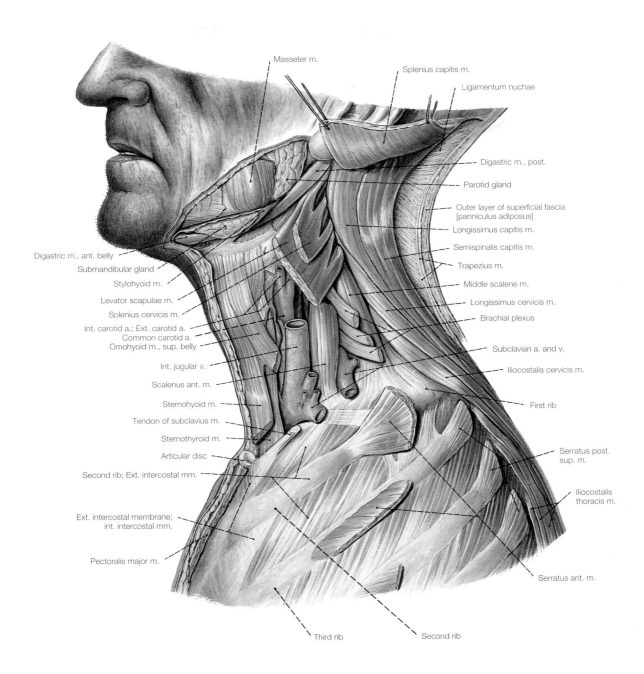

Masseter m.

Splenius capitis m.

Ligamentum nuchae

Digastric m., post.

Parotid gland

Outer layer of superficial fascia
[panniculus adiposus]

Longissimus capitis m.

Semispinalis capitis m.

Trapezius m.

Middle scalene m.

Longissimus cervicis m.

Brachial plexus

Subclavian a. and v.

Iliocostalis cervicis m.

First rib

Serratus post.
sup. m.

Iliocostalis
thoracis m.

Serratus ant. m.

Digastric m., ant. belly

Submandibular gland

Stylohyoid m.

Levator scapulae m.

Splenius cervicis m.

Int. carotid a.; Ext. carotid a.

Common carotid a.

Omohyoid m., sup. belly

Int. jugular v.

Scalenus ant. m.

Sternohyoid m.

Tendon of subclavius m.

Sternothyroid m.

Articular disc

Second rib; Ext. intercostal mm.

Ext. intercostal membrane;
int. intercostal mm.

Pectoralis major m.

Third rib

Second rib

Fig. 274 Vessels and nerves of the lateral region of
the neck. Deep layer after removal of the shoulder
girdle, lateral view of the right side (80%). The
splenius capitis muscle has been reflected upwards,
the splenius cervicis and levator scapulae muscles
have been reflected anteriorly.

Note the course of the subclavian vein in front of the
anterior scalene muscle and the subclavian artery
and brachial plexus in the space between the anterior
and middle scalene muscles.

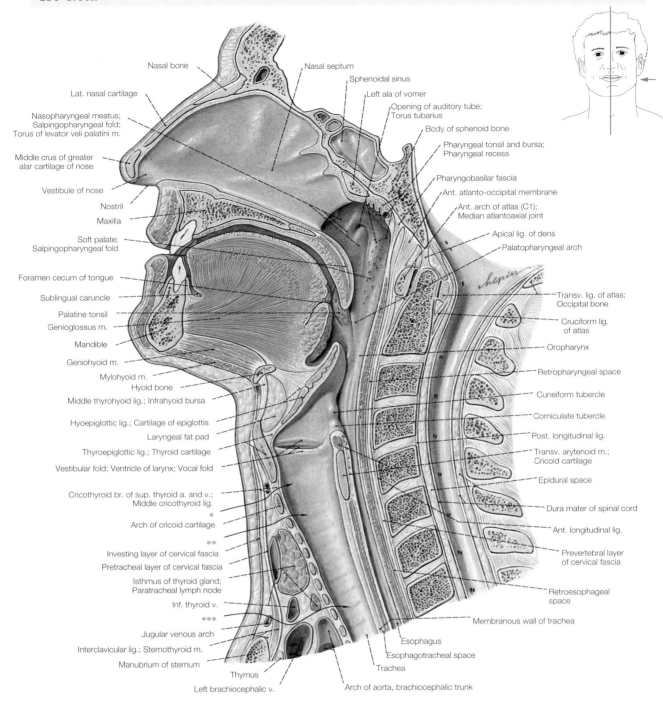

Nasal bone

Lat. nasal cartilage

Nasopharyngeal meatus;
Salpingopharyngeal fold;
Torus of levator veli palatini m.

Middle crus of greater
alar cartilage of nose

Vestibule of nose

Nostril

Maxilla

Soft palate;
Salpingopharyngeal fold

Foramen cecum of tongue

Sublingual caruncle

Palatine tonsil

Genioglossus m.

Mandible

Geniohyoid m.

Mylohyoid m.

Hyoid bone

Middle thyrohyoid lig.; Infrahyoid bursa

Hyoepiglottic lig.; Cartilage of epiglottis

Laryngeal fat pad

Thyroepiglottic lig.; Thyroid cartilage

Vestibular fold; Ventricle of larynx; Vocal fold

Cricothyroid br. of sup. thyroid a. and v.;
Middle cricothyroid lig.

*

Arch of cricoid cartilage

**

Investing layer of cervical fascia

Pretracheal layer of cervical fascia

Isthmus of thyroid gland;
Paratracheal lymph node

Inf. thyroid v.

***

Jugular venous arch

Interclavicular lig.; Sternothyroid m.

Manubrium of sternum

Thymus

Left brachiocephalic v.

Nasal septum

Sphenoidal sinus

Left ala of vomer

Opening of auditory tube;
Torus tubarius

Body of sphenoid bone

Pharyngeal tonsil and bursa;
Pharyngeal recess

Pharyngobasilar fascia

Ant. atlanto-occipital membrane

Ant. arch of atlas (C1);
Median atlantoaxial joint

Apical lig. of dens

Palatopharyngeal arch

Transv. lig. of atlas;
Occipital bone

Cruciform lig.
of atlas

Oropharynx

Retropharyngeal space

Cuneiform tubercle

Corniculate tubercle

Post. longitudinal lig.

Transv. arytenoid m.;
Cricoid cartilage

Epidural space

Dura mater of spinal cord

Ant. longitudinal lig.

Prevertebral layer
of cervical fascia

Retroesophageal
space

Membranous wall of trachea

Esophagus

Esophagotracheal space

Trachea

Arch of aorta, brachiocephalic trunk

Fig. 275 Head and neck. Paramedian section that
retains the nasal septum, medial view from the left
(80%). The arrows indicate the surgical approaches
to the trachea.

*   Coniotomy: through the middle cricothyroid lig.
**   High tracheotomy: above the isthmus of the thyroid gland
*** Low tracheotomy: below the isthmus of the thyroid gland

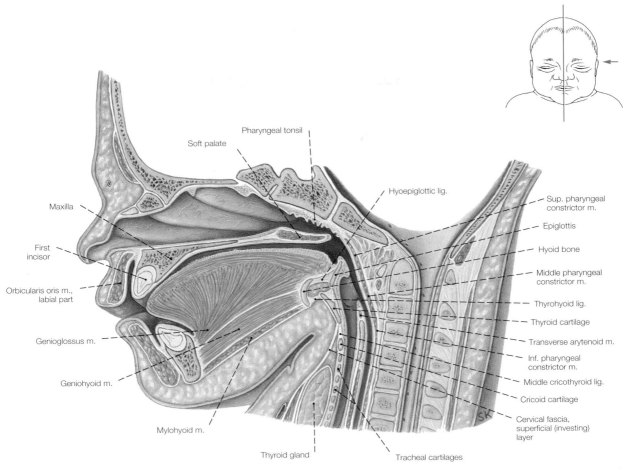

Fig. 276 Facial part of the head and neck. Median section through the head of a newborn, medial aspect (110%).

The larynx in the newborn and infant is positioned considerably higher than in the adult. Compare with Fig. 275.

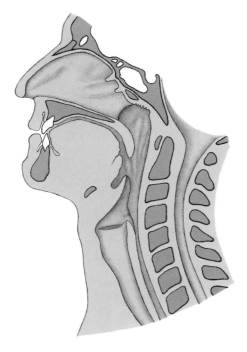

	Maxillary n. (V2)
	Glossopharyngeal n. (IX)
	Vagus n. (X)

Fig. 277 Sensory innervation of the pharynx, medial aspect.

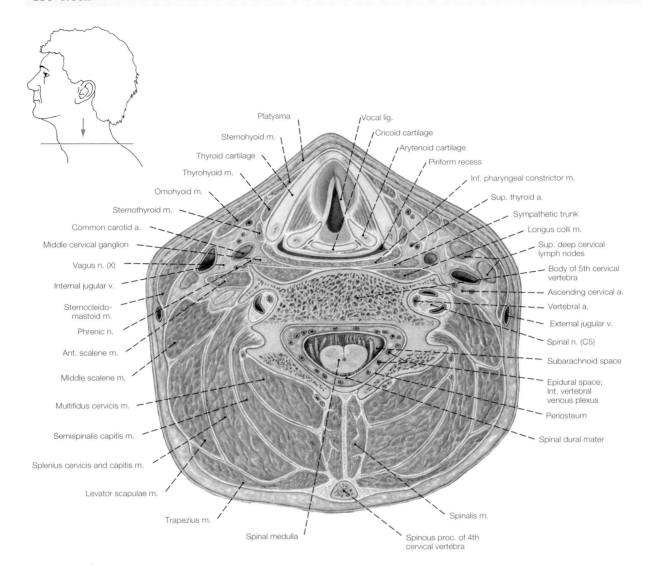

Platysma

Vocal lig.

Sternohyoid m.

Cricoid cartilage

Thyroid cartilage

Arytenoid cartilage

Thyrohyoid m.

Piriform recess

Omohyoid m.

Inf. pharyngeal constrictor m.

Sternothyroid m.

Sup. thyroid a.

Common carotid a.

Sympathetic trunk

Middle cervical ganglion

Longus colli m.

Vagus n. (X)

Sup. deep cervical
lymph nodes

Internal jugular v.

Body of 5th cervical
vertebra

Sternocleido-
mastoid m.

Ascending cervical a.

Phrenic n.

Vertebral a.

Ant. scalene m.

External jugular v.

Middle scalene m.

Spinal n. (C5)

Multifidus cervicis m.

Subarachnoid space

Semispinalis capitis m.

Epidural space;
Int. vertebral
venous plexus

Splenius cervicis and capitis m.

Periosteum

Levator scapulae m.

Spinal dural mater

Trapezius m.

Spinalis m.

Spinal medulla

Spinous proc. of 4th
cervical vertebra

Fig. 278   The neck. Transverse section at the level
of the rima glottidis, viewed from above. Note the
central position of the spinal canal in the middle of
the neck.

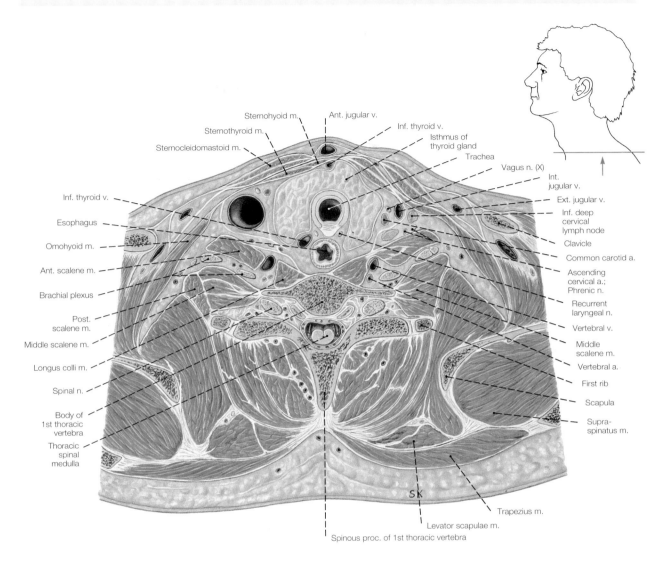

Sternohyoid m.

Ant. jugular v.

Sternothyroid m.

Inf. thyroid v.

Sternocleidomastoid m.

Isthmus of thyroid gland

Trachea

Vagus n. (X)

Int. jugular v.

Inf. thyroid v.

Esophagus

Ext. jugular v.

Inf. deep cervical lymph node

Omohyoid m.

Clavicle

Ant. scalene m.

Common carotid a.

Brachial plexus

Ascending cervical a.; Phrenic n.

Recurrent laryngeal n.

Post. scalene m.

Vertebral v.

Middle scalene m.

Middle scalene m.

Longus colli m.

Vertebral a.

Spinal n.

First rib

Body of 1st thoracic vertebra

Scapula

Thoracic spinal medulla

Supra- spinatus m.

Trapezius m.

Levator scapulae m.

Spinous proc. of 1st thoracic vertebra

Fig. 279 The neck. Transverse section at the level of the first thoracic vertebra in an elderly person, viewed from below (80%).

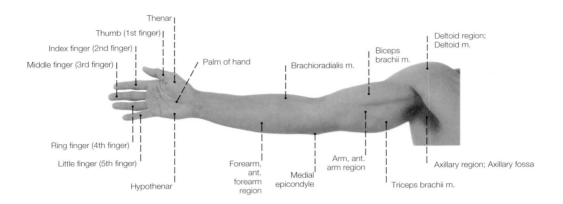

Thenar

Thumb (1st finger)

Index finger (2nd finger)

Middle finger (3rd finger)

Palm of hand

Brachioradialis m.

Biceps brachii m.

Deltoid region; Deltoid m.

Ring finger (4th finger)

Little finger (5th finger)

Forearm, ant. forearm region

Medial epicondyle

Arm, ant. arm region

Axillary region; Axillary fossa

Hypothenar

Triceps brachii m.

Fig. 280　The arm. Surface anatomy, anterior view of the right arm (10%).

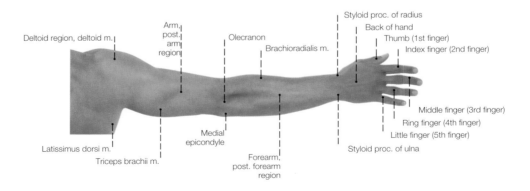

Deltoid region, deltoid m.

Arm, post. arm region

Olecranon

Brachioradialis m.

Styloid proc. of radius

Back of hand

Thumb (1st finger)

Index finger (2nd finger)

Middle finger (3rd finger)

Ring finger (4th finger)

Little finger (5th finger)

Latissimus dorsi m.

Medial epicondyle

Forearm, post. forearm region

Styloid proc. of ulna

Triceps brachii m.

Fig. 281　The arm. Surface anatomy, posterior view of the right arm (10%).

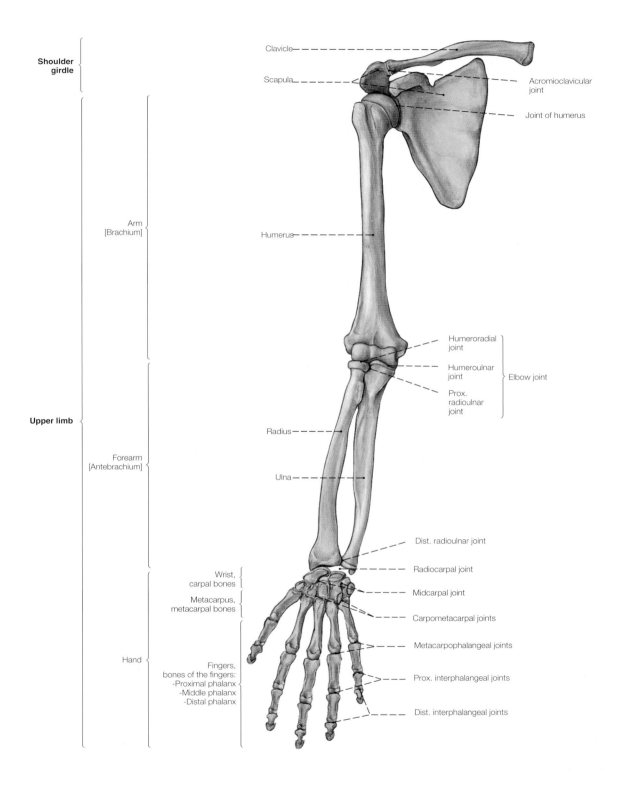

Shoulder girdle

Upper limb

Arm [Brachium]

Forearm [Antebrachium]

Hand

Clavicle

Scapula

Acromioclavicular joint

Joint of humerus

Humerus

Humeroradial joint

Humeroulnar joint

Prox. radioulnar joint

Elbow joint

Radius

Ulna

Dist. radioulnar joint

Radiocarpal joint

Wrist, carpal bones

Metacarpus, metacarpal bones

Fingers, bones of the fingers:
-Proximal phalanx
-Middle phalanx
-Distal phalanx

Midcarpal joint

Carpometacarpal joints

Metacarpophalangeal joints

Prox. interphalangeal joints

Dist. interphalangeal joints

Fig. 282 The right upper limb. Schema of the skeleton and joints, anterior view (25%).

Articulations of the Upper Limb (Fig. 282)
Articulations of the Shoulder Girdle

Joint	Type of Joint	Movement
Sternoclavicular joint	Double gliding; special feature: articular disc	Rotation on axis through articular facet (elevation, depression of shoulder); rotation on vertical axis of sternum (protraction, retraction of shoulder); rotation of clavicle on articular disc (circumduction of arm)
Acromioclavicular joint	Plane or gliding	Gliding motion of articular end of clavicle on acromion; rotation of scapula forward and backward on clavicle

Articulations of the Free Upper Limb

Joint	Type of Joint	Movement		
Shoulder joint	Ball-and-socket	Flexion (protraction) Extension (retraction) Abduction Adduction Medial rotation Lateral rotation Circumduction (combining flexion, extension, abduction, adduction)		
Elbow joint a) Humeroulnar joint	Hinge	Flexion Extension		
b) Humeroradial joint	Ball-and-socket (functionally restricted)	Flexion Extension Rotation		
c) Proximal radioulnar joint	Pivot	Pronation Supination		
Distal radioulnar joint	Pivot			
Carpal joints a) Radiocarpal joint	Ellipsoid	Flexion, Extension Abduction, Adduction Circumduction		
b) Midcarpal joint	Compound: saddle, gliding	Flexion, Extension Abduction Rotation		
Carpometacarpal joints of the medial four fingers	Plane or gliding	Various distinct movements		
Carpometacarpal joint of the thumb	Saddle	Flexion Extension	Abduction Adduction	Opposition Rotation Circumduction
Metacarpophalangeal joints	Ball-and-socket (functionally restricted)	Flexion Extension (*with respect to the middle finger)	Abduction* Adduction*	Circumduction
Interphalangeal joints	Hinge	Flexion Extension		

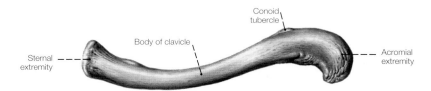

Fig. 283 The left clavicle, viewed from above (50%).

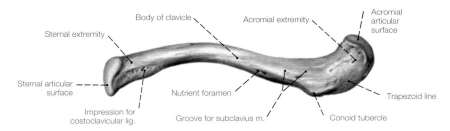

Fig. 284 The left clavicle, viewed from below (50%).

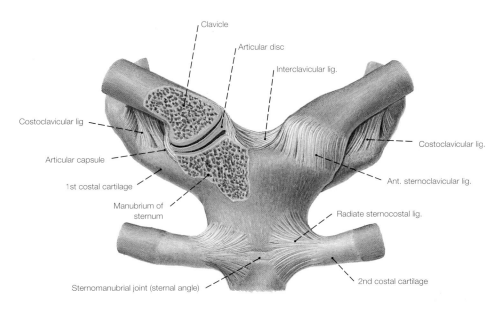

Fig. 285 The sternoclavicular joint, anterior view (70%). The right joint has been opened by a frontal cut.

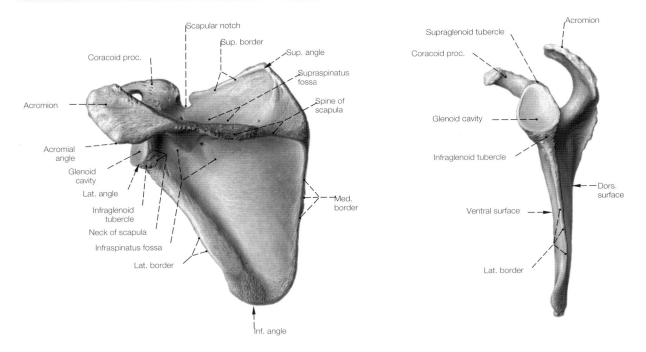

Fig. 286 The left scapula, posterior view (35%).

Fig. 287 The left scapula, lateral view (40%).

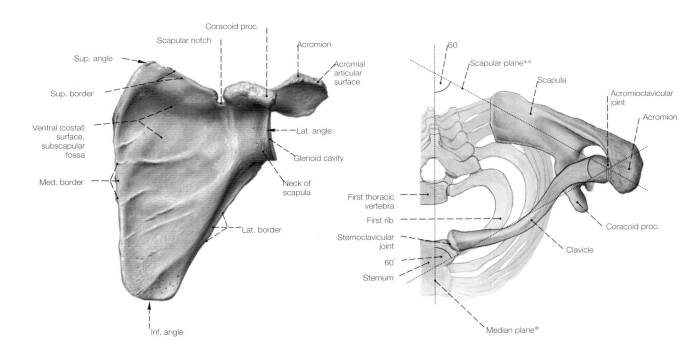

Fig. 288 The left scapula, anterior view (35%).

Fig. 289 The left shoulder girdle, cranial view. The angles refer to the average relations in the adult.

* Median plane
** Scapular plane

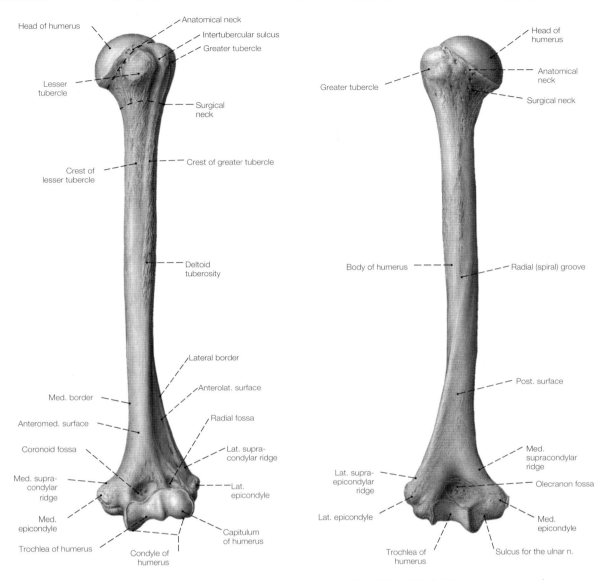

Head of humerus

Anatomical neck

Intertubercular sulcus

Greater tubercle

Lesser tubercle

Surgical neck

Crest of lesser tubercle

Crest of greater tubercle

Deltoid tuberosity

Lateral border

Anterolat. surface

Med. border

Anteromed. surface

Radial fossa

Coronoid fossa

Lat. supra- condylar ridge

Med. supra- condylar ridge

Lat. epicondyle

Med. epicondyle

Trochlea of humerus

Condyle of humerus

Capitulum of humerus

Fig. 290 The left humerus, anterior view (45%).

Head of humerus

Anatomical neck

Surgical neck

Greater tubercle

Body of humerus

Radial (spiral) groove

Post. surface

Med. supracondylar ridge

Lat. supra- epicondylar ridge

Olecranon fossa

Lat. epicondyle

Med. epicondyle

Trochlea of humerus

Sulcus for the ulnar n.

Fig. 291 The left humerus, posterior view (45%).

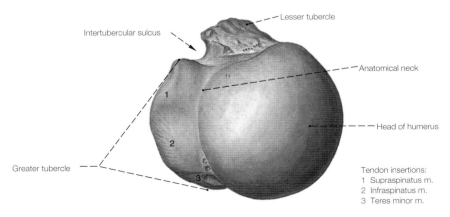

Intertubercular sulcus

Lesser tubercle

Anatomical neck

Head of humerus

Greater tubercle

1

2

3

Tendon insertions:
1 Supraspinatus m.
2 Infraspinatus m.
3 Teres minor m.

Fig. 292 The left humerus, view of the proximal end (100%).

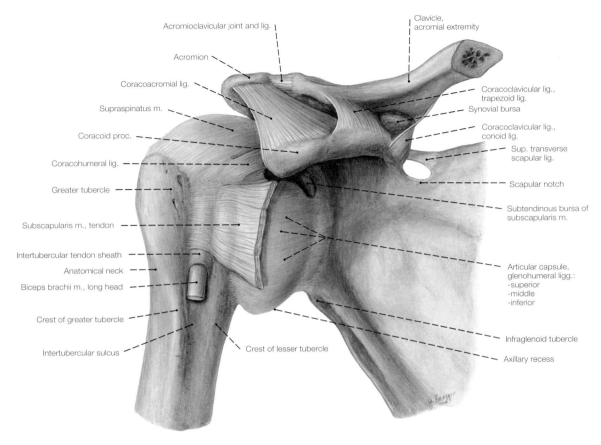

Acromioclavicular joint and lig.

Acromion

Coracoacromial lig.

Supraspinatus m.

Coracoid proc.

Coracohumeral lig.

Greater tubercle

Subscapularis m., tendon

Intertubercular tendon sheath

Anatomical neck

Biceps brachii m., long head

Crest of greater tubercle

Intertubercular sulcus

Crest of lesser tubercle

Clavicle, acromial extremity

Coracoclavicular lig., trapezoid lig.

Synovial bursa

Coracoclavicular lig., conoid lig.

Sup. transverse scapular lig.

Scapular notch

Subtendinous bursa of subscapularis m.

Articular capsule, glenohumeral ligg.:
-superior
-middle
-inferior

Infraglenoid tubercle

Axillary recess

Fig. 293   The left shoulder joint, anterior view (85%).

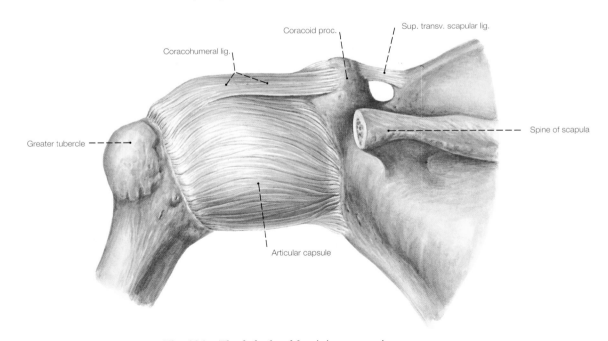

Coracohumeral lig.

Coracoid proc.

Sup. transv. scapular lig.

Greater tubercle

Spine of scapula

Articular capsule

Fig. 294   The left shoulder joint, posterior view (85%). The acromion has been removed.

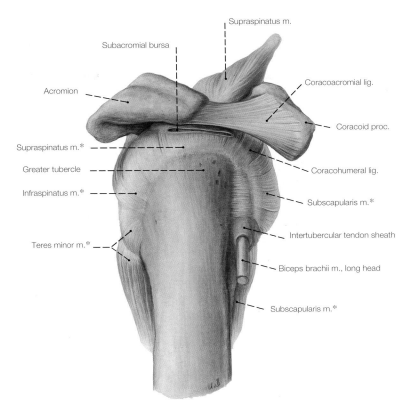

Supraspinatus m.

Subacromial bursa

Coracoacromial lig.

Acromion

Coracoid proc.

Supraspinatus m.*

Greater tubercle

Coracohumeral lig.

Infraspinatus m.*

Subscapularis m.*

Teres minor m.*

Intertubercular tendon sheath

Biceps brachii m., long head

Subscapularis m.*

Fig. 295 The right shoulder joint, lateral view (70%). The deltoid muscle has been removed.

The muscle tendons marked with asterisks (*) together form the rotator cuff.

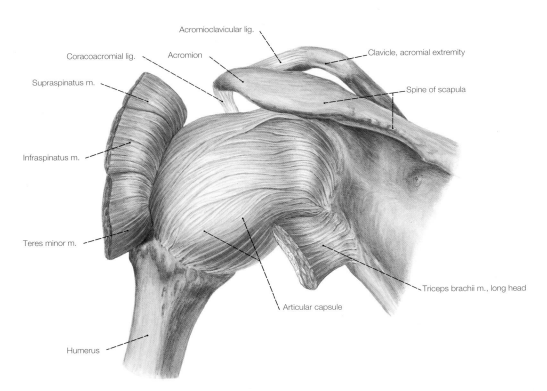

Acromioclavicular lig.

Coracoacromial lig.

Acromion

Clavicle, acromial extremity

Supraspinatus m.

Spine of scapula

Infraspinatus m.

Teres minor m.

Triceps brachii m., long head

Articular capsule

Humerus

Fig. 296 The left shoulder joint, posterior view (80%).

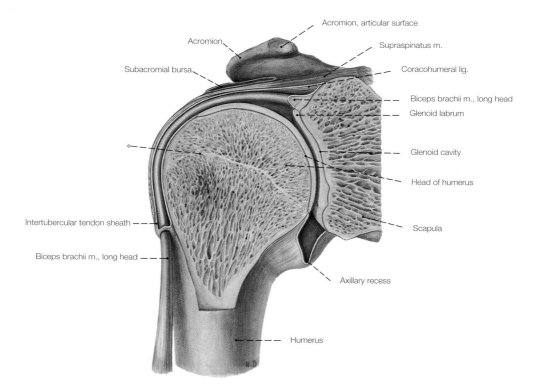

Fig. 297   The right shoulder joint, sectioned in the scapular plane, anterior view (80%).

* Ossified epiphyseal plate

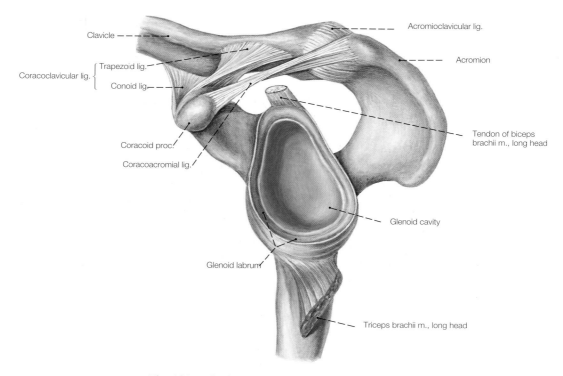

Fig. 298   The left shoulder joint, lateral view (80%). The articular capsule has been separated at the glenoid labrum and the head of the humerus removed.

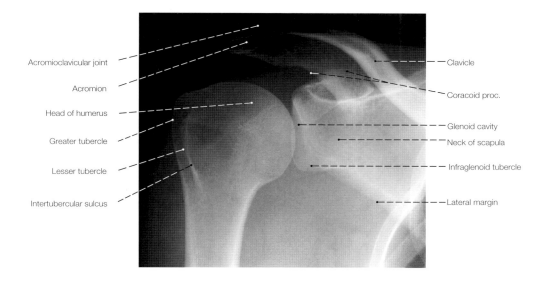

Acromioclavicular joint

Acromion

Head of humerus

Greater tubercle

Lesser tubercle

Intertubercular sulcus

Clavicle

Coracoid proc.

Glenoid cavity

Neck of scapula

Infraglenoid tubercle

Lateral margin

Fig. 299 The right shoulder joint, anterior view. AP radiograph with the subject in the upright position, arm hanging loose, and scapula nearly parallel to the plane of the film (the joint is in the neutral position with reference to all three major planes of movement).

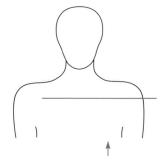

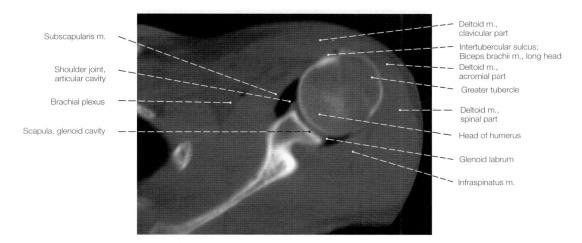

Subscapularis m.

Shoulder joint, articular cavity

Brachial plexus

Scapula, glenoid cavity

Deltoid m., clavicular part

Intertubercular sulcus; Biceps brachii m., long head

Deltoid m., acromial part

Greater tubercle

Deltoid m., spinal part

Head of humerus

Glenoid labrum

Infraspinatus m.

Fig. 300 The left shoulder joint, viewed from below. Computer tomographic (CT) cross section at the level of the center of curvature of the head of the humerus, with the arm in the midposition and the joint cavity filled with air (pneumo-CT).

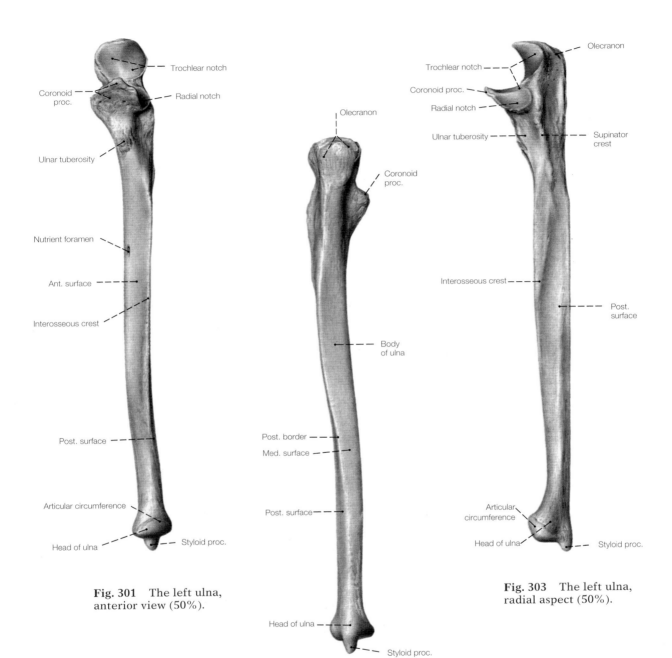

Coronoid proc.

Trochlear notch

Radial notch

Ulnar tuberosity

Nutrient foramen

Ant. surface

Interosseous crest

Post. surface

Articular circumference

Head of ulna

Styloid proc.

Fig. 301 The left ulna, anterior view (50%).

Olecranon

Coronoid proc.

Body of ulna

Post. border

Med. surface

Post. surface

Head of ulna

Styloid proc.

Fig. 302 The left ulna, posterior view (50%).

Trochlear notch

Olecranon

Coronoid proc.

Radial notch

Ulnar tuberosity

Supinator crest

Interosseous crest

Post. surface

Articular circumference

Head of ulna

Styloid proc.

Fig. 303 The left ulna, radial aspect (50%).

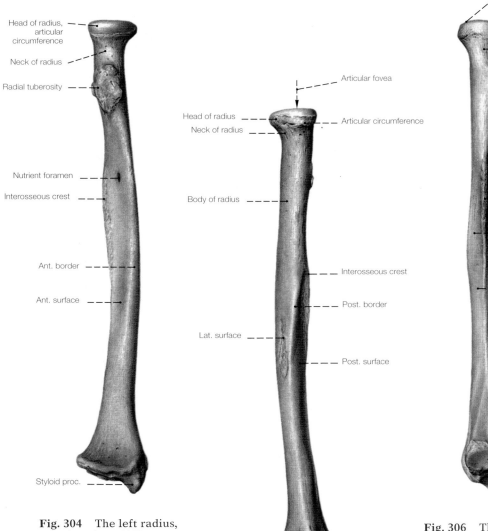

Head of radius,
articular
circumference

Neck of radius

Radial tuberosity

Nutrient foramen

Interosseous crest

Ant. border

Ant. surface

Styloid proc.

Fig. 304 The left radius,
anterior view (50%).

Articular fovea

Head of radius

Neck of radius

Articular circumference

Body of radius

Interosseous crest

Post. border

Lat. surface

Post. surface

*

Dors. tubercle

Styloid proc.

Fig. 305 The left radius,
posterior view (50%).

* Grooves and crests for the
attachment of the extensor
tendons

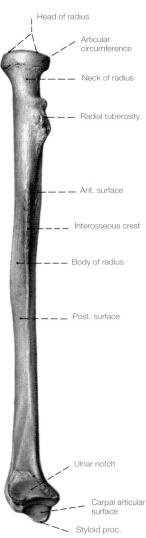

Head of radius

Articular
circumference

Neck of radius

Radial tuberosity

Ant. surface

Interosseous crest

Body of radius

Post. surface

Ulnar notch

Carpal articular
surface

Styloid proc.

Fig. 306 The left radius,
ulnar aspect (50%).

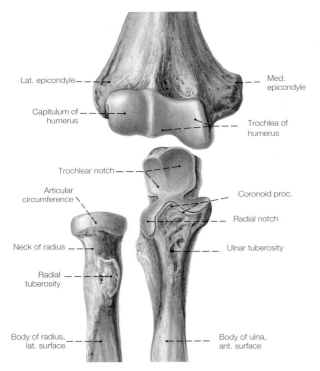

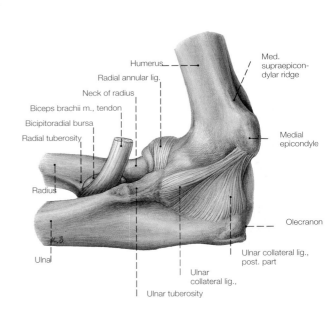

Fig. 307   The right elbow joint, anterior view (55%). The joint has been disarticulated for didactic purposes.

Fig. 308   The right elbow joint in 90° flexion and 90° supination, medial view (55%).

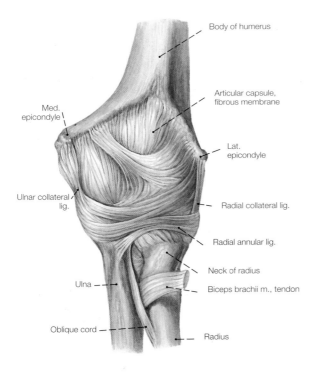

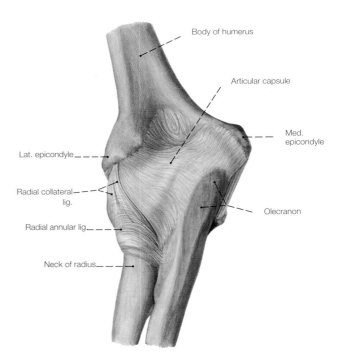

Fig. 309   The left elbow joint, anterior view (55%).

Fig. 310   The left elbow joint, posterior view (55%).

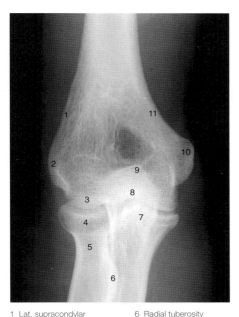

1 Lat. supracondylar ridge
2 Lat. epicondyle
3 Capitulum of humerus
4 Head of radius
5 Neck of radius
6 Radial tuberosity
7 Coronoid proc.
8 Trochlea of humerus
9 Olecranon
10 Med. epicondyle
11 Med. supracondylar ridge

Fig. 311 The elbow joint, AP radiograph.

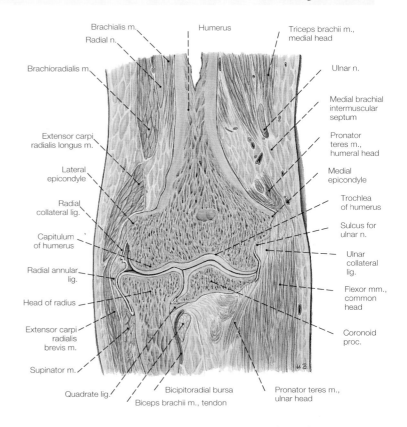

Fig. 312 The right elbow joint, frontal section, anterior view (55%).

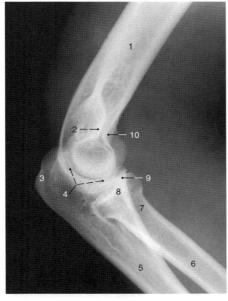

1 Humerus
2 Olecranon fossa
3 Olecranon
4 Trochlear notch
5 Ulna
6 Radius
7 Neck of radius
8 Head of radius
9 Coronoid proc.
10 Coronoid fossa

Fig. 313 The elbow joint, lateral radiograph.

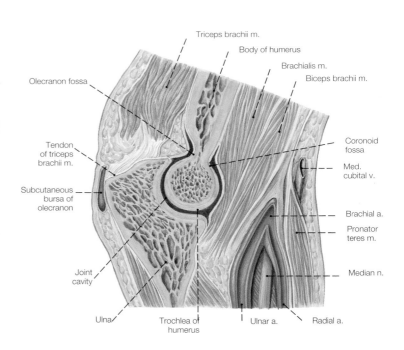

Fig. 314 The left elbow joint, sagittal section, medial view (60%).

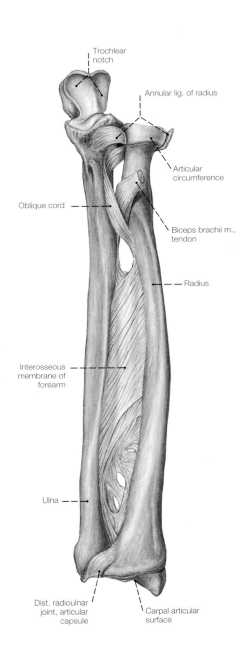

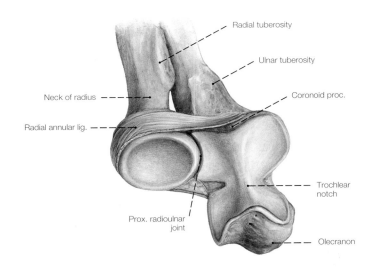

Fig. 315 Ligaments of the bones of the left forearm, anterior view (50%). The annular ligament has been cut.

Fig. 316 The right proximal radioulnar joint, anterior view of the proximal end (85%).

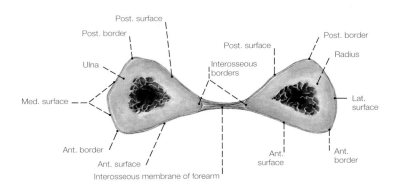

Fig. 317 Cross section through the bones of the left forearm, viewed from the distal end (115%).

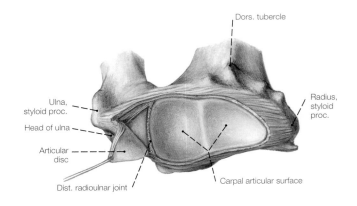

Fig. 318 The left distal radioulnar joint, posterior view of the distal end (85%). The articular disc has been separated from the radius and reflected toward the ulnar side.

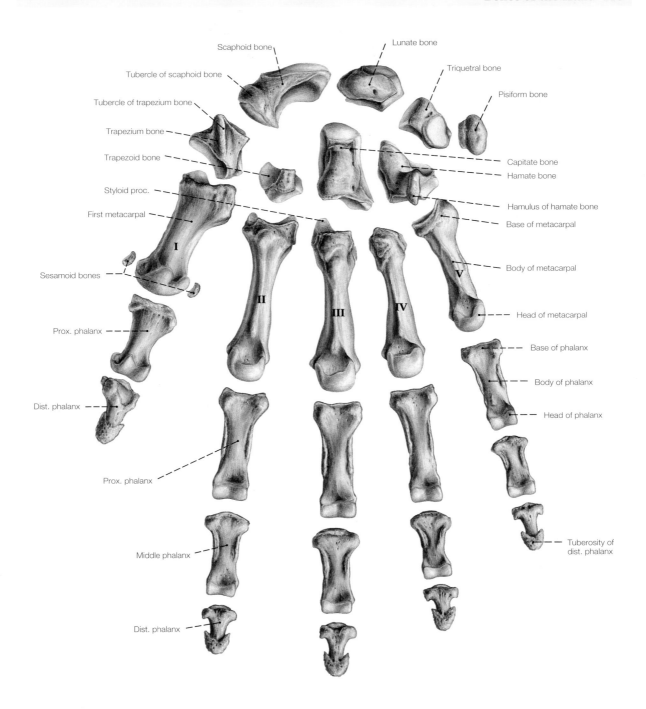

Scaphoid bone

Tubercle of scaphoid bone

Tubercle of trapezium bone

Trapezium bone

Trapezoid bone

Styloid proc.

First metacarpal

Sesamoid bones

Prox. phalanx

Dist. phalanx

Prox. phalanx

Middle phalanx

Dist. phalanx

Lunate bone

Triquetral bone

Pisiform bone

Capitate bone

Hamate bone

Hamulus of hamate bone

Base of metacarpal

Body of metacarpal

Head of metacarpal

Base of phalanx

Body of phalanx

Head of phalanx

Tuberosity of dist. phalanx

I   First finger (thumb)
II Second finger (index finger)
III Third finger (middle finger)
IV Fourth finger (ring finger)
V   Fifth finger (little finger)

Fig. 319   The bones of the right hand, palmar view (70%). The bones have been disarticulated for didactic purposes.

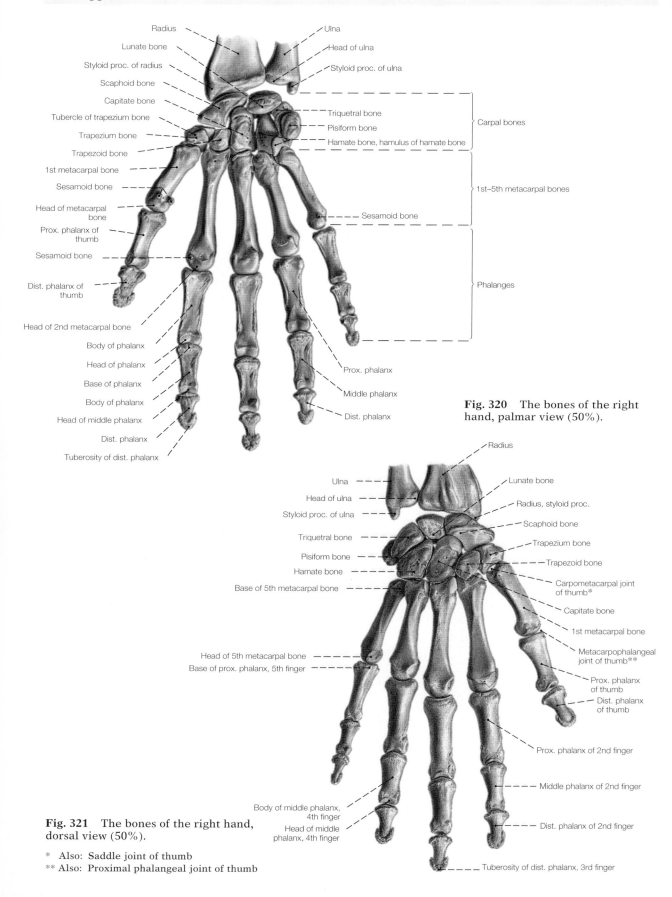

Radius
Lunate bone
Styloid proc. of radius
Scaphoid bone
Capitate bone
Tubercle of trapezium bone
Trapezium bone
Trapezoid bone
1st metacarpal bone
Sesamoid bone
Head of metacarpal bone
Prox. phalanx of thumb
Sesamoid bone
Dist. phalanx of thumb
Head of 2nd metacarpal bone
Body of phalanx
Head of phalanx
Base of phalanx
Body of phalanx
Head of middle phalanx
Dist. phalanx
Tuberosity of dist. phalanx

Ulna
Head of ulna
Styloid proc. of ulna

Triquetral bone
Pisiform bone
Hamate bone, hamulus of hamate bone

Sesamoid bone

Prox. phalanx
Middle phalanx
Dist. phalanx

Carpal bones
1st–5th metacarpal bones
Phalanges

Fig. 320   The bones of the right hand, palmar view (50%).

Radius
Ulna
Head of ulna
Styloid proc. of ulna
Triquetral bone
Pisiform bone
Hamate bone
Base of 5th metacarpal bone

Lunate bone
Radius, styloid proc.
Scaphoid bone
Trapezium bone
Trapezoid bone
Carpometacarpal joint of thumb*
Capitate bone
1st metacarpal bone
Metacarpophalangeal joint of thumb**
Prox. phalanx of thumb
Dist. phalanx of thumb

Head of 5th metacarpal bone
Base of prox. phalanx, 5th finger

Prox. phalanx of 2nd finger

Middle phalanx of 2nd finger

Dist. phalanx of 2nd finger

Body of middle phalanx, 4th finger
Head of middle phalanx, 4th finger

Tuberosity of dist. phalanx, 3rd finger

Fig. 321   The bones of the right hand, dorsal view (50%).

*   Also: Saddle joint of thumb
** Also: Proximal phalangeal joint of thumb

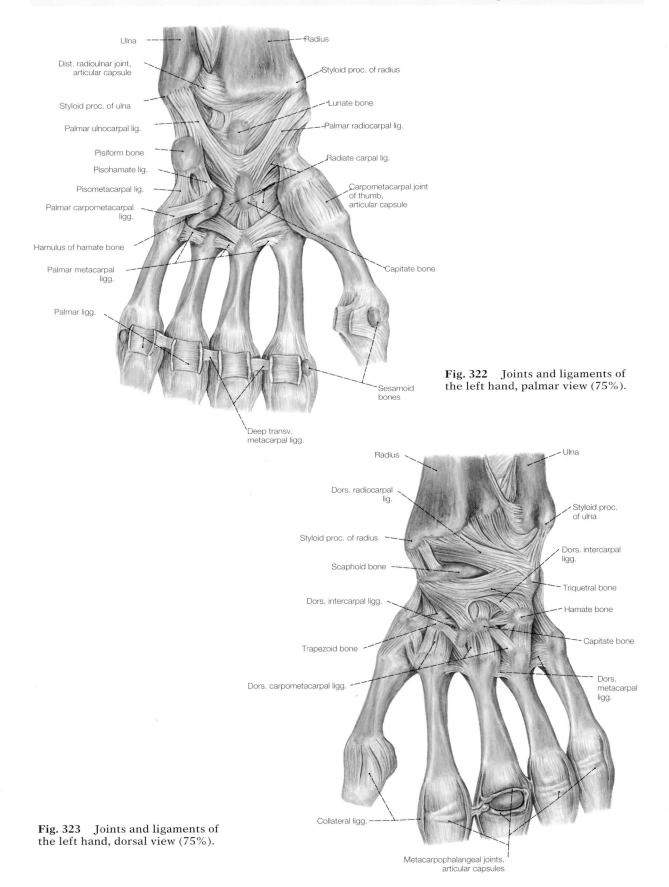

Ulna

Dist. radioulnar joint,
articular capsule

Styloid proc. of ulna

Palmar ulnocarpal lig.

Pisiform bone

Pisohamate lig.

Pisometacarpal lig.

Palmar carpometacarpal
ligg.

Hamulus of hamate bone

Palmar metacarpal
ligg.

Palmar ligg.

Radius

Styloid proc. of radius

Lunate bone

Palmar radiocarpal lig.

Radiate carpal lig.

Carpometacarpal joint
of thumb,
articular capsule

Capitate bone

Sesamoid
bones

Deep transv.
metacarpal ligg.

Fig. 322 Joints and ligaments of
the left hand, palmar view (75%).

Radius

Dors. radiocarpal
lig.

Styloid proc. of radius

Scaphoid bone

Dors. intercarpal ligg.

Trapezoid bone

Dors. carpometacarpal ligg.

Collateral ligg.

Ulna

Styloid proc.
of ulna

Dors. intercarpal
ligg.

Triquetral bone

Hamate bone

Capitate bone

Dors.
metacarpal
ligg.

Metacarpophalangeal joints,
articular capsules

Fig. 323 Joints and ligaments of
the left hand, dorsal view (75%).

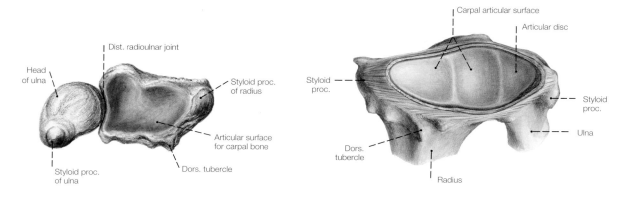

Dist. radioulnar joint

Head
of ulna

Styloid proc.
of radius

Styloid proc.
of ulna

Articular surface
for carpal bone

Dors. tubercle

Fig. 324 The left radius and ulna, view of the
distal ends (75%).

Carpal articular surface

Articular disc

Styloid
proc.

Styloid
proc.

Ulna

Dors.
tubercle

Radius

Fig. 325 The right proximal radiocarpal joint,
view of the distal end (85%).

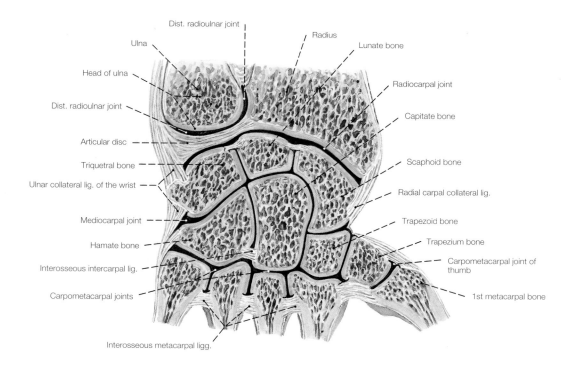

Dist. radioulnar joint

Ulna

Radius

Lunate bone

Head of ulna

Radiocarpal joint

Dist. radioulnar joint

Capitate bone

Articular disc

Scaphoid bone

Triquetral bone

Ulnar collateral lig. of the wrist

Radial carpal collateral lig.

Mediocarpal joint

Trapezoid bone

Hamate bone

Trapezium bone

Interosseous intercarpal lig.

Carpometacarpal joint of
thumb

Carpometacarpal joints

1st metacarpal bone

Interosseous metacarpal ligg.

Fig. 326 The joints of the wrist in a longitudinal
section parallel to the dorsum of the hand.

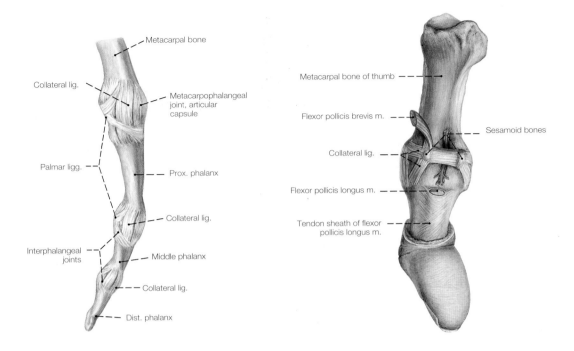

Fig. 327 labels: Metacarpal bone; Collateral lig.; Metacarpophalangeal joint, articular capsule; Palmar ligg.; Prox. phalanx; Collateral lig.; Interphalangeal joints; Middle phalanx; Collateral lig.; Dist. phalanx

Fig. 328 labels: Metacarpal bone of thumb; Flexor pollicis brevis m.; Sesamoid bones; Collateral lig.; Flexor pollicis longus m.; Tendon sheath of flexor pollicis longus m.

Fig. 327 The finger joints, lateral view.

Fig. 328 The metacarpophalangeal joint of the right thumb, radial palmar view. The radial and ulnar collateral ligaments are integrated by a transverse ligament between the sesamoid bones, forming a bracing system that limits extension at the joint.

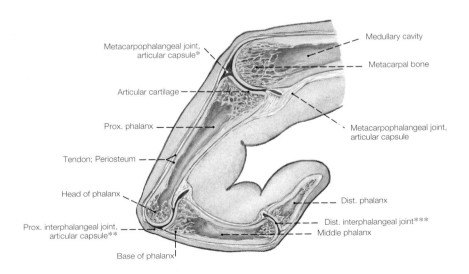

Fig. 329 labels: Metacarpophalangeal joint, articular capsule*; Medullary cavity; Metacarpal bone; Articular cartilage; Prox. phalanx; Metacarpophalangeal joint, articular capsule; Tendon; Periosteum; Head of phalanx; Dist. phalanx; Prox. interphalangeal joint, articular capsule**; Dist. interphalangeal joint***; Middle phalanx; Base of phalanx

Fig. 329 The finger joints, sagittal section, lateral view. Note the position of the flexion creases in relation to the corresponding joints.

* Clinically: **MP** (= **m**etacar**p**ophalangeal joint)
** Clinically: **PIP** (= **p**roximal **i**nter**p**halangeal joint)
*** Clinically: **DIP** (= **d**istal **i**nter**p**halangeal joint)

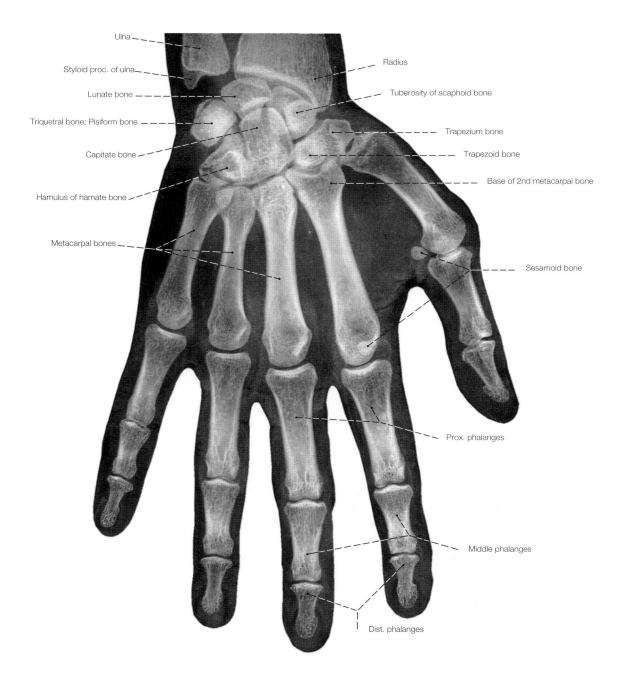

Ulna

Styloid proc. of ulna

Lunate bone

Triquetral bone; Pisiform bone

Capitate bone

Hamulus of hamate bone

Metacarpal bones

Radius

Tuberosity of scaphoid bone

Trapezium bone

Trapezoid bone

Base of 2nd metacarpal bone

Sesamoid bone

Prox. phalanges

Middle phalanges

Dist. phalanges

Fig. 330   The hand, PA radiograph.
Note: The pisiform bone is projected onto
the triquetral bone.

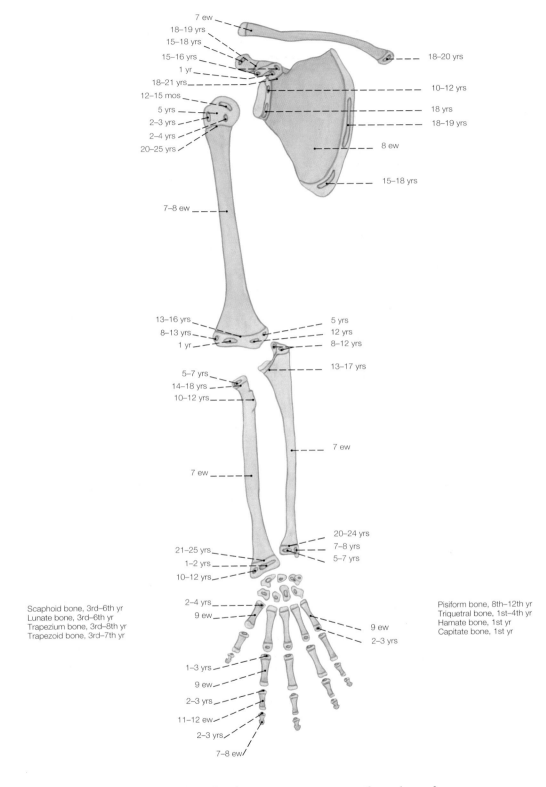

7 ew
18–19 yrs
15–18 yrs
15–16 yrs
1 yr
18–21 yrs
12–15 mos
5 yrs
2–3 yrs
2–4 yrs
20–25 yrs

18–20 yrs
10–12 yrs
18 yrs
18–19 yrs
8 ew
15–18 yrs

7–8 ew

13–16 yrs
8–13 yrs
1 yr

5 yrs
12 yrs
8–12 yrs

13–17 yrs

5–7 yrs
14–18 yrs
10–12 yrs

7 ew

7 ew

20–24 yrs
7–8 yrs
5–7 yrs

21–25 yrs
1–2 yrs
10–12 yrs

Scaphoid bone, 3rd–6th yr
Lunate bone, 3rd–6th yr
Trapezium bone, 3rd–8th yr
Trapezoid bone, 3rd–7th yr

2–4 yrs
9 ew

9 ew
2–3 yrs

Pisiform bone, 8th–12th yr
Triquetral bone, 1st–4th yr
Hamate bone, 1st yr
Capitate bone, 1st yr

1–3 yrs
9 ew
2–3 yrs
11–12 ew
2–3 yrs

7–8 ew

Fig. 331 Appearance of endochondral ossification centers and the ossification of the epiphyseal plates of the upper limb (average ages according to LANZ, 1956).

ew = embryonic week
mos = age in months
yrs = age in years

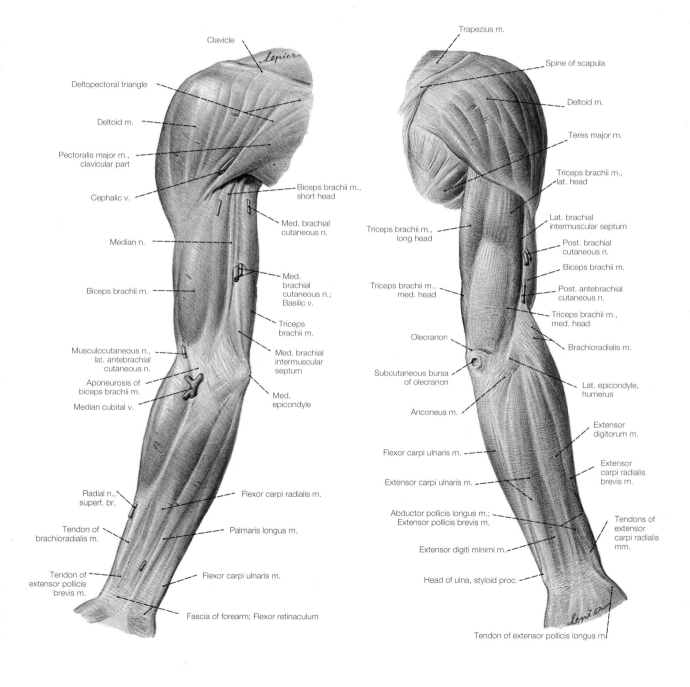

Clavicle

Deltopectoral triangle

Deltoid m.

Pectoralis major m., clavicular part

Cephalic v.

Median n.

Biceps brachii m.

Musculocutaneous n., lat. antebrachial cutaneous n.

Aponeurosis of biceps brachii m.

Median cubital v.

Radial n., superf. br.

Tendon of brachioradialis m.

Tendon of extensor pollicis brevis m.

Biceps brachii m., short head

Med. brachial cutaneous n.

Med. brachial cutaneous n.; Basilic v.

Triceps brachii m.

Med. brachial intermuscular septum

Med. epicondyle

Flexor carpi radialis m.

Palmaris longus m.

Flexor carpi ulnaris m.

Fascia of forearm; Flexor retinaculum

Trapezius m.

Spine of scapula

Deltoid m.

Teres major m.

Triceps brachii m., lat. head

Triceps brachii m., long head

Lat. brachial intermuscular septum

Post. brachial cutaneous n.

Biceps brachii m.

Post. antebrachial cutaneous n.

Triceps brachii m., med. head

Triceps brachii m., med. head

Brachioradialis m.

Olecranon

Subcutaneous bursa of olecranon

Anconeus m.

Flexor carpi ulnaris m.

Extensor carpi ulnaris m.

Abductor pollicis longus m.; Extensor pollicis brevis m.

Extensor digiti minimi m.

Head of ulna, styloid proc.

Lat. epicondyle, humerus

Extensor digitorum m.

Extensor carpi radialis brevis m.

Tendons of extensor carpi radialis mm.

Tendon of extensor pollicis longus m.

Fig. 332 The fascia of the flexor aspect of the right upper limb (25%).

Fig. 333 The fascia of the extensor aspect of the right upper limb (25%).

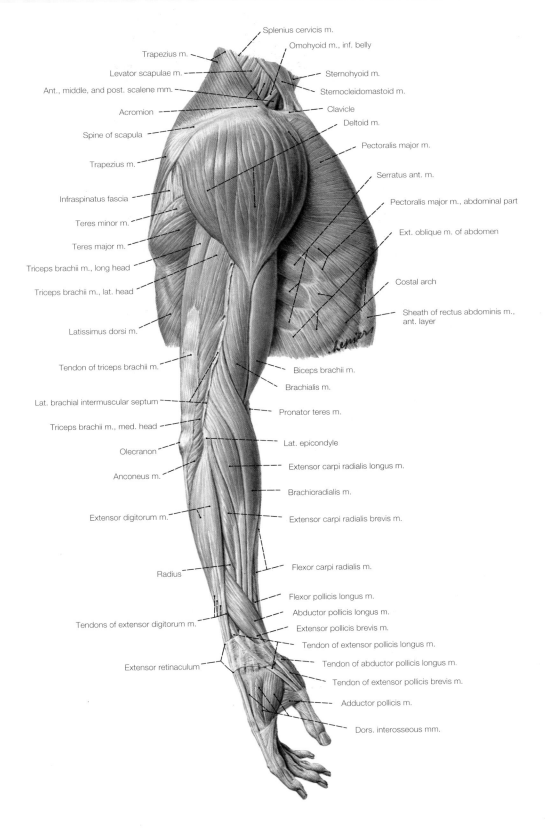

Splenius cervicis m.
Omohyoid m., inf. belly
Trapezius m.
Levator scapulae m.
Sternohyoid m.
Ant., middle, and post. scalene mm.
Sternocleidomastoid m.
Acromion
Clavicle
Spine of scapula
Deltoid m.
Pectoralis major m.
Trapezius m.
Serratus ant. m.
Infraspinatus fascia
Pectoralis major m., abdominal part
Teres minor m.
Ext. oblique m. of abdomen
Teres major m.
Triceps brachii m., long head
Triceps brachii m., lat. head
Costal arch
Latissimus dorsi m.
Sheath of rectus abdominis m., ant. layer
Tendon of triceps brachii m.
Biceps brachii m.
Brachialis m.
Lat. brachial intermuscular septum
Pronator teres m.
Triceps brachii m., med. head
Olecranon
Lat. epicondyle
Anconeus m.
Extensor carpi radialis longus m.
Brachioradialis m.
Extensor digitorum m.
Extensor carpi radialis brevis m.
Radius
Flexor carpi radialis m.
Flexor pollicis longus m.
Abductor pollicis longus m.
Tendons of extensor digitorum m.
Extensor pollicis brevis m.
Tendon of extensor pollicis longus m.
Extensor retinaculum
Tendon of abductor pollicis longus m.
Tendon of extensor pollicis brevis m.
Adductor pollicis m.
Dors. interosseous mm.

Fig. 334 Muscles of the right upper limb,
thorax and lower neck region,
lateral view (23%).

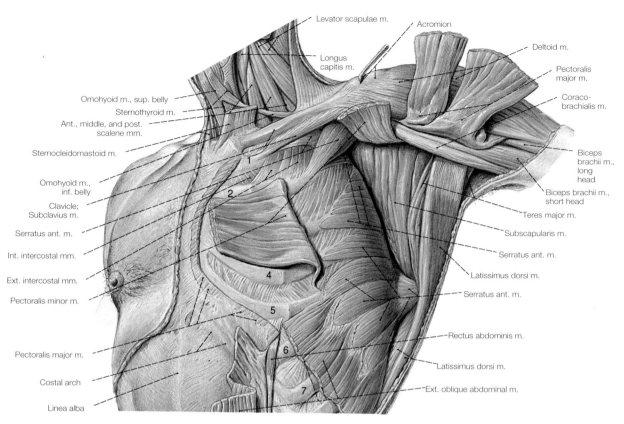

Fig. 335 Muscles of the left arm, thorax and lower neck region, anterolateral view (30%). The left shoulder has been retracted.

1, 2, 4–7 indicate the corresponding ribs.

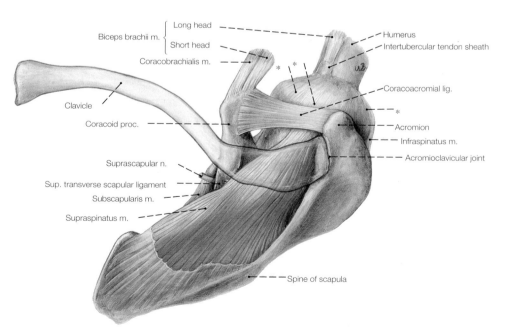

Fig. 336 The right shoulder and shoulder muscles, viewed from above (60%). The deltoid muscle has been removed and part of the clavicle has been made transparent.

The tendons marked with an asterisk (*) form the "rotator cuff" (compare with Fig. 295).

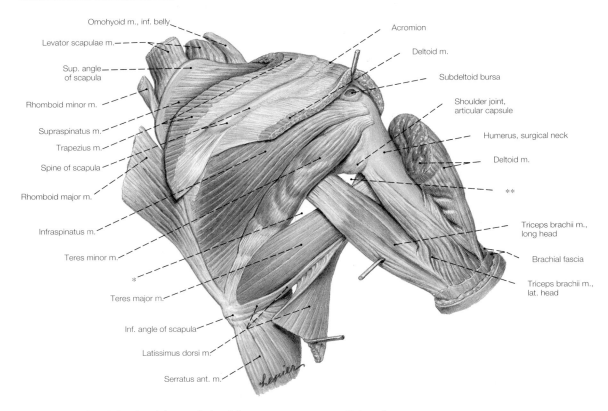

Coracoclavicular lig., conoid lig.
Deltoid m.
Articular capsule of acromioclavicular joint
Acromion
Coracoacromial lig.
Subacromial bursa
Coracoclavicular lig., trapezoid lig.
Coracoid proc.
Bursa of coracobrachialis m.; Coracobrachialis m.
Biceps brachii m., short head
Deltoid m.
Intertubercular tendon sheath
Pectoralis major m.
Pectoralis minor m.
Tendon of latissimus dorsi m.
Biceps brachii m., long head
Coracobrachialis m.
Biceps brachii m., short head
Triceps brachii m., lat. head
Triceps brachii m., long head

Clavicle
Trapezius m.
Subclavius m.
Sup. transv. scapular lig.
Omohyoid m., inf. belly
Levator scapulae m.
Serratus ant. m.
Rhomboid minor m.
Supraspinatus m.
Subscapularis m.
Rhomboid major m.
Med. border of scapula
Teres major m.
Serratus ant. m.
Articular capsule (axillary recess)

Fig. 337 The right shoulder and its muscles, anterior view (45%). Several of the superficial muscles have been removed.

* Triangular space
** Quadrangular space

Omohyoid m., inf. belly
Levator scapulae m.
Sup. angle of scapula
Rhomboid minor m.
Supraspinatus m.
Trapezius m.
Spine of scapula
Rhomboid major m.
Infraspinatus m.
Teres minor m.
Teres major m.
Inf. angle of scapula
Latissimus dorsi m.
Serratus ant. m.

Acromion
Deltoid m.
Subdeltoid bursa
Shoulder joint, articular capsule
Humerus, surgical neck
Deltoid m.
Triceps brachii m., long head
Brachial fascia
Triceps brachii m., lat. head

Fig. 338 The right shoulder and shoulder muscles, posterior view (45%).

* Triangular space
** Quadrangular space

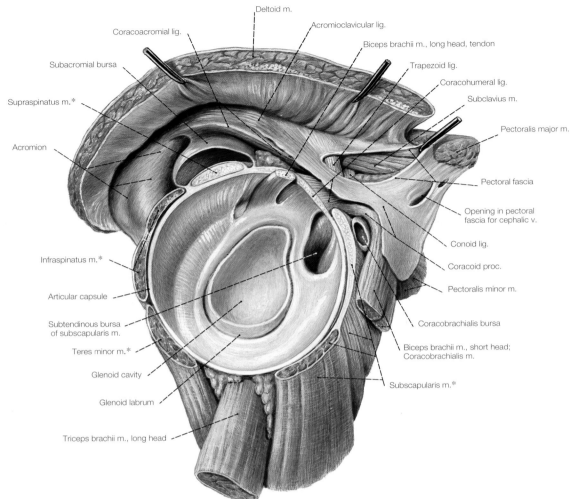

Coracoacromial lig.

Subacromial bursa

Supraspinatus m.*

Acromion

Infraspinatus m.*

Articular capsule

Subtendinous bursa
of subscapularis m.

Teres minor m.*

Glenoid cavity

Glenoid labrum

Triceps brachii m., long head

Deltoid m.

Acromioclavicular lig.

Biceps brachii m., long head, tendon

Trapezoid lig.

Coracohumeral lig.

Subclavius m.

Pectoralis major m.

Pectoral fascia

Opening in pectoral
fascia for cephalic v.

Conoid lig.

Coracoid proc.

Pectoralis minor m.

Coracobrachialis bursa

Biceps brachii m., short head;
Coracobrachialis m.

Subscapularis m.*

Fig. 339 The right shoulder joint, lateral view
after removal of the head of the humerus (90%).

The tendons of the muscles marked with an asterisk
(*) form the "rotator cuff."

Muscles of the Shoulder

Name *Innervation*	Origin	Insertion	Function
Deltoid muscle *Axillary n.* Clavicular part Acromial part Spinal part	Clavicular part: acromial third of clavicle; acromial part: acromion; spinal part: spine of scapula	Deltoid tuberosity (subdeltoid bursa between muscle and greater tubercle)	*Shoulder joint* Abduction of the arm, effected primarily by acromial part, with anterior and posterior fibers bracing the limb; clavicular part assists pectoralis major m. in flexing arm; spinal part assists latissimus dorsi m. in extending arm; all parts support the weight of the arm
Supraspinatus m. *Suprascapularis n.* from brachial plexus, supraclavicular part	Supraspinatus fossa	Proximal facet of the greater tubercle	*Shoulder joint* Abduction of the arm, lateral rotation of humerus; as part of rotator cuff holds head of humerus in glenoid cavity

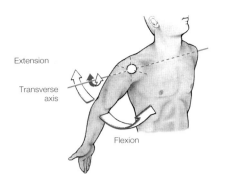

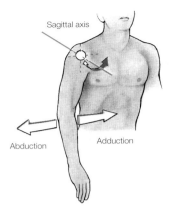

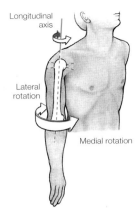

Fig. 340 Shoulder joint, movement in the sagittal plane.

Fig. 341 Shoulder joint, movement in the frontal plane.

Fig. 342 Shoulder joint, movement in the transverse plane.

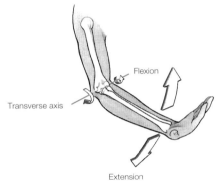

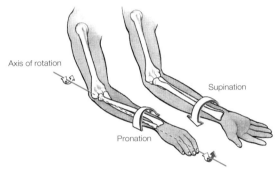

Fig. 343 Elbow joint, movement in the sagittal plane.

Fig. 344 Elbow joint, rotation movements of the hand.

Muscles of the Shoulder (continued)

Name *Innervation*	Origin	Insertion	Function
Infraspinatus m. *Suprascapular n.*	Caudal margin of the spine of the scapula, infraspinatus fossa	Middle facet of the greater tubercle	*Shoulder joint* Lateral rotation, of humerus; as part of rotator cuff holds head of humerus in glenoid cavity
Teres minor m. *Axillary n.*	Caudal section of the infraspinatus fossa and lateral border of the scapula (middle third)	Distal facet of the greater tubercle	*Shoulder joint* Lateral rotation and weak adduction of the arm; as part of rotator cuff draws humerus toward glenoid cavity
Teres major m. *Subscapular nn.* of the brachial plexus, infraclavicular part or *Thoracodorsal n.*	Lateral border and inferior angle of the scapula	Tendon on crest of lesser tubercle (humerus), dorsal to the latissimus dorsi m. (the 2 tendons separated by a subtendinous bursa)	*Shoulder joint* Adduction and extension of a flexed arm, medial rotation
Subscapularis m. *Subscapular nn.* of the brachial plexus, infraclavicular part	Costal fascia, subscapular fossa	Short, broad tendon into the lesser tubercle and its adjacent crest. Under the insertion is the subtendinous bursa of the subscapular m.	*Shoulder joint* Medial rotation of the adducted arm; as part of rotator cuff maintains head of humerus in glenoid cavity

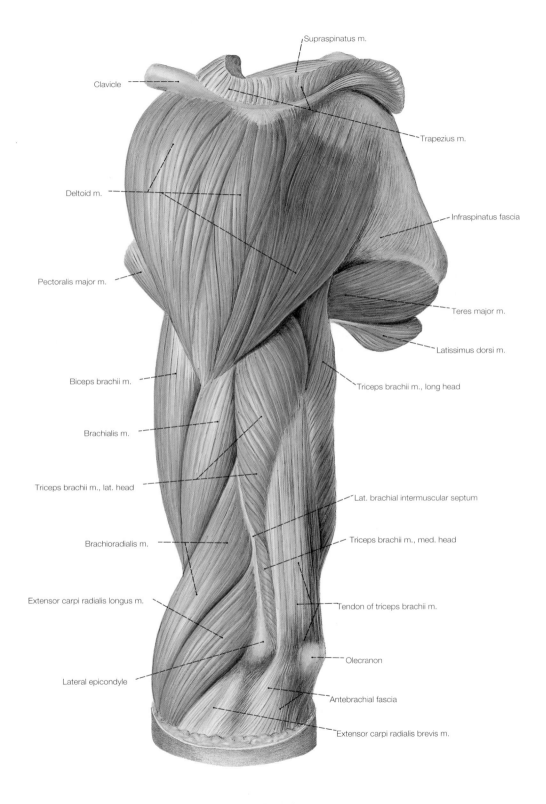

Supraspinatus m.

Clavicle

Trapezius m.

Deltoid m.

Infraspinatus fascia

Pectoralis major m.

Teres major m.

Latissimus dorsi m.

Biceps brachii m.

Triceps brachii m., long head

Brachialis m.

Triceps brachii m., lat. head

Lat. brachial intermuscular septum

Brachioradialis m.

Triceps brachii m., med. head

Extensor carpi radialis longus m.

Tendon of triceps brachii m.

Olecranon

Lateral epicondyle

Antebrachial fascia

Extensor carpi radialis brevis m.

Fig. 345 Muscles of the left arm,
posterolateral view (45%).

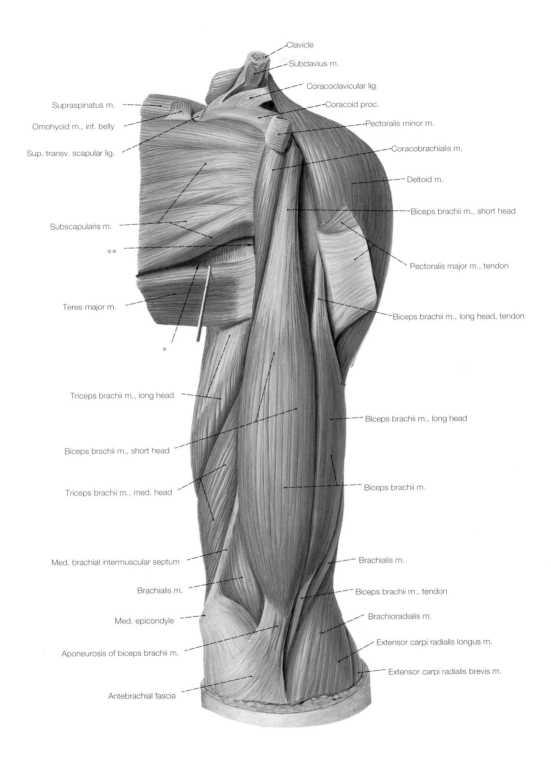

Clavicle

Subclavius m.

Coracoclavicular lig.

Coracoid proc.

Pectoralis minor m.

Coracobrachialis m.

Deltoid m.

Biceps brachii m., short head

Pectoralis major m., tendon

Biceps brachii m., long head, tendon

Biceps brachii m., long head

Biceps brachii m.

Brachialis m.

Biceps brachii m., tendon

Brachioradialis m.

Extensor carpi radialis longus m.

Extensor carpi radialis brevis m.

Supraspinatus m.

Omohyoid m., inf. belly

Sup. transv. scapular lig.

Subscapularis m.

**

Teres major m.

*

Triceps brachii m., long head

Biceps brachii m., short head

Triceps brachii m., med. head

Med. brachial intermuscular septum

Brachialis m.

Med. epicondyle

Aponeurosis of biceps brachii m.

Antebrachial fascia

Fig. 346 Muscles of the left arm, anterior view (40%).

* Triangular space
** Quadrangular space

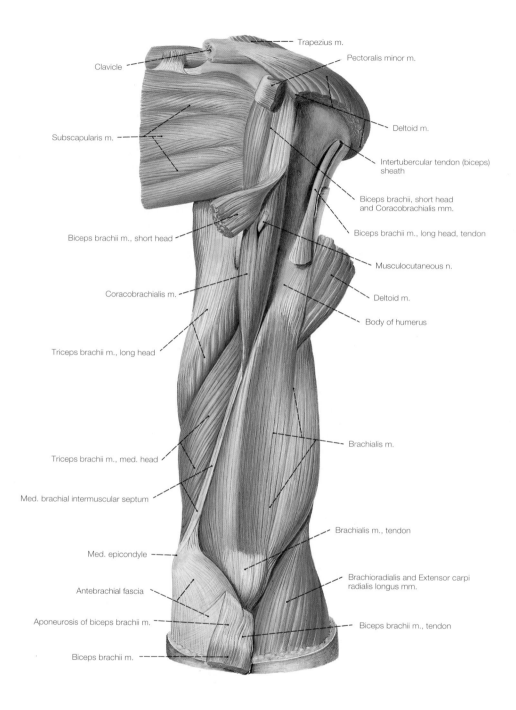

Trapezius m.

Pectoralis minor m.

Clavicle

Deltoid m.

Subscapularis m.

Intertubercular tendon (biceps) sheath

Biceps brachii, short head and Coracobrachialis mm.

Biceps brachii m., short head

Biceps brachii m., long head, tendon

Musculocutaneous n.

Coracobrachialis m.

Deltoid m.

Body of humerus

Triceps brachii m., long head

Brachialis m.

Triceps brachii m., med. head

Med. brachial intermuscular septum

Brachialis m., tendon

Med. epicondyle

Brachioradialis and Extensor carpi radialis longus mm.

Antebrachial fascia

Aponeurosis of biceps brachii m.

Biceps brachii m., tendon

Biceps brachii m.

Fig. 347 Muscles of the left arm, anterior view
(40%). The deep layer after partial removal of the
deltoid and biceps brachii muscles.

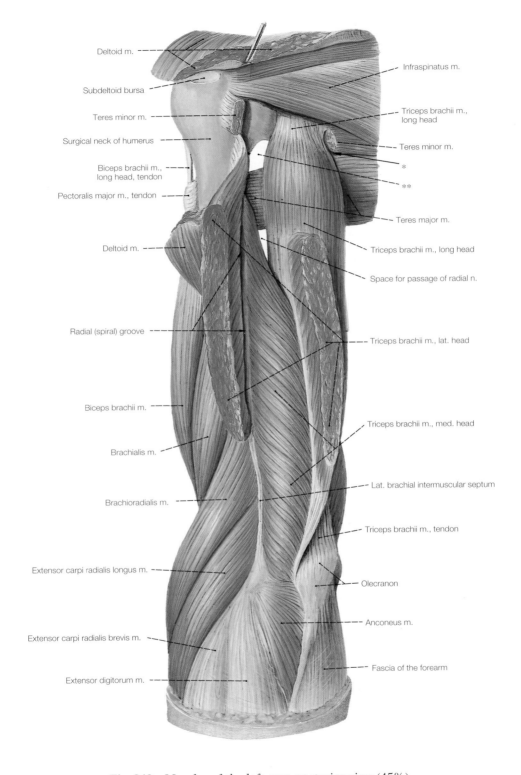

Deltoid m.

Subdeltoid bursa

Teres minor m.

Surgical neck of humerus

Biceps brachii m.,
long head, tendon

Pectoralis major m., tendon

Deltoid m.

Radial (spiral) groove

Biceps brachii m.

Brachialis m.

Brachioradialis m.

Extensor carpi radialis longus m.

Extensor carpi radialis brevis m.

Extensor digitorum m.

Infraspinatus m.

Triceps brachii m.,
long head

Teres minor m.

*

**

Teres major m.

Triceps brachii m., long head

Space for passage of radial n.

Triceps brachii m., lat. head

Triceps brachii m., med. head

Lat. brachial intermuscular septum

Triceps brachii m., tendon

Olecranon

Anconeus m.

Fascia of the forearm

Fig. 348 Muscles of the left arm, posterior view (45%).
The deep layer after partial removal of the
deltoid muscle.

*   Triangular space
** Quadrangular space

Extensor Muscles of the Arm

Name *Innervation*	Origin	Insertion	Function
1. Triceps brachii m. *Radial n.* Long head (operates two joints)	Infraglenoidal tubercle of scapula; separates the two axillary spaces; forms a distinct tendon	Fibers pass distally joining common tendon of insertion on the olecranon	*Shoulder joint* Extension of humerus by long head; *Elbow joint* Extension of forearm; braces extended elbow joint (when pushing an object)
Lateral head (operates one joint)	Lateral and posterior surface of body of humerus, posterior 2/3 of lateral intermuscular septum	Joins the common tendon of insertion on the olecranon	
Medial head (operates one joint)	Whole length of medial intermuscular septum; dorsal surface of body of humerus (distal to crest of greater tubercle and groove for radial nerve); distal third of lateral intermuscular septum (to lateral epicondyle)	Posterior aspect of olecranon and into deep fascia on both sides of the forearm	
2. Anconeus m. (situated in the forearm) *Radial n.*	Lateral epicondyle of humerus; continuation of the lateral side of the medial head of the triceps brachii muscle	Posterior surface of ulna, slightly distal to olecranon	*Elbow joint* Extension

Flexor Muscles of the Arm

Name *Innervation*	Origin	Insertion	Function
1. Biceps brachii m. *Musclocutaneous n.* Long head	Tendon through shoulder joint to supraglenoid tubercle of scapula (long tendon)	Posterior surface of radial tuberosity. Bicipital aponeurosis to antebrachial fascia	*Shoulder joint* Long head: aids in abduction and holds head of humerus in place; Short head: aids in adduction
Short head	Short tendon from tip of coracoid process of scapula		Both parts: support weight of arm *Elbow joint* Flexion and supination of forearm
2. Coracobrachialis m. *Musculocutaneous n.* (usually pierces the muscle)	Apex of coracoid process (fused with short head of biceps)	Ventral and medial surface of humerus near its middle	*Shoulder joint* Flexion and adduction of the arm
3. Brachialis m. *Musculocutaneous n.*	Distal half of anterior aspect of humerus, distal to deltoid tuberosity and the medial and lateral intermuscular septa	As a thick muscle mass extends over the anterior surface of the capsule of the elbow joint to the ulnar tuberosity	*Elbow joint* Flexion of the forearm (exclusively!)

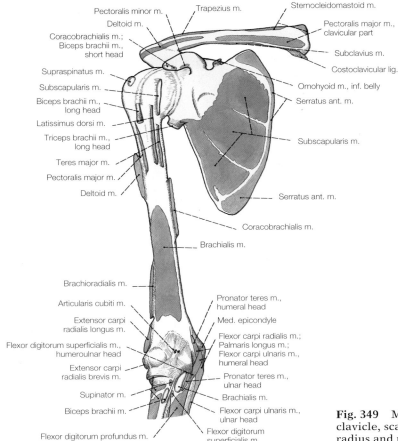

Pectoralis minor m.
Deltoid m.
Coracobrachialis m.;
Biceps brachii m.,
short head
Supraspinatus m.
Subscapularis m.
Biceps brachii m.,
long head
Latissimus dorsi m.
Triceps brachii m.,
long head
Teres major m.
Pectoralis major m.
Deltoid m.

Trapezius m.
Sternocleidomastoid m.
Pectoralis major m.,
clavicular part
Subclavius m.
Costoclavicular lig.
Omohyoid m., inf. belly
Serratus ant. m.
Subscapularis m.
Serratus ant. m.
Coracobrachialis m.

Brachialis m.

Brachioradialis m.
Articularis cubiti m.
Extensor carpi
radialis longus m.
Flexor digitorum superficialis m.,
humeroulnar head
Extensor carpi
radialis brevis m.
Supinator m.
Biceps brachii m.
Flexor digitorum profundus m.

Pronator teres m.,
humeral head
Med. epicondyle
Flexor carpi radialis m.;
Palmaris longus m.;
Flexor carpi ulnaris m.,
humeral head
Pronator teres m.,
ulnar head
Brachialis m.
Flexor carpi ulnaris m.,
ulnar head
Flexor digitorum
superficialis m.

Fig. 349 Muscle origins and insertions on the right clavicle, scapula, humerus, and proximal parts of the radius and ulna, anterior view.

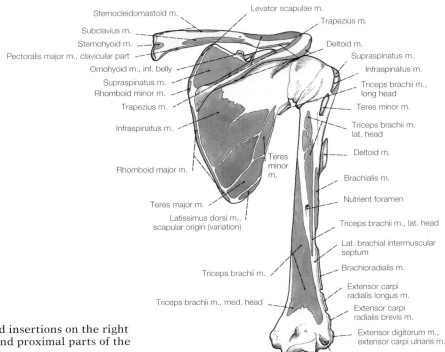

Sternocleidomastoid m.
Subclavius m.
Sternohyoid m.
Pectoralis major m., clavicular part
Omohyoid m., inf. belly
Supraspinatus m.
Rhomboid minor m.
Trapezius m.
Infraspinatus m.
Rhomboid major m.
Teres major m.
Latissimus dorsi m.,
scapular origin (variation)
Triceps brachii m.
Triceps brachii m., med. head

Levator scapulae m.
Trapezius m.
Deltoid m.
Supraspinatus m.
Infraspinatus m.
Triceps brachii m.,
long head
Teres minor m.
Triceps brachii m.
lat. head
Deltoid m.
Brachialis m.
Nutrient foramen
Triceps brachii m., lat. head
Lat. brachial intermuscular
septum
Brachioradialis m.
Extensor carpi
radialis longus m.
Extensor carpi
radialis brevis m.
Extensor digitorum m.,
extensor carpi ulnaris m.
Anconeus m.
Teres minor m.

Fig. 350 Muscle origins and insertions on the right clavicle, scapula, humerus and proximal parts of the radius and ulna, posterior view.

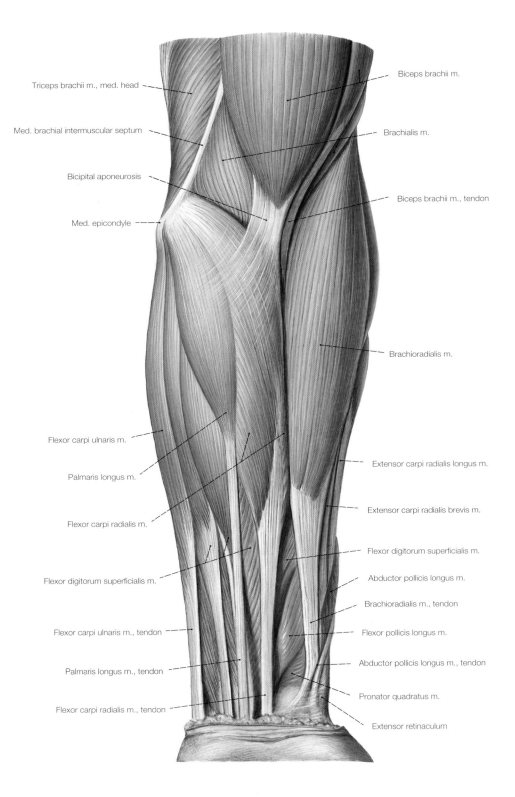

Triceps brachii m., med. head

Med. brachial intermuscular septum

Bicipital aponeurosis

Med. epicondyle

Flexor carpi ulnaris m.

Palmaris longus m.

Flexor carpi radialis m.

Flexor digitorum superficialis m.

Flexor carpi ulnaris m., tendon

Palmaris longus m., tendon

Flexor carpi radialis m., tendon

Biceps brachii m.

Brachialis m.

Biceps brachii m., tendon

Brachioradialis m.

Extensor carpi radialis longus m.

Extensor carpi radialis brevis m.

Flexor digitorum superficialis m.

Abductor pollicis longus m.

Brachioradialis m., tendon

Flexor pollicis longus m.

Abductor pollicis longus m., tendon

Pronator quadratus m.

Extensor retinaculum

Fig. 351 Muscles of the left forearm, anterior view (50%).

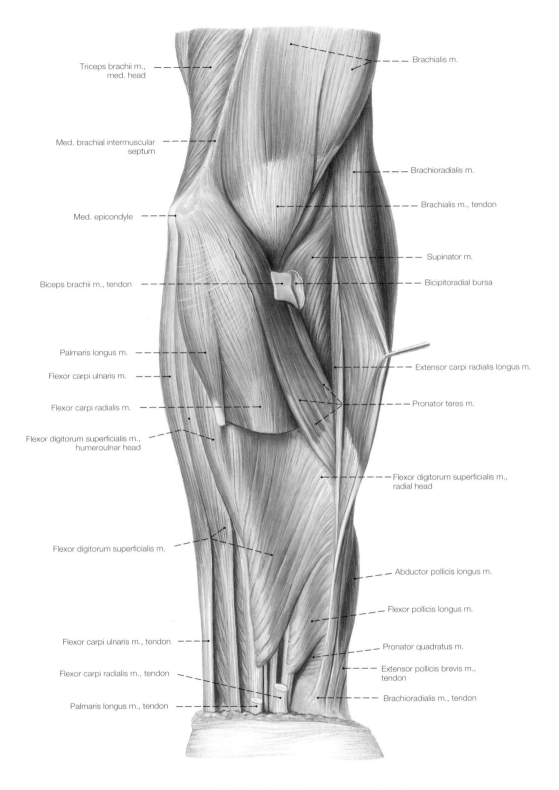

Triceps brachii m.,
med. head

Med. brachial intermuscular
septum

Med. epicondyle

Biceps brachii m., tendon

Palmaris longus m.

Flexor carpi ulnaris m.

Flexor carpi radialis m.

Flexor digitorum superficialis m.,
humeroulnar head

Flexor digitorum superficialis m.

Flexor carpi ulnaris m., tendon

Flexor carpi radialis m., tendon

Palmaris longus m., tendon

Brachialis m.

Brachioradialis m.

Brachialis m., tendon

Supinator m.

Bicipitoradial bursa

Extensor carpi radialis longus m.

Pronator teres m.

Flexor digitorum superficialis m.,
radial head

Abductor pollicis longus m.

Flexor pollicis longus m.

Pronator quadratus m.

Extensor pollicis brevis m.,
tendon

Brachioradialis m., tendon

Fig. 352 Muscles of the left forearm, anterior view
(50%). The middle layer after partial removal of the
palmaris longus and the flexor carpi radialis
muscles.

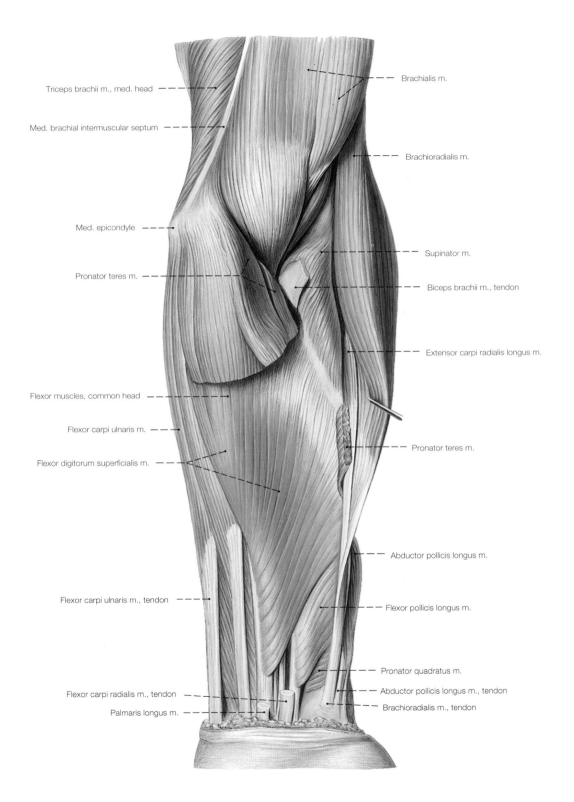

Triceps brachii m., med. head

Med. brachial intermuscular septum

Med. epicondyle

Pronator teres m.

Flexor muscles, common head

Flexor carpi ulnaris m.

Flexor digitorum superficialis m.

Flexor carpi ulnaris m., tendon

Flexor carpi radialis m., tendon

Palmaris longus m.

Brachialis m.

Brachioradialis m.

Supinator m.

Biceps brachii m., tendon

Extensor carpi radialis longus m.

Pronator teres m.

Abductor pollicis longus m.

Flexor pollicis longus m.

Pronator quadratus m.

Abductor pollicis longus m., tendon

Brachioradialis m., tendon

Fig. 353 Muscles of the left forearm, anterior view (50%). The middle layer after partial removal of the superficial flexors.

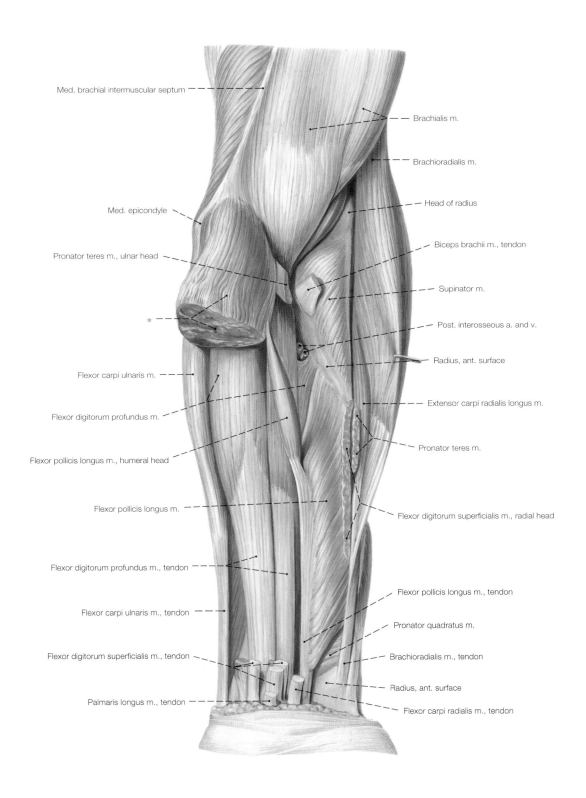

Med. brachial intermuscular septum

Brachialis m.

Brachioradialis m.

Head of radius

Med. epicondyle

Pronator teres m., ulnar head

Biceps brachii m., tendon

Supinator m.

*

Post. interosseous a. and v.

Radius, ant. surface

Flexor carpi ulnaris m.

Flexor digitorum profundus m.

Extensor carpi radialis longus m.

Flexor pollicis longus m., humeral head

Pronator teres m.

Flexor pollicis longus m.

Flexor digitorum superficialis m., radial head

Flexor digitorum profundus m., tendon

Flexor pollicis longus m., tendon

Flexor carpi ulnaris m., tendon

Pronator quadratus m.

Flexor digitorum superficialis m., tendon

Brachioradialis m., tendon

Radius, ant. surface

Palmaris longus m., tendon

Flexor carpi radialis m., tendon

Fig. 354 Muscles of the left forearm, anterior view (50%). The deep layer after partial removal of the superficial flexors.

* Common head of the superficial flexor muscles

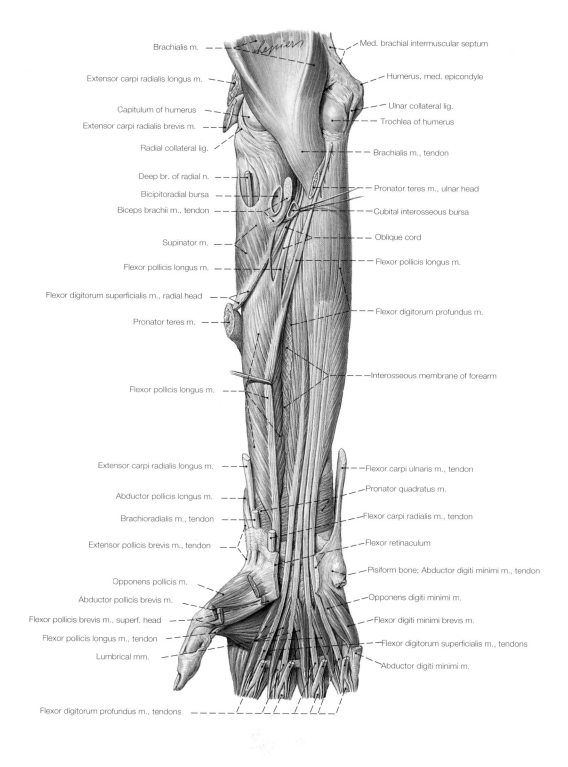

Brachialis m.

Extensor carpi radialis longus m.

Capitulum of humerus

Extensor carpi radialis brevis m.

Radial collateral lig.

Deep br. of radial n.

Bicipitoradial bursa

Biceps brachii m., tendon

Supinator m.

Flexor pollicis longus m.

Flexor digitorum superficialis m., radial head

Pronator teres m.

Flexor pollicis longus m.

Extensor carpi radialis longus m.

Abductor pollicis longus m.

Brachioradialis m., tendon

Extensor pollicis brevis m., tendon

Opponens pollicis m.

Abductor pollicis brevis m.

Flexor pollicis brevis m., superf. head

Flexor pollicis longus m., tendon

Lumbrical mm.

Flexor digitorum profundus m., tendons

Med. brachial intermuscular septum

Humerus, med. epicondyle

Ulnar collateral lig.

Trochlea of humerus

Brachialis m., tendon

Pronator teres m., ulnar head

Cubital interosseous bursa

Oblique cord

Flexor pollicis longus m.

Flexor digitorum profundus m.

Interosseous membrane of forearm

Flexor carpi ulnaris m., tendon

Pronator quadratus m.

Flexor carpi radialis m., tendon

Flexor retinaculum

Pisiform bone; Abductor digiti minimi m., tendon

Opponens digiti minimi m.

Flexor digiti minimi brevis m.

Flexor digitorum superficialis m., tendons

Abductor digiti minimi m.

Fig. 355   Muscles of the right forearm and hand,
anterior view (45%). The deep layer after removal of
the superficial flexors.

Flexor Muscles of the Forearm

Name *Innervation*	Origin	Insertion	Function
Superficial Group			
Pronator teres m. *Median n.*	Medial epicondyle of the humerus, antebrachial fascia Coronoid process of the ulna	On the lateral and dorsal surface of radius (middle $^1/_3$)	*Elbow joint* Humeral head: pronation, flexion Ulnar head: pronation
Flexor carpi radialis m. *Median n.*	Medial epicondyle of the humerus, antebrachial fascia	Base of 2nd metacarpal bone, palmar surface	*Elbow joint* Flexion, pronation *Wrist and carpal joints* Flexion (palmar flexion) and abduction (radial flexion)
Palmaris longus m. (variable) *Median n.*	Medial epicondyle of humerus, antebrachial fascia	Palmar aponeurosis	*Elbow joint* Flexion *Wrist and carpal joints* Flexion (palmar flexion), tension of palmar aponeurosis
Flexor digitorum superficialis m. *Median n.* Humeroulnar head	Medial epicondyle of the humerus and coronoid process of ulna	4 long tendons to the middle phalanges of fingers 2–5	*Elbow joint* Flexion *Wrist and carpal joints* Flexion (palmar flexion), *Metacarpophalangeal joints (digits 2–5)* Flexion, adduction *Interphalangeal joints (digits 2–5)* Flexion
Radial head	Upper half, anterior border of radius		
Flexor carpi ulnaris m. *Ulnar n.* Humeral head Ulnar head	Medial epicondyle of the humerus Olecranon and, via the antebrachial fascia, posterior border of ulna (upper $^2/_3$)	Pisiform bone and, by ligaments, to 5th metacarpal and hamate bones	*Elbow joint* Flexion *Wrist and carpal joints* Flexion (palmar flexion), adduction (ulnar flexion)
Deep Group			
Flexor digitorum profundus m. *Ulnar n.* for the ulnar side, *Median n.* for the radial side	Anterior and medial surface of ulna; interosseous membrane	Distal phalanges of fingers 2 to 5	*Wrist and carpal joints* Flexion (palmar flexion) *Metacarpophalangeal joints (digits 2–5)* Flexion, adduction *Interphalangeal joints (digits 2–5)* Flexion
Flexor pollicis longus m. *Median n.* Radial head Humeral head	Anterior surface of radius (distal to insertion of supinator muscle); interosseus membrane Medial epicondyle of humerus	Terminal phalanx of thumb	*Wrist and carpal joints* Flexion (palmar flexion) *Carpometacarpal joint of thumb* Adduction, opposition *Metacarpophalangeal joint of thumb* Flexion
Pronator quadratus m. *Median n.* *Interosseus anterior m.*	Anterior border of ulna, distal $^1/_4$	Anterior border and surface of radius	*Radioulnar joint* Pronation
Supinator m. *Radial n.* (The deep branch of the radial n. pierces the muscle and divides it into a superficial and a deep layer)	Lat. epicondyle humerus, radial collateral and radioulnar annular ligg., supinator crest of ulna	Superficial fibers: Lat. edge of radial tuberosity and oblique line of radii Deep fibers: Back part of medial surface of radial tuberosity and dors. and lat. aspects of upper third of radial shaft	*Radioulnar joint* Supination

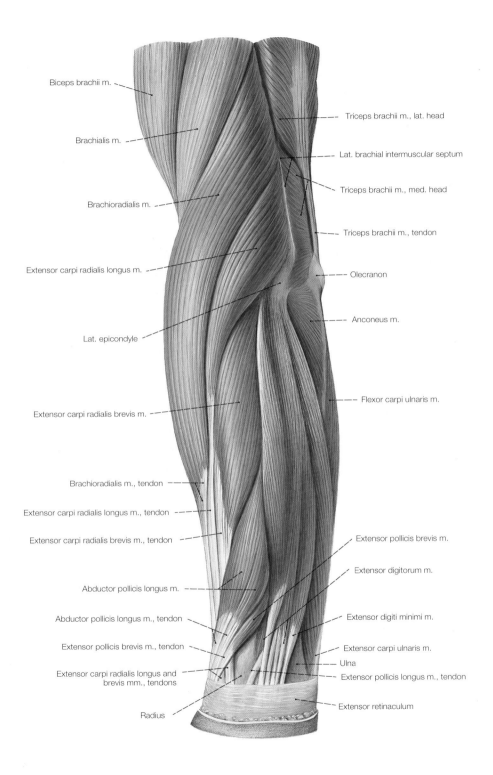

Biceps brachii m.

Brachialis m.

Brachioradialis m.

Extensor carpi radialis longus m.

Lat. epicondyle

Extensor carpi radialis brevis m.

Brachioradialis m., tendon

Extensor carpi radialis longus m., tendon

Extensor carpi radialis brevis m., tendon

Abductor pollicis longus m.

Abductor pollicis longus m., tendon

Extensor pollicis brevis m., tendon

Extensor carpi radialis longus and brevis mm., tendons

Radius

Triceps brachii m., lat. head

Lat. brachial intermuscular septum

Triceps brachii m., med. head

Triceps brachii m., tendon

Olecranon

Anconeus m.

Flexor carpi ulnaris m.

Extensor pollicis brevis m.

Extensor digitorum m.

Extensor digiti minimi m.

Extensor carpi ulnaris m.

Ulna

Extensor pollicis longus m., tendon

Extensor retinaculum

Fig. 356 Muscles of the left forearm and distal
parts of the arm, viewed from the lateral (radial)
side (45%). The forearm is positioned midway
between supination and pronation.

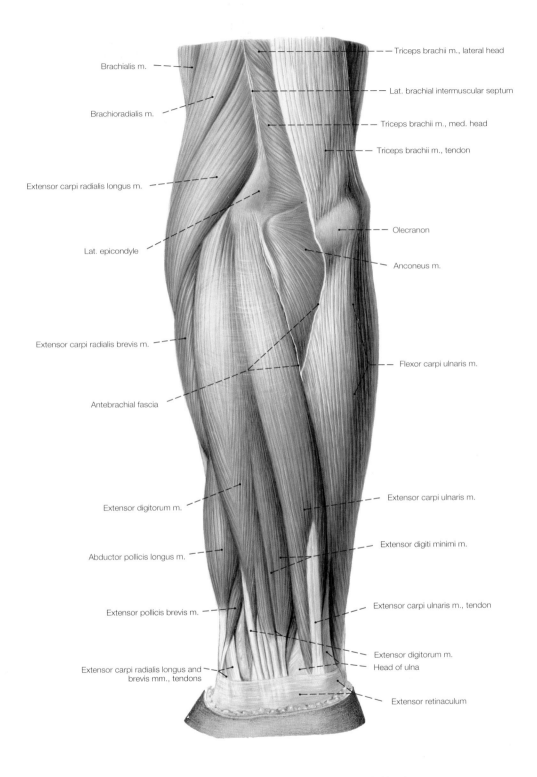

Brachialis m.

Brachioradialis m.

Extensor carpi radialis longus m.

Lat. epicondyle

Extensor carpi radialis brevis m.

Antebrachial fascia

Extensor digitorum m.

Abductor pollicis longus m.

Extensor pollicis brevis m.

Extensor carpi radialis longus and brevis mm., tendons

Triceps brachii m., lateral head

Lat. brachial intermuscular septum

Triceps brachii m., med. head

Triceps brachii m., tendon

Olecranon

Anconeus m.

Flexor carpi ulnaris m.

Extensor carpi ulnaris m.

Extensor digiti minimi m.

Extensor carpi ulnaris m., tendon

Extensor digitorum m.
Head of ulna

Extensor retinaculum

Fig. 357 Muscles of the left forearm and distal parts of the arm, posterolateral view (50%). The forearm is positioned midway between supination and pronation.

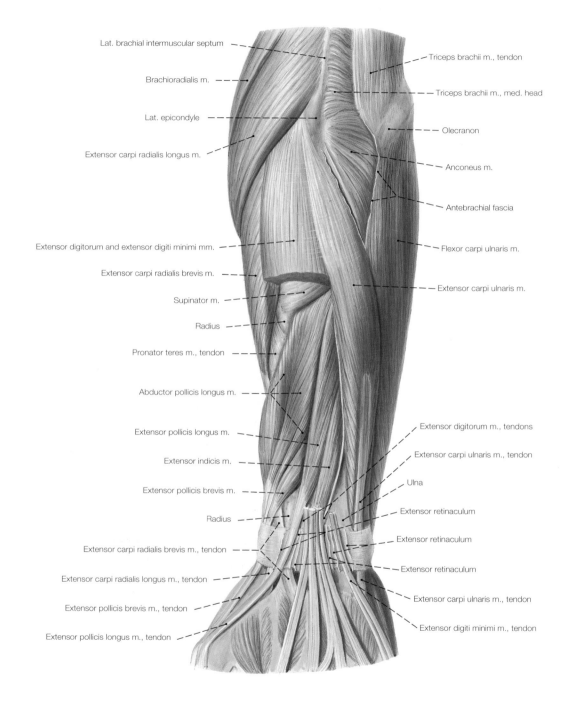

Lat. brachial intermuscular septum

Brachioradialis m.

Lat. epicondyle

Extensor carpi radialis longus m.

Extensor digitorum and extensor digiti minimi mm.

Extensor carpi radialis brevis m.

Supinator m.

Radius

Pronator teres m., tendon

Abductor pollicis longus m.

Extensor pollicis longus m.

Extensor indicis m.

Extensor pollicis brevis m.

Radius

Extensor carpi radialis brevis m., tendon

Extensor carpi radialis longus m., tendon

Extensor pollicis brevis m., tendon

Extensor pollicis longus m., tendon

Triceps brachii m., tendon

Triceps brachii m., med. head

Olecranon

Anconeus m.

Antebrachial fascia

Flexor carpi ulnaris m.

Extensor carpi ulnaris m.

Extensor digitorum m., tendons

Extensor carpi ulnaris m., tendon

Ulna

Extensor retinaculum

Extensor retinaculum

Extensor retinaculum

Extensor carpi ulnaris m., tendon

Extensor digiti minimi m., tendon

Fig. 358 Muscles of the left forearm, posterolateral
view (45%). The extensor digitorum and extensor digiti
minimi muscles have been partially removed.
The forearm is positioned midway between supination
and pronation.

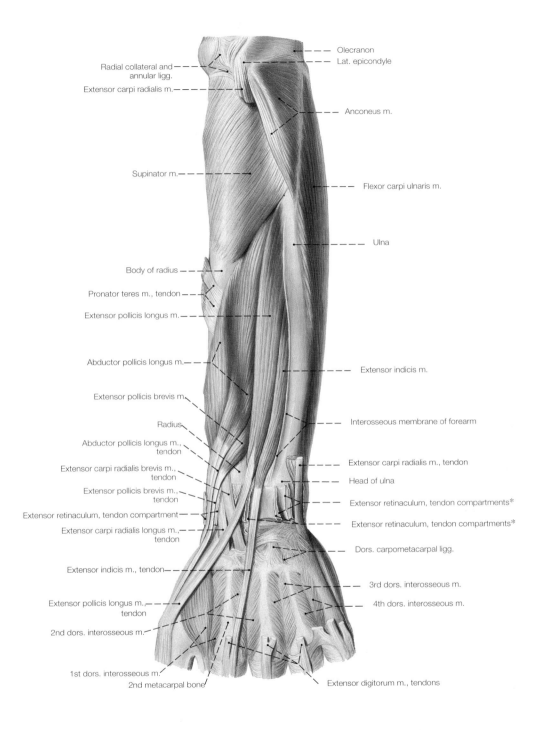

Olecranon

Lat. epicondyle

Radial collateral and
annular ligg.

Extensor carpi radialis m.

Anconeus m.

Supinator m.

Flexor carpi ulnaris m.

Ulna

Body of radius

Pronator teres m., tendon

Extensor pollicis longus m.

Abductor pollicis longus m.

Extensor indicis m.

Extensor pollicis brevis m.

Radius

Interosseous membrane of forearm

Abductor pollicis longus m.,
tendon

Extensor carpi radialis brevis m.,
tendon

Extensor pollicis brevis m.,
tendon

Extensor carpi radialis m., tendon

Head of ulna

Extensor retinaculum, tendon compartments*

Extensor retinaculum, tendon compartment

Extensor carpi radialis longus m.,
tendon

Extensor retinaculum, tendon compartments*

Dors. carpometacarpal ligg.

Extensor indicis m., tendon

3rd dors. interosseous m.

Extensor pollicis longus m.,
tendon

4th dors. interosseous m.

2nd dors. interosseous m.

1st dors. interosseous m.

2nd metacarpal bone

Extensor digitorum m., tendons

Fig. 359 Muscles of the left forearm and hand, posterolateral view (45%). The deep layer after removal of the superficial extensors. The forearm is positioned midway between supination and pronation.

* The tendon compartments of the extensor retinaculum have been opened.

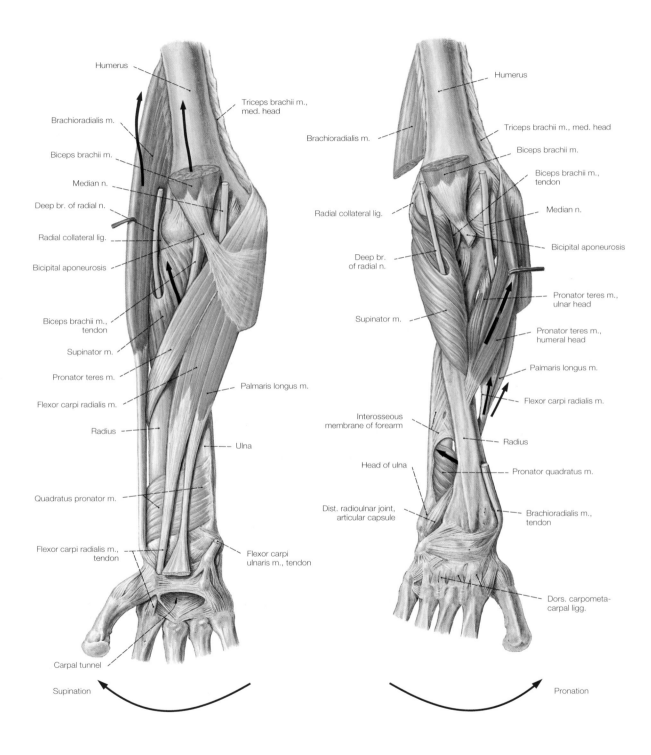

Humerus

Brachioradialis m.

Biceps brachii m.

Median n.

Deep br. of radial n.

Radial collateral lig.

Bicipital aponeurosis

Biceps brachii m., tendon

Supinator m.

Pronator teres m.

Flexor carpi radialis m.

Radius

Quadratus pronator m.

Flexor carpi radialis m., tendon

Carpal tunnel

Supination

Triceps brachii m., med. head

Palmaris longus m.

Ulna

Flexor carpi ulnaris m., tendon

Humerus

Brachioradialis m.

Triceps brachii m., med. head

Biceps brachii m.

Biceps brachii m., tendon

Radial collateral lig.

Median n.

Bicipital aponeurosis

Deep br. of radial n.

Pronator teres m., ulnar head

Supinator m.

Pronator teres m., humeral head

Palmaris longus m.

Flexor carpi radialis m.

Interosseous membrane of forearm

Radius

Head of ulna

Pronator quadratus m.

Dist. radioulnar joint, articular capsule

Brachioradialis m., tendon

Dors. carpometa-carpal ligg.

Pronation

Fig. 360   The right forearm in supination, anterior (palmar) view (40%). The arrows indicate the direction of force generated by the main supinator muscles.

Fig. 361   The right forearm in pronation (40%). Anterior view of the elbow region, dorsal view of the hand region. The arrows indicate the direction of force generated by the main pronator muscles.

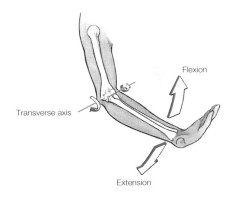

Fig. 362   Elbow joint: Flexion
and extension of the forearm.

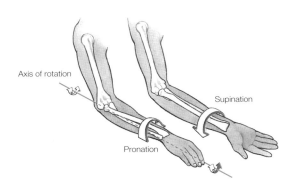

Fig. 363   Elbow joint:
Rotation of the hand.

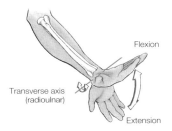

Fig. 364   Wrist and carpal joints: Flexion (palmar)
and extension (dorsiflexion) of the hand.

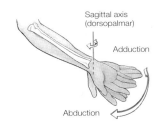

Fig. 365   Wrist and carpal joints: Adduction (ulnar
flexion) and abduction (radial flexion) of the hand.

Extensor Muscles of the Forearm, Superficial (Radial) Group

Name *Innervation*	Origin	Insertion	Function
Brachioradialis m. *Radial n.*	Lateral supracondylar ridge of humerus; lateral intermuscular septum	Lateral side of base of styloid process of radius	*Elbow joint* Flexion, when forearm in semipronated position and flexion is against resistance
Extensor carpi radialis longus m. *Radial n.*	Distal $\frac{1}{3}$ of lateral supracondylar ridge of humerus and lateral intermuscular septum	Dorsal surface of base of 2nd metacarpal bone	*Elbow joint* Flexion, although weak *Wrist and carpal joints* Extension (dorsiflexion), abduction (radial flexion) of hand
Extensor carpi radialis brevis m. *Radial n.*	Lateral epicondyle of humerus; radial collateral ligament of elbow joint	Dorsal surface of base of 3rd metacarpal bone	Same as above

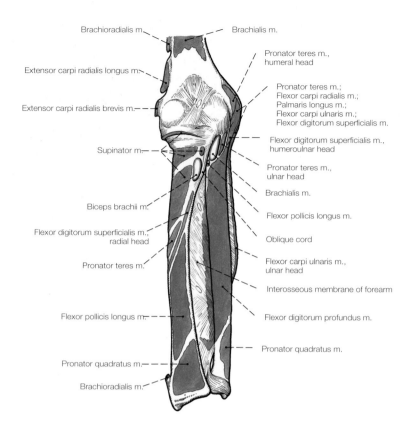

Brachioradialis m.

Brachialis m.

Extensor carpi radialis longus m.

Pronator teres m., humeral head

Extensor carpi radialis brevis m.

Pronator teres m.; Flexor carpi radialis m.; Palmaris longus m.; Flexor carpi ulnaris m.; Flexor digitorum superficialis m.

Flexor digitorum superficialis m., humeroulnar head

Supinator m.

Pronator teres m., ulnar head

Brachialis m.

Biceps brachii m.

Flexor pollicis longus m.

Flexor digitorum superficialis m., radial head

Oblique cord

Pronator teres m.

Flexor carpi ulnaris m., ulnar head

Interosseous membrane of forearm

Flexor pollicis longus m.

Flexor digitorum profundus m.

Pronator quadratus m.

Pronator quadratus m.

Brachioradialis m.

Fig. 366 Muscle origins and insertions of the right radius, ulna and distal end of the humerus, anterior aspect.

Extensor Muscles of the Forearm, Superficial (Posterior) Group

Name *Innervation*	Origin	Insertion	Function
Extensor digitorum m. *Radial n.*	Lateral epicondyle of humerus; antebrachial fascia	By 4 tendons to middle and distal phalanges of the fingers	*Elbow joint* Extension *Wrist and carpal joints* Extension (dorsiflexion), adduction (ulnar flexion) *Carpometacarpal joints (digits 2–5)* Extension *Metacarpophalangeal and interphalangeal joints (digits 2–5)* Extension
Extensor digiti minimi m. *Radial n.*	same as above	Joins extensor digitorum tendon to little finger	*Elbow joint* Extension *Wrist and carpal joints* Extension (dorsiflexion), adduction (ulnar flexion) *Carpometacarpal joints (digit 5)* Extension *Metacarpophalangeal and interphalangeal joints (digit 5)* Extension
Extensor carpi ulnaris m. (separated from the extensor digitorum and extensor digiti minimi mm. by a distinct intermuscular septum) *Radial n.*	Lateral epicondyle of humerus; antebrachial fascia	Base of 5th metacarpal, dorsal surface	*Elbow joint* Extension *Wrist and carpal joints* Extension (dorsiflexion), adduction (ulnar flexion)

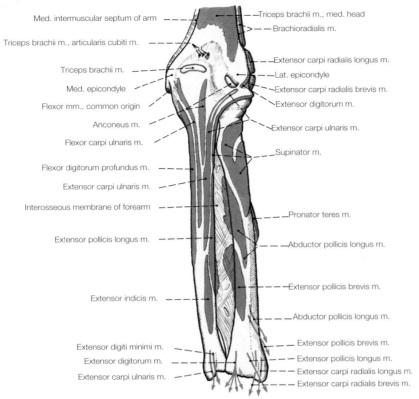

Med. intermuscular septum of arm — Triceps brachii m., med. head

Brachioradialis m.

Triceps brachii m., articularis cubiti m. —

Triceps brachii m. — Extensor carpi radialis longus m.

Lat. epicondyle

Med. epicondyle — Extensor carpi radialis brevis m.

Flexor mm., common origin — Extensor digitorum m.

Anconeus m. — Extensor carpi ulnaris m.

Flexor carpi ulnaris m. —

Supinator m.

Flexor digitorum profundus m. —

Extensor carpi ulnaris m. —

Interosseous membrane of forearm — Pronator teres m.

Extensor pollicis longus m. — Abductor pollicis longus m.

Extensor pollicis brevis m.

Abductor pollicis longus m.

Extensor indicis m. —

Extensor pollicis brevis m.

Extensor digiti minimi m. — Extensor pollicis longus m.

Extensor digitorum m. — Extensor carpi radialis longus m.

Extensor carpi ulnaris m. — Extensor carpi radialis brevis m.

Fig. 367 Muscle origins and insertions of the right radius, ulna and distal end of the humerus, posterior

Extensor Muscles of the Forearm, Deep (Ulnar) Group

Name Innervation	Origin	Insertion	Function
Extensor pollicis longus m. *Radial n.*	Posterior surface of ulna; interosseous membrane	Base of distal phalanx of thumb	*Wrist and carpal joints* Extension (dorsiflexion), abduction (radial flexion) *Carpometacarpal joint of thumb* Extension *Metacarpophalangeal and interphalangeal joints of thumb* Extension
Extensor indicis m. *Radial n.*	same as above	Extensor hood of the index finger	*Wrist and carpal joints* Extension (dorsiflexion), abduction (radial flexion) *Carpometacarpal joints (digit 2)* Extension, adduction *Metacarpophalangeal and interphalangeal joints of index finger (digit 2)* Extension

Extensor Muscles of the Forearm, Deep (Radial) Group

Abductor pollicis longus m. *Radial n.*	Posterior surfaces of ulna and radius; interosseous membrane	Base of 1st metacarpal of thumb, radial side	*Radioulnar joints* Supination *Wrist and carpal joints* Flexion (palmar flexion), abduction (radial flexion) *Metacarpophalangeal joint of thumb* Extension
Extensor pollicis brevis m. *Radial n.*	Posterior surface of radius; interosseous membrane	Base of proximal phalanx of thumb	*Wrist and carpal joints* Flexion (palmar flexion), abduction (radial flexion) *Carpometacarpal joint of thumb* Extension *Metacarpophalangeal joint of thumb* Extension

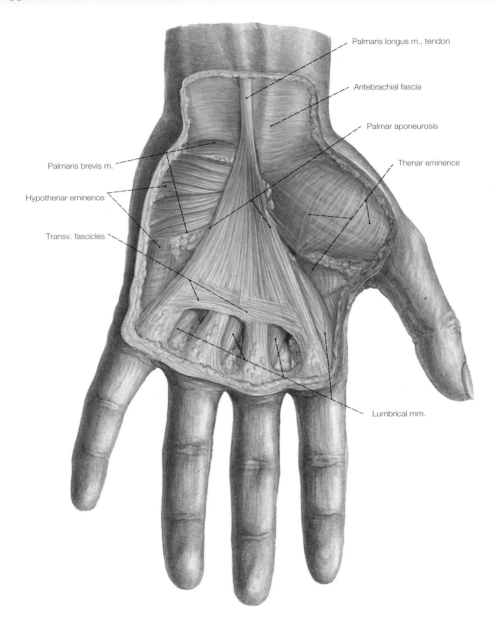

Fig. 368 Muscles of the left hand, palmar aspect (70%). When the palmaris longus muscle is absent (in 20% of cases) the palmar aponeurosis blends proximally with the flexor retinaculum.

Palmaris Brevis Muscle

Name *Innervation*	Origin	Insertion	Function
Palmaris brevis m. (Superficial muscle beneath the skin; several separate bundles) *Ulnar n.,* *Superficial branch*	Palmar aponeurosis, medial margin (occasionally trapezium bone)	Skin over medial border of palm	Tenses skin of the hypothenar region

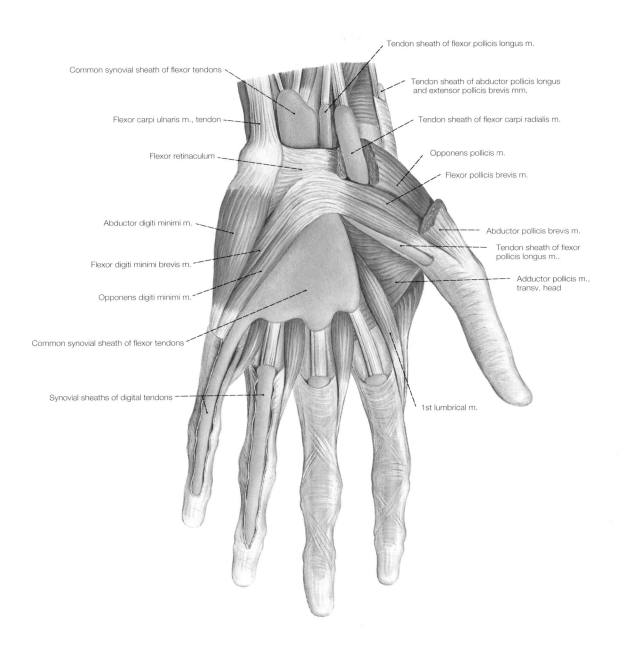

Tendon sheath of flexor pollicis longus m.

Common synovial sheath of flexor tendons

Tendon sheath of abductor pollicis longus
and extensor pollicis brevis mm.

Flexor carpi ulnaris m., tendon

Tendon sheath of flexor carpi radialis m.

Flexor retinaculum

Opponens pollicis m.

Flexor pollicis brevis m.

Abductor digiti minimi m.

Abductor pollicis brevis m.

Tendon sheath of flexor
pollicis longus m..

Flexor digiti minimi brevis m.

Adductor pollicis m.,
transv. head

Opponens digiti minimi m.

Common synovial sheath of flexor tendons

Synovial sheaths of digital tendons

1st lumbrical m.

Fig. 369 Tendon sheaths of the left hand,
palmar aspect (70%).

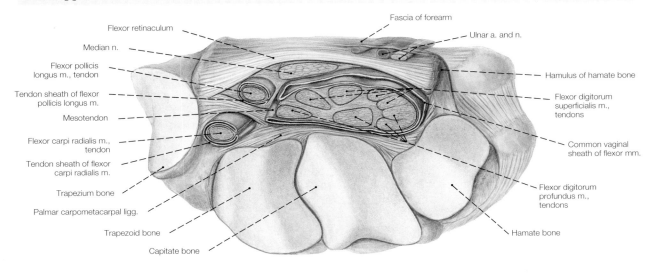

Fig. 370 Palmar carpal tendon sheaths of the right hand (175%). Transverse section through the carpal tunnel at the level of the carpometacarpal joints.

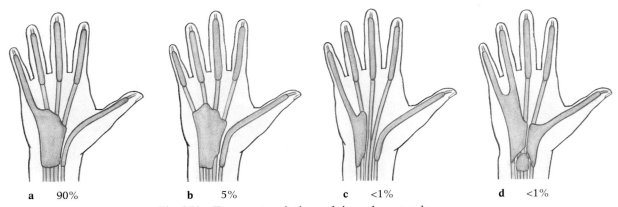

a   90%   **b**   5%   **c**   <1%   **d**   <1%

Fig. 371 Frequent variations of the palmar tendon sheaths of the hand. Because inflammation can readily spread within the synovial sheaths, extreme care is essential during surgical intervention.

Hypothenar Muscles

Name *Innervation*	Origin	Insertion	Function
Abductor digiti minimi m. *Ulnar n.,* *Deep branch*	Pisiform bone and tendon of flexor carpi ulnaris m.	Base of proximal phalanx of little finger, ulnar side of dorsal aponeurosis of little finger	*Carpometacarpal joint (5th)* Opposition *Metacarpophalangeal joint (5th)* Abduction *Interphalangeal joints (digit 5)* Extension
Flexor digiti minimi brevis m. (variable) *Ulnar n.,* *Deep branch*	Flexor retinaculum; hamulus of hamate bone	Ulnar side of base of proximal phalanx of little finger	*Carpometacarpal joint (5th)* Opposition *Metacarpophalangeal joint (5th)* Flexion, abduction
Opponens digiti minimi m. *Ulnar n.,* *Deep branch*	Flexor retinaculum; hamulus of hamate bone	Ulnar margin of 5th metacarpal bone	*Carpometacarpal joint (5th)* Opposition
Palmaris brevis m. (See page 208)			

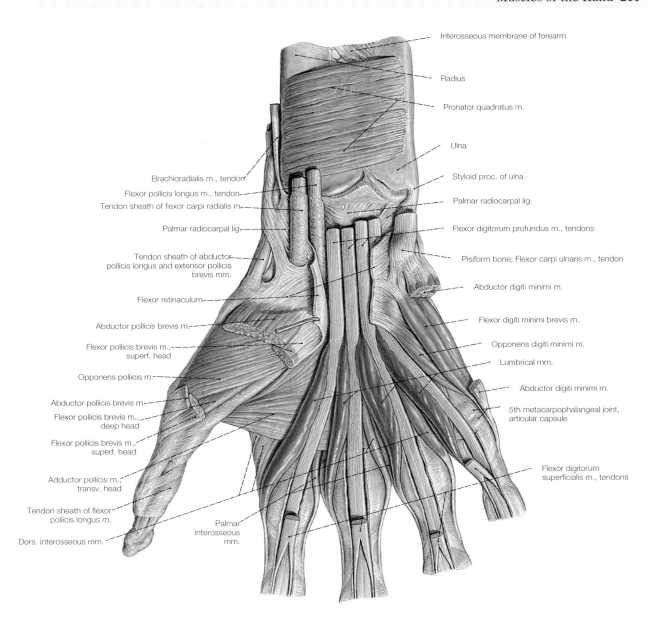

Interosseous membrane of forearm

Radius

Pronator quadratus m.

Ulna

Styloid proc. of ulna

Palmar radiocarpal lig.

Flexor digitorum profundus m., tendons

Pisiform bone; Flexor carpi ulnaris m., tendon

Abductor digiti minimi m.

Flexor digiti minimi brevis m.

Opponens digiti minimi m.

Lumbrical mm.

Abductor digiti minimi m.

5th metacarpophalangeal joint, articular capsule

Flexor digitorum superficialis m., tendons

Brachioradialis m., tendon

Flexor pollicis longus m., tendon

Tendon sheath of flexor carpi radialis m.

Palmar radiocarpal lig.

Tendon sheath of abductor pollicis longus and extensor pollicis brevis mm.

Flexor retinaculum

Abductor pollicis brevis m.

Flexor pollicis brevis m., superf. head

Opponens pollicis m.

Abductor pollicis brevis m.

Flexor pollicis brevis m., deep head

Flexor pollicis brevis m., superf. head

Adductor pollicis m., transv. head

Tendon sheath of flexor pollicis longus m.

Dors. interosseous mm.

Palmar interosseous mm.

Fig. 372 Muscles of the right hand, palmar aspect (90%). The deep layer with the flexor retinaculum severed and several superficial muscles removed.

Lumbrical Muscles of the Hand

Name *Innervation*	Origin	Insertion	Function
Lumbrical mm. *Median n. (1st, 2nd),* *Ulnar n. (3rd, 4th)* (1st and 2nd lumbrical mm. have one head; 3rd and 4th lumbrical mm. have two heads)	Radial side of the tendons of flexor digitorum profundus m.	Dorsal aponeurosis of digits 2–5	*Metacarpophalangeal joints (2nd–5th)* Flexion, abduction *Interphalangeal joints* Extension

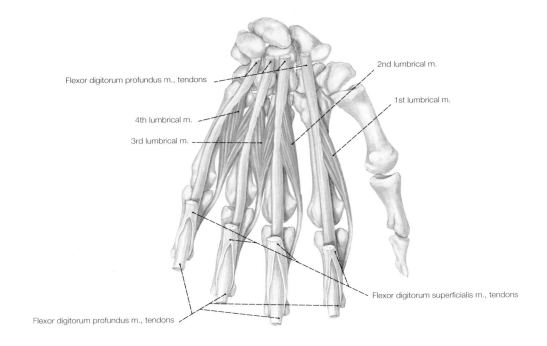

Flexor digitorum profundus m., tendons

2nd lumbrical m.

1st lumbrical m.

4th lumbrical m.

3rd lumbrical m.

Flexor digitorum superficialis m., tendons

Flexor digitorum profundus m., tendons

Fig. 373   The lumbrical muscles of the left hand, palmar aspect (55%).

Thenar Muscles

The superficial layer is formed by the abductor pollicis brevis, opponens pollicis and the superficial head of the flexor pollicis brevis muscles, while the deep layer is formed by the deep head of the flexor pollicis brevis and the adductor pollicis muscles.

Name *Innervation*	Origin	Insertion	Function
Abductor pollicis brevis m. *Median n.*	Flexor retinaculum: tuberosity of scaphoid: ridge of trapezium (accessory slips from abductor pollicis longus m.)	Radial side of base of proximal phalanx of thumb: radial sesamoid bone	*Carpometacarpal joint (1st)* Abduction, opposition *Metacarpophalangeal joint (1st)* Flexion
Opponens pollicis m. *Median n.*	Flexor retinaculum: ridge of trapezium	Entire length of radial border of metacarpal of thumb	*Carpometacarpal joint (1st)* Opposition, adduction
Flexor pollicis brevis m. Superficial head *Median n.*	Distal border of flexor retinaculum: distal part of tubercule of trapezium.	Radial side of base of proximal phalanx of thumb with radial sesamoid bone in its tendon	*Carpometacarpal joint (1st)* Opposition, adduction *Metacarpophalangeal joint (1st)* Flexion
Deep head *Ulnar n., deep palmar br.*	Trapezoid and capitate bones		
Adductor pollicis m. *Ulnar n., deep palmar br.* Oblique head	Capitate bone: bases of 2nd and 3rd metacarpals, intercarpal ligaments, sheath of flexor carpi radialis	Medial (ulnar) side of base of proximal phalanx of thumb, sesamoid bone	*Carpometacarpal joint (1st)* Adduction, opposition *Metacarpophalangeal joint (1st)* Flexion
Traverse head	Palmar surface of 3rd metacarpal		

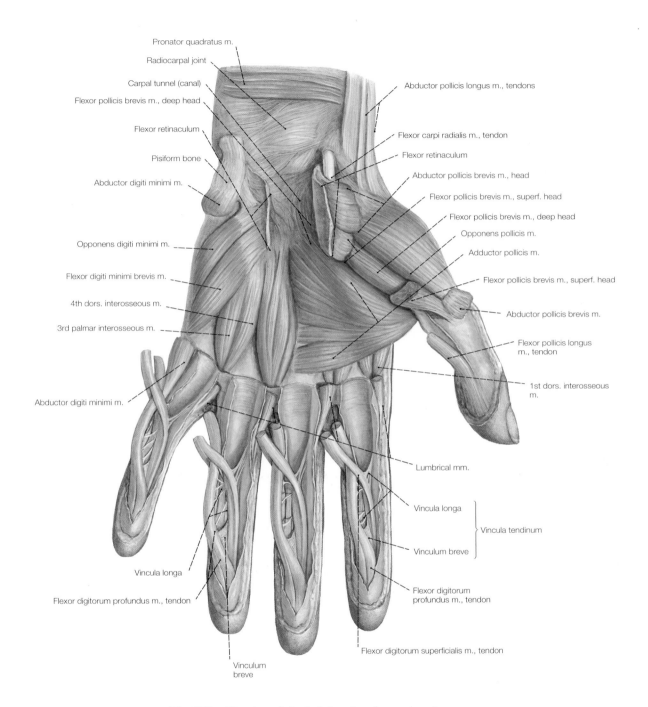

Pronator quadratus m.

Radiocarpal joint

Carpal tunnel (canal)

Flexor pollicis brevis m., deep head

Flexor retinaculum

Pisiform bone

Abductor digiti minimi m.

Opponens digiti minimi m.

Flexor digiti minimi brevis m.

4th dors. interosseous m.

3rd palmar interosseous m.

Abductor digiti minimi m.

Abductor pollicis longus m., tendons

Flexor carpi radialis m., tendon

Flexor retinaculum

Abductor pollicis brevis m., head

Flexor pollicis brevis m., superf. head

Flexor pollicis brevis m., deep head

Opponens pollicis m.

Adductor pollicis m.

Flexor pollicis brevis m., superf. head

Abductor pollicis brevis m.

Flexor pollicis longus m., tendon

1st dors. interosseous m.

Lumbrical mm.

Vincula longa

Vinculum breve

Vincula tendinum

Vincula longa

Flexor digitorum profundus m., tendon

Vinculum breve

Flexor digitorum profundus m., tendon

Flexor digitorum superficialis m., tendon

Fig. 374 Muscles of the left hand, palmar aspect (70%). The deep layer after removal of the superficial and deep flexors of the fingers along with several thenar and hypothenar muscles.

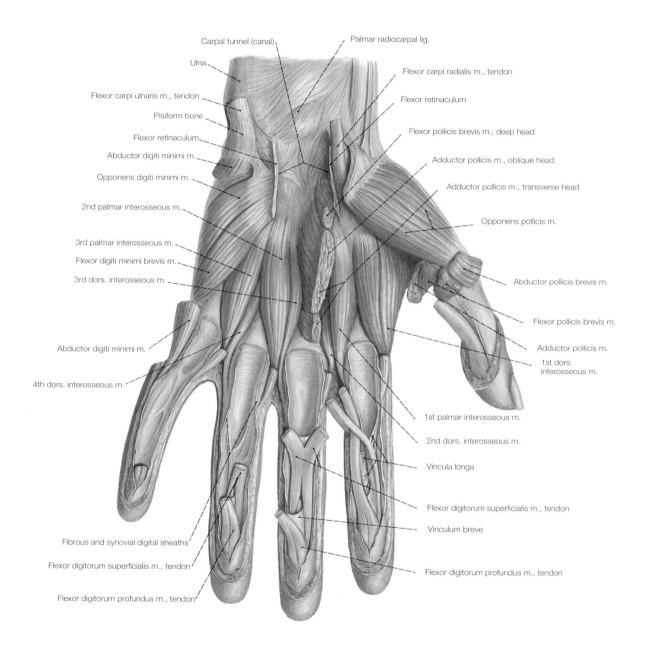

Carpal tunnel (canal)

Palmar radiocarpal lig.

Ulna

Flexor carpi radialis m., tendon

Flexor carpi ulnaris m., tendon

Flexor retinaculum

Pisiform bone

Flexor pollicis brevis m., deep head

Flexor retinaculum

Adductor pollicis m., oblique head

Abductor digiti minimi m.

Adductor pollicis m., transverse head

Opponens digiti minimi m.

Opponens pollicis m.

2nd palmar interosseous m.

3rd palmar interosseous m.

Flexor digiti minimi brevis m.

3rd dors. interosseous m.

Abductor pollicis brevis m.

Flexor pollicis brevis m.

Adductor pollicis m.

Abductor digiti minimi m.

1st dors. interosseous m.

4th dors. interosseous m.

1st palmar interosseous m.

2nd dors. interosseous m.

Vincula longa

Flexor digitorum superficialis m., tendon

Vinculum breve

Fibrous and synovial digital sheaths

Flexor digitorum superficialis m., tendon

Flexor digitorum profundus m., tendon

Flexor digitorum profundus m., tendon

Fig. 375 Muscles of the left hand, palmar aspect (70%). The deepest layer with both heads of the adductor pollicis muscle sectioned.

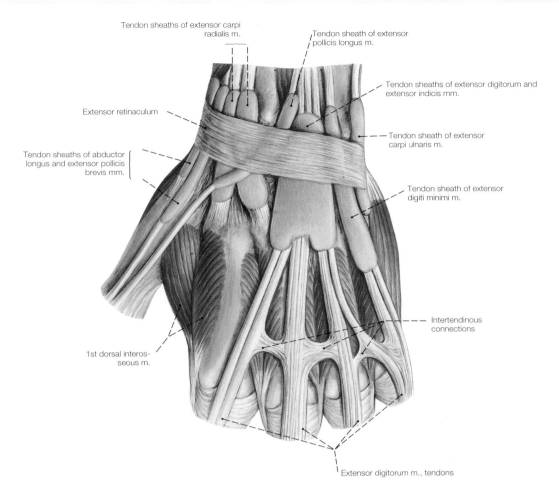

Tendon sheaths of extensor carpi radialis m.

Tendon sheath of extensor pollicis longus m.

Tendon sheaths of extensor digitorum and extensor indicis mm.

Extensor retinaculum

Tendon sheath of extensor carpi ulnaris m.

Tendon sheaths of abductor longus and extensor pollicis brevis mm.

Tendon sheath of extensor digiti minimi m.

Intertendinous connections

1st dorsal interosseous m.

Extensor digitorum m., tendons

Fig. 376 The dorsal carpal tendon sheaths of the left hand (80%), dorsal aspect.

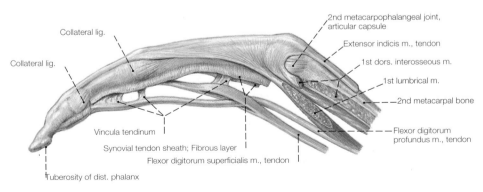

Collateral lig.

2nd metacarpophalangeal joint, articular capsule

Collateral lig.

Extensor indicis m., tendon

1st dors. interosseous m.

1st lumbrical m.

2nd metacarpal bone

Vincula tendinum

Synovial tendon sheath; Fibrous layer

Flexor digitorum profundus m., tendon

Flexor digitorum superficialis m., tendon

Tuberosity of dist. phalanx

Fig. 377 The tendon insertions of the right index finger, viewed from the lateral (radial) aspect (85%). The tendons of both flexors of the finger have been dissected from the tendon sheath.

The tendons of the interosseous and lumbrical muscles along with the tendons of the digital

extensor muscles radiate into the dorsal aponeurosis (extensor hood) of the finger. Note the course of these tendons in relation to the axis of the metacarpophalangeal joint.

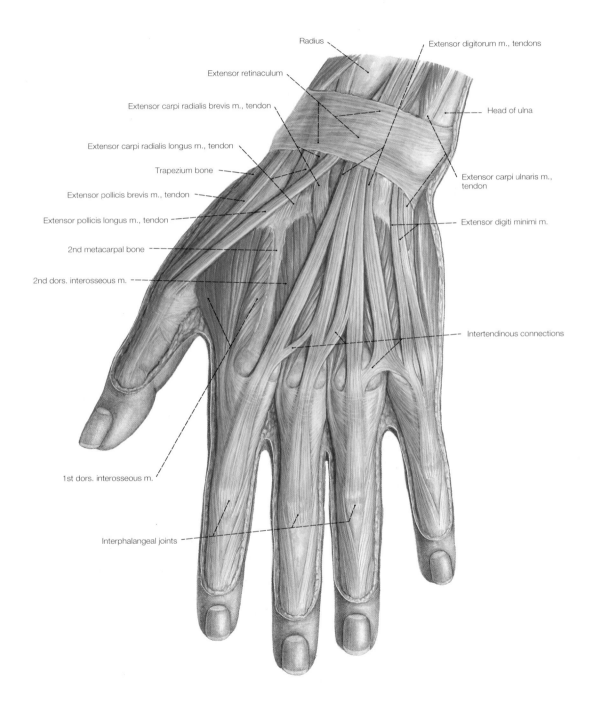

Radius

Extensor digitorum m., tendons

Extensor retinaculum

Head of ulna

Extensor carpi radialis brevis m., tendon

Extensor carpi radialis longus m., tendon

Trapezium bone

Extensor carpi ulnaris m., tendon

Extensor pollicis brevis m., tendon

Extensor pollicis longus m., tendon

Extensor digiti minimi m.

2nd metacarpal bone

2nd dors. interosseous m.

Intertendinous connections

1st dors. interosseous m.

Interphalangeal joints

Fig. 378 The muscles of left hand, dorsal aspect (80%).

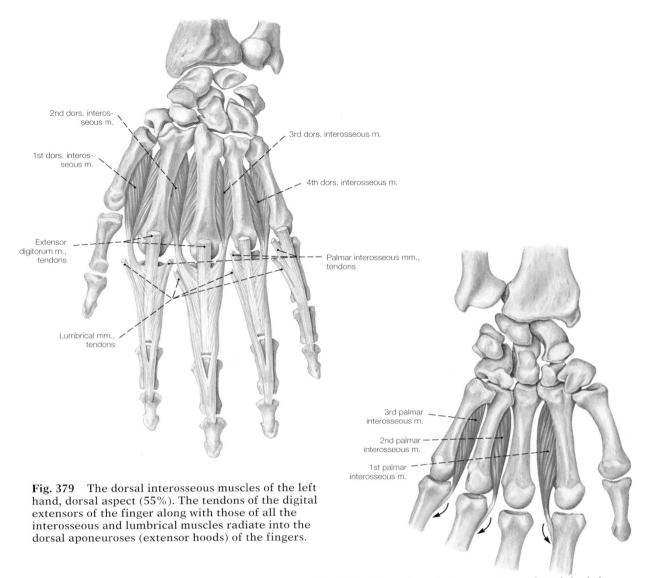

Fig. 379 The dorsal interosseous muscles of the left hand, dorsal aspect (55%). The tendons of the digital extensors of the finger along with those of all the interosseous and lumbrical muscles radiate into the dorsal aponeuroses (extensor hoods) of the fingers.

Fig. 380 The palmar interosseous muscles of the left hand, palmar aspect (55%). The tendons of the palmar interosseous muscles also radiate into the dorsal aponeuroses (extensor hoods) of the fingers (indicated by the arrows).

Interosseous Muscles of the Hand

Name *Innervation*	Origin	Insertion	Function
Dorsal interosseous mm. *Ulnar n.*	By two heads from 1st–5th metacarpal bones	Extensor hood of 2nd–4th fingers	*Metacarpophalangeal joints (2nd–4th)* Flexion, abduction (in relation to middle finger) *Interphalangeal joints (digits 2–5)* Extension
Palmar interosseous mm. *Ulnar n.*	By one head from 2nd–5th metacarpal bones	Extensor hood of 2nd–5th fingers	*Metacarpophalangeal joints (2nd–4th)* Flexion, adduction (In relation to middle finger) *Interphalangeal joints (digits 2–5)* Extension

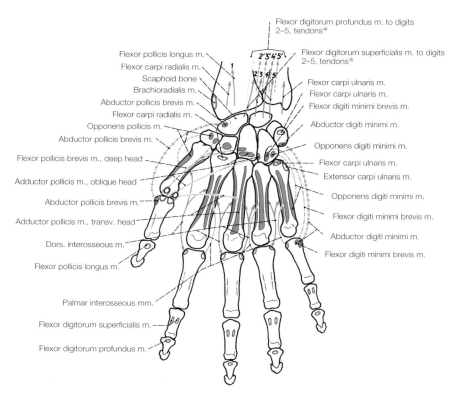

Flexor digitorum profundus m. to digits 2–5, tendons*

Flexor pollicis longus m.
Flexor carpi radialis m.
Scaphoid bone
Brachioradialis m.
Abductor pollicis brevis m.
Flexor carpi radialis m.
Opponens pollicis m.
Abductor pollicis brevis m.
Flexor pollicis brevis m., deep head
Adductor pollicis m., oblique head
Abductor pollicis brevis m.
Adductor pollicis m., transv. head
Dors. interosseous m.
Flexor pollicis longus m.

Flexor digitorum superficialis m. to digits 2–5, tendons*
Flexor carpi ulnaris m.
Flexor carpi ulnaris m.
Flexor digiti minimi brevis m.
Abductor digiti minimi m.
Opponens digiti minimi m.
Flexor carpi ulnaris m.
Extensor carpi ulnaris m.
Opponens digiti minimi m.
Flexor digiti minimi brevis m.
Abductor digiti minimi m.
Flexor digiti minimi brevis m.

Palmar interosseous mm.
Flexor digitorum superficialis m.
Flexor digitorum profundus m.

Fig. 381 Muscle origins and insertions on the bones of the right hand, palmar aspect.

* The flexors supply digits 2–5

Innervation of the Muscles of the Upper Limb

Thoracodorsal n.	Latissimus dorsi m. Teres major m. (Var.)	*Median n.*	Pronator teres m. Flexor carpi radialis m. Palmaris longus m.
Suprascapular n.	Supraspinatus m. Infraspinatus m.		Flexor digitorum superficialis m. Flexor digitorum profundus m. (radial part)
Subscapular n.	Subscapularis m. Teres major m.		Flexor pollicis longus m. Pronator quadratus m. Palmaris brevis m.
Axillary n.	Deltoid m. Teres minor m.		Opponens pollicis m. Abductor pollicis brevis m. 1st and 2nd lumbrical mm.
Radial n.	Triceps brachii m. Anconeus m. Brachioradialis m. Extensor carpi radialis longus m. Extensor carpi radialis brevis m. Extensor carpi ulnaris m. Extensor digitorum m. Extensor digiti minimi m. Extensor pollicis longus m. Abductor pollicis longus m. Extensor pollicis brevis m. Supinator m.	*Ulnar n.*	3rd and 4th lumbrical mm. Dorsal interosseous mm. Palmar interosseous mm. Flexor carpi ulnaris m. Flexor digitorum profundus m. (ulnar part) Abductor digiti minimi m. Flexor digiti minimi brevis m. Opponens digiti minimi m. Opponens pollicis m. Flexor pollicis brevis m. Adductor pollicis m.
Musculocutaneous n.	Biceps brachii m. Brachialis m. Coracobrachialis m.		

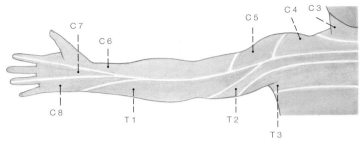

Fig. 382 Segmental cutaneous innervation (dermatomes) of the upper limb, anterior aspect.

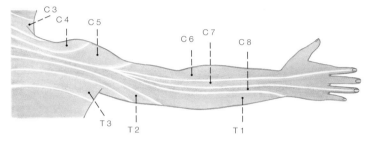

Fig. 383 Segmental cutaneous innervation (dermatomes) of the upper limb, posterior aspect.

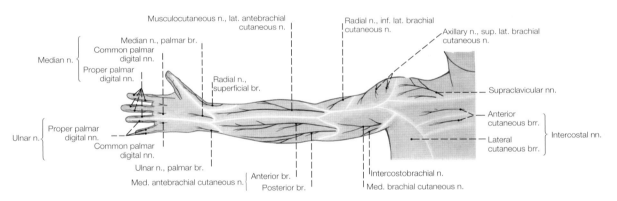

Fig. 384 Cutaneous nerves of the upper limb, anterior aspect.

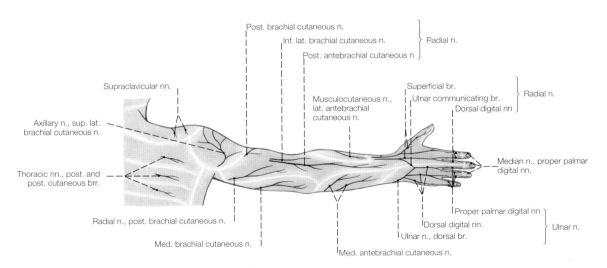

Fig. 385 Cutaneous nerves of the upper limb, posterior aspect.

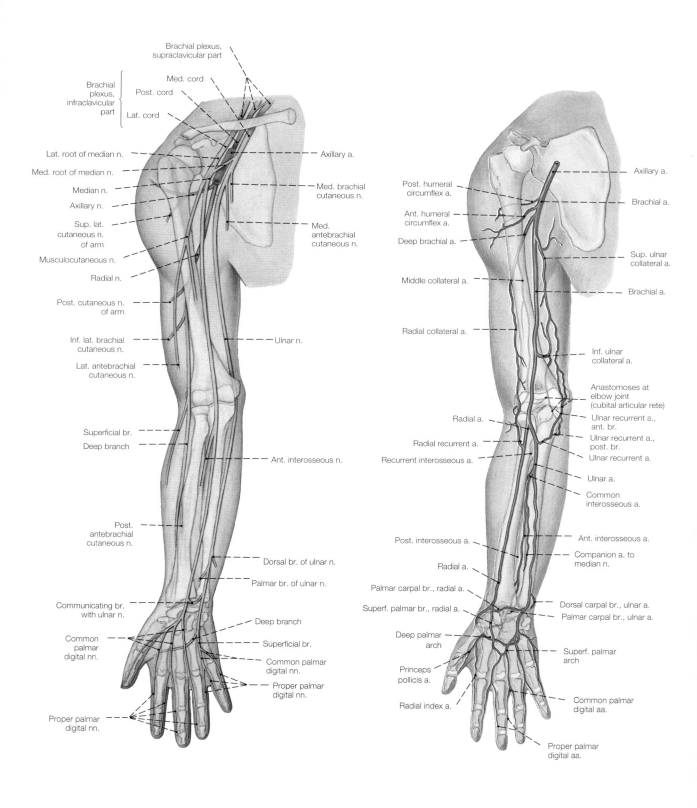

Brachial plexus, supraclavicular part

Brachial plexus, infraclavicular part

Med. cord

Post. cord

Lat. cord

Lat. root of median n.

Med. root of median n.

Median n.

Axillary n.

Sup. lat. cutaneous n. of arm

Musculocutaneous n.

Radial n.

Post. cutaneous n. of arm

Inf. lat. brachial cutaneous n.

Lat. antebrachial cutaneous n.

Superficial br.

Deep branch

Post. antebrachial cutaneous n.

Communicating br. with ulnar n.

Common palmar digital nn.

Proper palmar digital nn.

Axillary a.

Med. brachial cutaneous n.

Med. antebrachial cutaneous n.

Ulnar n.

Ant. interosseous n.

Dorsal br. of ulnar n.

Palmar br. of ulnar n.

Deep branch

Superficial br.

Common palmar digital nn.

Proper palmar digital nn.

Fig. 386 Nerves of the upper limb; Survey, anterior aspect.

Post. humeral circumflex a.

Ant. humeral circumflex a.

Deep brachial a.

Middle collateral a.

Radial collateral a.

Radial a.

Radial recurrent a.

Recurrent interosseous a.

Post. interosseous a.

Radial a.

Palmar carpal br., radial a.

Superf. palmar br., radial a.

Deep palmar arch

Princeps pollicis a.

Radial index a.

Axillary a.

Brachial a.

Sup. ulnar collateral a.

Brachial a.

Inf. ulnar collateral a.

Anastomoses at elbow joint (cubital articular rete)

Ulnar recurrent a., ant. br.

Ulnar recurrent a., post. br.

Ulnar recurrent a.

Ulnar a.

Common interosseous a.

Ant. interosseous a.

Companion a. to median n.

Dorsal carpal br., ulnar a.

Palmar carpal br., ulnar a.

Superf. palmar arch

Common palmar digital aa.

Proper palmar digital aa.

Fig. 387 Arteries of the upper limb; Survey, anterior aspect.

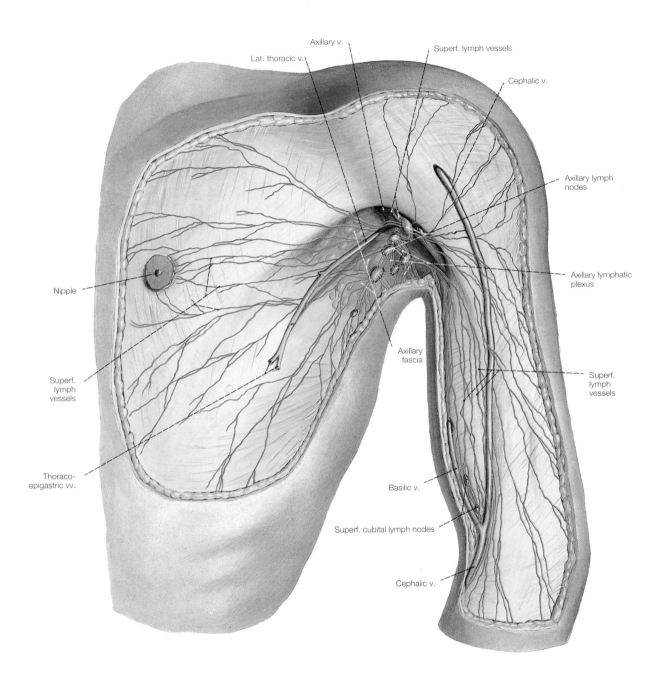

Fig. 388 Superficial lymphatic vessels, lymph
nodes, and veins of the left arm, lateral thoracic
wall and axilla, anterior view (50%).

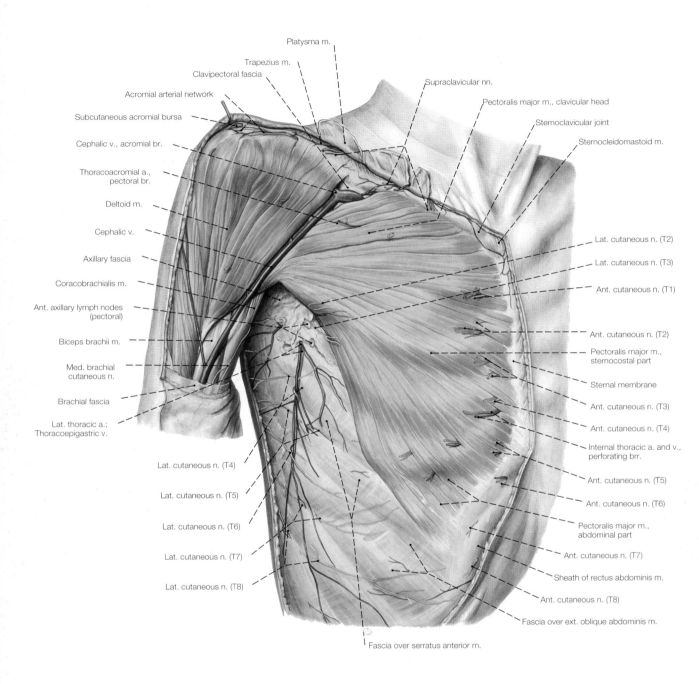

Platysma m.

Trapezius m.

Clavipectoral fascia

Supraclavicular nn.

Acromial arterial network

Pectoralis major m., clavicular head

Subcutaneous acromial bursa

Sternoclavicular joint

Cephalic v., acromial br.

Sternocleidomastoid m.

Thoracoacromial a.,
pectoral br.

Deltoid m.

Lat. cutaneous n. (T2)

Cephalic v.

Lat. cutaneous n. (T3)

Axillary fascia

Ant. cutaneous n. (T1)

Coracobrachialis m.

Ant. axillary lymph nodes
(pectoral)

Ant. cutaneous n. (T2)

Biceps brachii m.

Pectoralis major m.,
sternocostal part

Med. brachial
cutaneous n.

Sternal membrane

Brachial fascia

Ant. cutaneous n. (T3)

Ant. cutaneous n. (T4)

Lat. thoracic a.;
Thoracoepigastric v.

Internal thoracic a. and v.,
perforating brr.

Lat. cutaneous n. (T4)

Ant. cutaneous n. (T5)

Lat. cutaneous n. (T5)

Ant. cutaneous n. (T6)

Lat. cutaneous n. (T6)

Pectoralis major m.,
abdominal part

Lat. cutaneous n. (T7)

Ant. cutaneous n. (T7)

Lat. cutaneous n. (T8)

Sheath of rectus abdominis m.

Ant. cutaneous n. (T8)

Fascia over ext. oblique abdominis m.

Fascia over serratus anterior m.

Fig. 389 Vessels and nerves of the right arm and
shoulder and the deltopectoral triangle,
anterolateral view (45%).

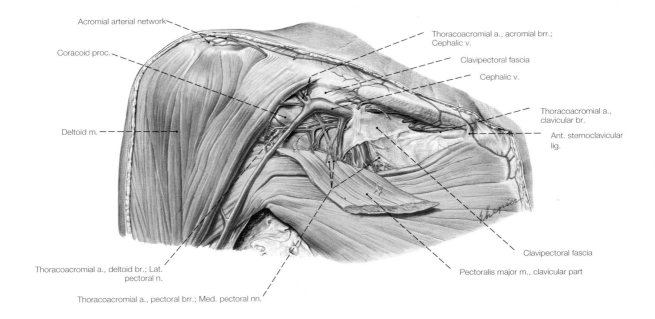

Acromial arterial network

Coracoid proc.

Deltoid m.

Thoracoacromial a., deltoid br.; Lat. pectoral n.

Thoracoacromial a., pectoral brr.; Med. pectoral nn.

Thoracoacromial a., acromial brr.; Cephalic v.

Clavipectoral fascia

Cephalic v.

Thoracoacromial a., clavicular br.

Ant. sternoclavicular lig.

Clavipectoral fascia

Pectoralis major m., clavicular part

Fig. 390 The right deltopectoral triangle, anterior view (45%). The clavicular part of the pectoralis major muscle has been removed.

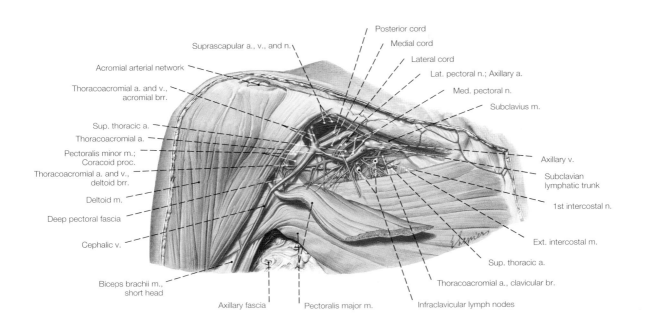

Suprascapular a., v., and n.

Acromial arterial network

Thoracoacromial a. and v., acromial brr.

Sup. thoracic a.

Thoracoacromial a.

Pectoralis minor m.; Coracoid proc.

Thoracoacromial a. and v., deltoid brr.

Deltoid m.

Deep pectoral fascia

Cephalic v.

Biceps brachii m., short head

Axillary fascia

Pectoralis major m.

Posterior cord

Medial cord

Lateral cord

Lat. pectoral n.; Axillary a.

Med. pectoral n.

Subclavius m.

Axillary v.

Subclavian lymphatic trunk

1st intercostal n.

Ext. intercostal m.

Sup. thoracic a.

Thoracoacromial a., clavicular br.

Infraclavicular lymph nodes

Fig. 391 The right deltopectoral triangle, anterior view (45%). The clavipectoral fascia has been removed.

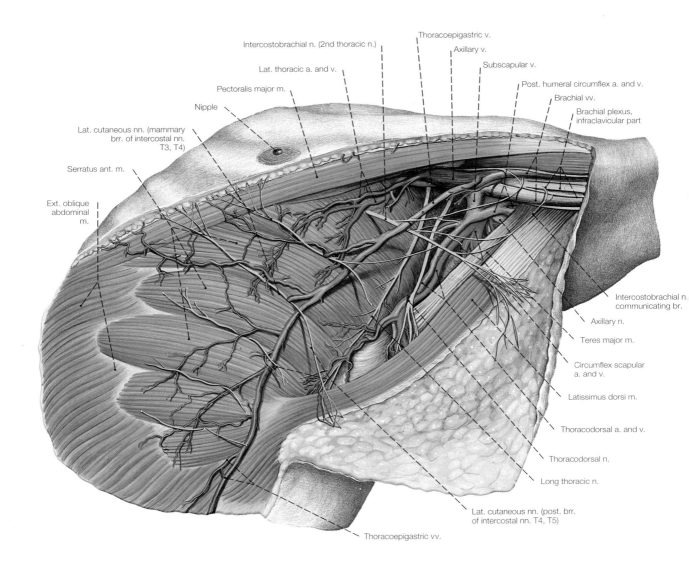

Intercostobrachial n. (2nd thoracic n.)

Thoracoepigastric v.

Axillary v.

Subscapular v.

Lat. thoracic a. and v.

Post. humeral circumflex a. and v.

Pectoralis major m.

Brachial vv.

Nipple

Brachial plexus, infraclavicular part

Lat. cutaneous nn. (mammary brr. of intercostal nn. T3, T4)

Serratus ant. m.

Ext. oblique abdominal m.

Intercostobrachial n. communicating br.

Axillary n.

Teres major m.

Circumflex scapular a. and v.

Latissimus dorsi m.

Thoracodorsal a. and v.

Thoracodorsal n.

Long thoracic n.

Lat. cutaneous nn. (post. brr. of intercostal nn. T4, T5)

Thoracoepigastric vv.

Fig. 392 The left axilla, viewed from below (50%). The axillary fascia and the fascia of the lateral thoracic wall have been removed.

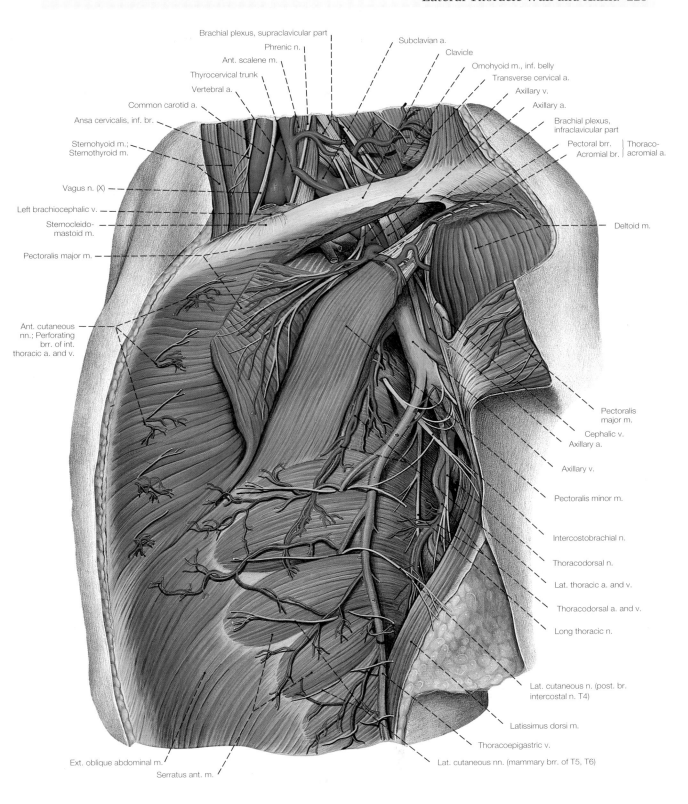

Fig. 393 The left lateral thoracic wall, infraclavicular fossa, and axilla, lateral aspect (60%). The pectoralis major and the sternocleidomastoid muscles have been sectioned.

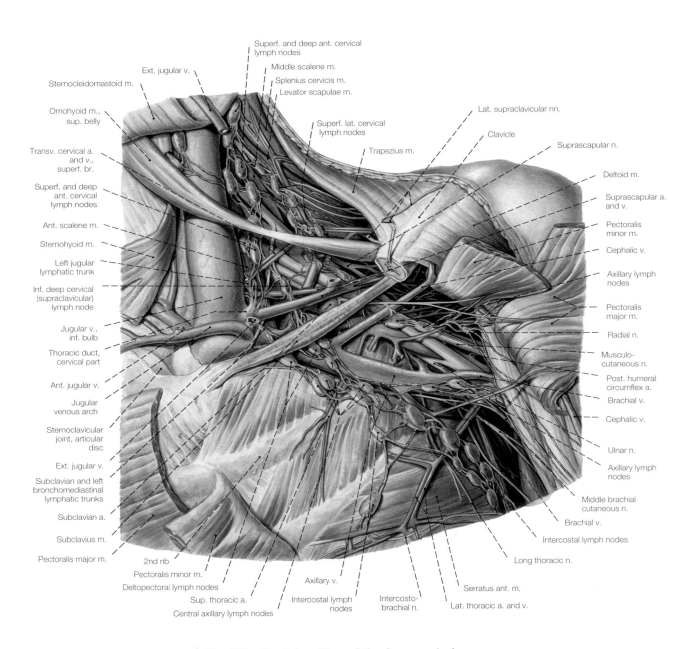

Superf. and deep ant. cervical lymph nodes

Ext. jugular v.

Middle scalene m.

Splenius cervicis m.

Levator scapulae m.

Sternocleidomastoid m.

Superf. lat. cervical lymph nodes

Lat. supraclavicular nn.

Omohyoid m., sup. belly

Clavicle

Suprascapular n.

Trapezius m.

Transv. cervical a. and v., superf. br.

Deltoid m.

Superf. and deep ant. cervical lymph nodes

Suprascapular a. and v.

Pectoralis minor m.

Ant. scalene m.

Cephalic v.

Sternohyoid m.

Axillary lymph nodes

Left jugular lymphatic trunk

Pectoralis major m.

Inf. deep cervical (supraclavicular) lymph node

Radial n.

Jugular v., inf. bulb

Musculo-cutaneous n.

Thoracic duct, cervical part

Post. humeral circumflex a.

Ant. jugular v.

Brachial v.

Jugular venous arch

Cephalic v.

Sternoclavicular joint, articular disc

Ulnar n.

Ext. jugular v.

Axillary lymph nodes

Subclavian and left bronchomediastinal lymphatic trunks

Middle brachial cutaneous n.

Subclavian a.

Brachial v.

Subclavius m.

Intercostal lymph nodes

Pectoralis major m.

2nd rib

Long thoracic n.

Pectoralis minor m.

Serratus ant. m.

Deltopectoral lymph nodes

Axillary v.

Lat. thoracic a. and v.

Sup. thoracic a.

Intercostal lymph nodes

Intercosto-brachial n.

Central axillary lymph nodes

Fig. 394 The left axilla and the deep cervical region, anterior view (60%). The clavicle has been partially removed and the pectoralis muscles have been sectioned.

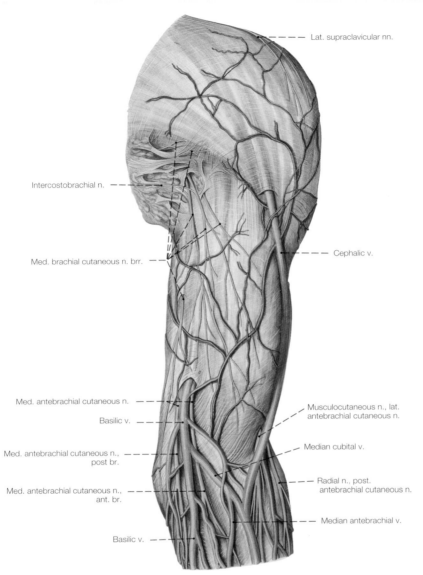

Lat. supraclavicular nn.

Intercostobrachial n.

Med. brachial cutaneous n. brr.

Cephalic v.

Med. antebrachial cutaneous n.

Basilic v.

Med. antebrachial cutaneous n., post br.

Med. antebrachial cutaneous n., ant. br.

Basilic v.

Musculocutaneous n., lat. antebrachial cutaneous n.

Median cubital v.

Radial n., post. antebrachial cutaneous n.

Median antebrachial v.

Fig. 395 Superficial veins and cutaneous nerves of the anterior aspect of the left arm and the cubital fossa (35%).

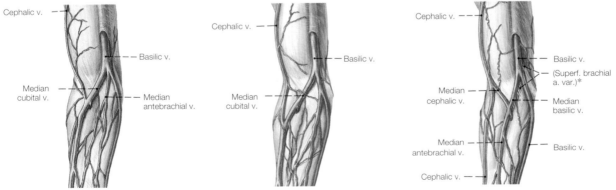

Cephalic v.

Basilic v.

Median cubital v.

Median antebrachial v.

Cephalic v.

Basilic v.

Median cubital v.

Cephalic v.

Basilic v.

(Superf. brachial a. var.)*

Median cephalic v.

Median basilic v.

Median antebrachial v.

Basilic v.

Cephalic v.

Fig. 396 Variations in the superficial veins of the region of the right elbow. The veins of the cubital fossa, being easily accessible, are preferred for blood draws and intravenous injections over those in other regions of the body.

* This variation can be particularly dangerous in the rare case when an intravenous injection mistakenly becomes intraarterial.

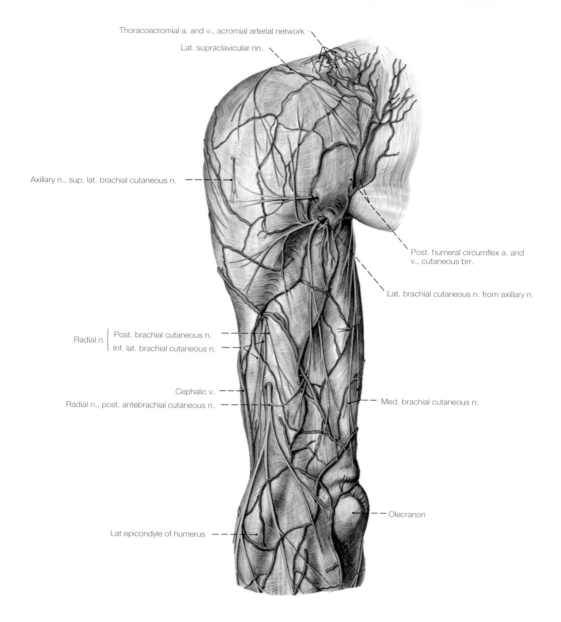

Thoracoacromial a. and v., acromial arterial network

Lat. supraclavicular nn.

Axillary n., sup. lat. brachial cutaneous n.

Post. humeral circumflex a. and v., cutaneous brr.

Lat. brachial cutaneous n. from axillary n.

Radial n. { Post. brachial cutaneous n.
Inf. lat. brachial cutaneous n.

Cephalic v.

Radial n., post. antebrachial cutaneous n.

Med. brachial cutaneous n.

Olecranon

Lat epicondyle of humerus

Fig. 397 Superficial blood vessels and cutaneous nerves of the posterior aspect of the left arm and elbow (35%).

Superficial Veins of the Upper Limb

The cephalic vein begins in the venous network on the radial side of the dorsum of the hand, receives tributaries from the palm of the hand via the intercapitular veins, courses proximally on the radial border of the forearm to the cubital fossa where it anastomoses with the basilic vein. It continues in the arm, generally smaller than in the forearm, in the lateral bicipital sulcus proximally to the deltopectoral triangle, where it pierces the clavipectoral fascia and enters the axillary vein.

The basilic vein originates in the venous network on the ulnar side of the dorsum of the hand, ascends on the posterior surface of the ulnar side of the forearm to the cubital fossa where it connects to the cephalic vein via the median cubital vein. Continuing proximally in the arm, it runs in the medial bicipital sulcus to somewhat below the middle of the arm where it perforates the deep fascia and joins the medial branch of the brachial vein.

The median cubital vein is the oblique, highly variable, anastomosis between the basilic and cephalic veins, and, in most instances, receives the median antebrachial vein which drains the superficial venous palmar arch of the hand and the forearm.

The median basilic and median cephalic veins form connections between the basilic, cephalic and median antebrachial veins.

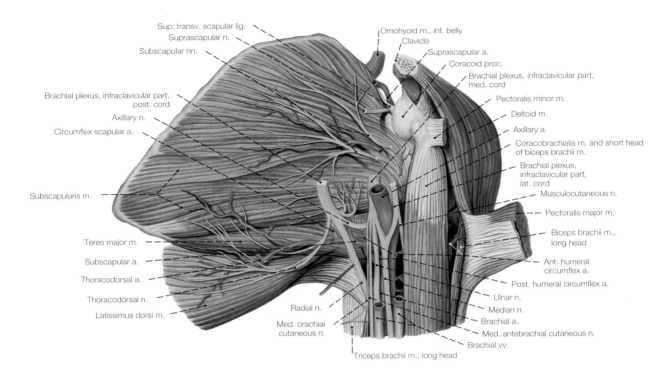

Sup. transv. scapular lig.
Suprascapular n.
Subscapular nn.
Omohyoid m., inf. belly
Clavicle
Suprascapular a.
Coracoid proc.
Brachial plexus, infraclavicular part, med. cord
Pectoralis minor m.
Deltoid m.
Axillary a.
Coracobrachialis m. and short head of biceps brachii m.
Brachial plexus, infraclavicular part, lat. cord
Musculocutaneous n.
Pectoralis major m.
Biceps brachii m., long head
Ant. humeral circumflex a.
Post. humeral circumflex a.
Ulnar n.
Median n.
Brachial a.
Med. antebrachial cutaneous n.
Brachial vv.
Brachial plexus, infraclavicular part, post. cord
Axillary n.
Circumflex scapular a.
Subscapularis m.
Teres major m.
Subscapular a.
Thoracodorsal a.
Thoracodorsal n.
Latissimus dorsi m.
Radial n.
Med. brachial cutaneous n.
Triceps brachii m., long head

Fig. 398 Blood vessels and nerves of the left axilla and shoulder, anterior aspect (60%). The clavicle has been sectioned and the arm detached from the body.

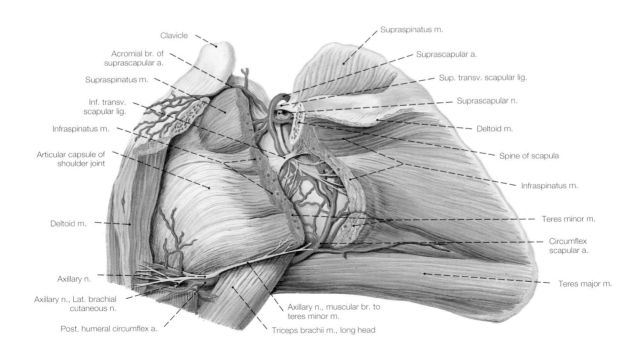

Clavicle
Acromial br. of suprascapular a.
Supraspinatus m.
Inf. transv. scapular lig.
Infraspinatus m.
Articular capsule of shoulder joint
Deltoid m.
Axillary n.
Axillary n., Lat. brachial cutaneous n.
Post. humeral circumflex a.
Supraspinatus m.
Suprascapular a.
Sup. transv. scapular lig.
Suprascapular n.
Deltoid m.
Spine of scapula
Infraspinatus m.
Teres minor m.
Circumflex scapular a.
Teres major m.
Axillary n., muscular br. to teres minor m.
Triceps brachii m., long head

Fig. 399 Blood vessels and nerves of the left shoulder, posterior aspect (60%). The deltoid and trapezius muscles have been partially removed.

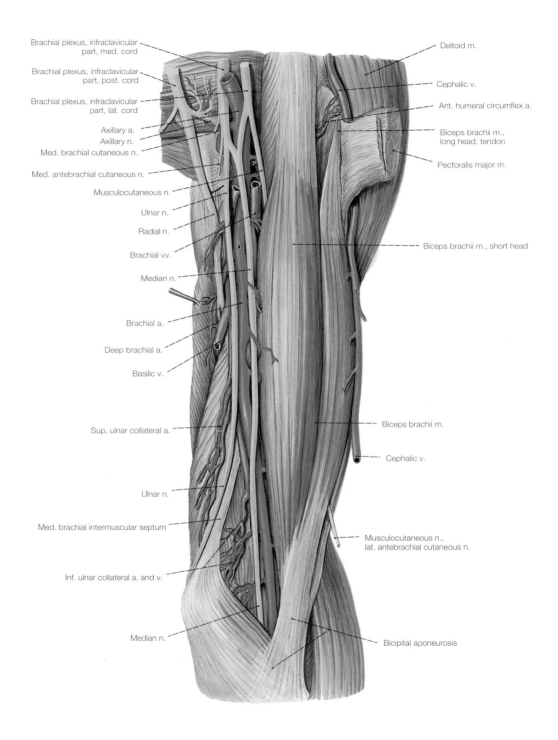

Brachial plexus, infraclavicular part, med. cord

Brachial plexus, infraclavicular part, post. cord

Brachial plexus, infraclavicular part, lat. cord

Axillary a.

Axillary n.

Med. brachial cutaneous n.

Med. antebrachial cutaneous n.

Musculocutaneous n.

Ulnar n.

Radial n.

Brachial vv.

Median n.

Brachial a.

Deep brachial a.

Basilic v.

Sup. ulnar collateral a.

Ulnar n.

Med. brachial intermuscular septum

Inf. ulnar collateral a. and v.

Median n.

Deltoid m.

Cephalic v.

Ant. humeral circumflex a.

Biceps brachii m., long head, tendon

Pectoralis major m.

Biceps brachii m., short head

Biceps brachii m.

Cephalic v.

Musculocutaneous n., lat. antebrachial cutaneous n.

Bicipital aponeurosis

Fig. 400 Blood vessels and nerves of the anterior aspect of the left arm, (45%).

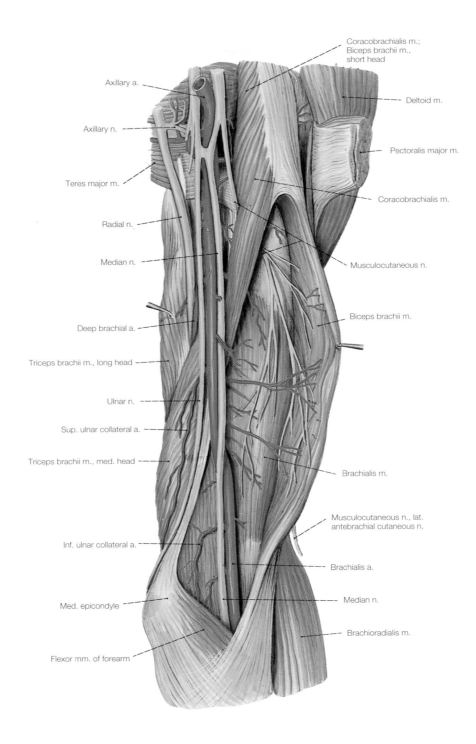

Coracobrachialis m.;
Biceps brachii m.,
short head

Axillary a.

Axillary n.

Deltoid m.

Pectoralis major m.

Teres major m.

Coracobrachialis m.

Radial n.

Median n.

Musculocutaneous n.

Biceps brachii m.

Deep brachial a.

Triceps brachii m., long head

Ulnar n.

Sup. ulnar collateral a.

Triceps brachii m., med. head

Brachialis m.

Musculocutaneous n., lat.
antebrachial cutaneous n.

Inf. ulnar collateral a.

Brachialis a.

Med. epicondyle

Median n.

Brachioradialis m.

Flexor mm. of forearm

Fig. 401 Arteries and nerves of the anterior aspect
of the left arm (45%). The musculocutaneus nerve
normally penetrates the coracobrachialis muscle.

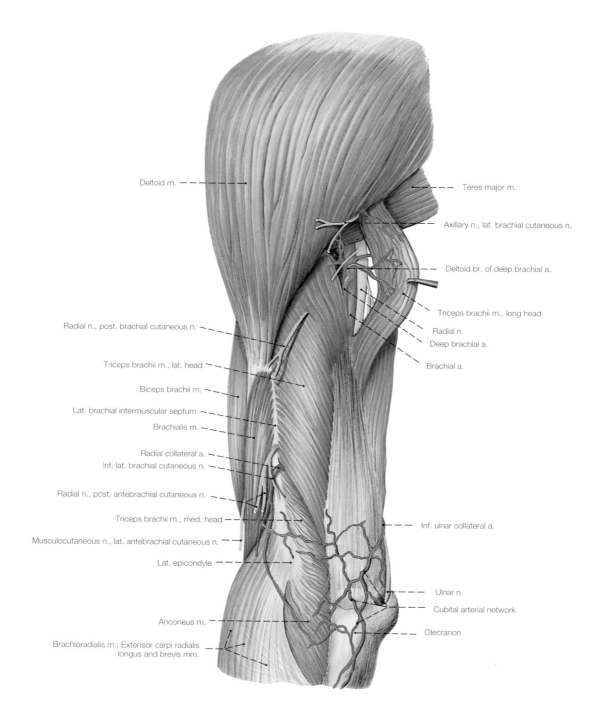

Deltoid m.

Teres major m.

Axillary n., lat. brachial cutaneous n.

Deltoid br. of deep brachial a.

Triceps brachii m., long head

Radial n.
Deep brachial a.

Brachial a.

Radial n., post. brachial cutaneous n.

Triceps brachii m., lat. head

Biceps brachii m.

Lat. brachial intermuscular septum

Brachialis m.

Radial collateral a.
Inf. lat. brachial cutaneous n.

Radial n., post. antebrachial cutaneous n.

Triceps brachii m., med. head

Inf. ulnar collateral a.

Musculocutaneous n., lat. antebrachial cutaneous n.

Lat. epicondyle

Ulnar n.
Cubital arterial network

Anconeus m.

Olecranon

Brachioradialis m.; Extensor carpi radialis
longus and brevis mm.

Fig. 402 Arteries and nerves of the
posterior aspect of the left arm (40%).

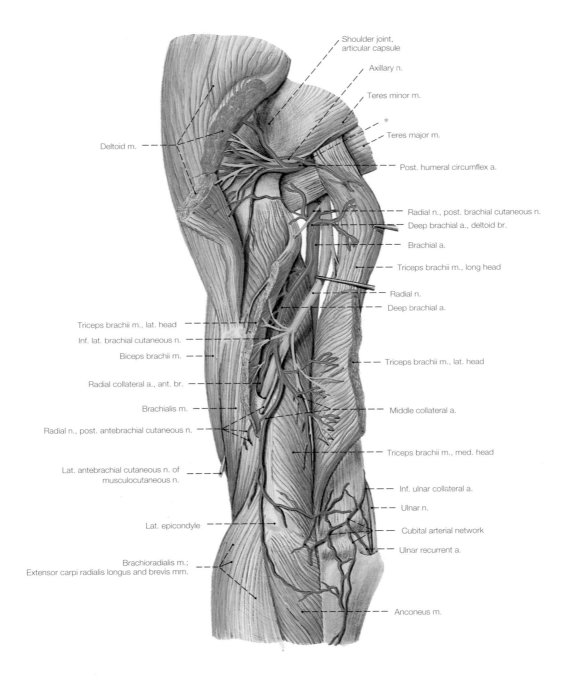

Shoulder joint, articular capsule

Axillary n.

Teres minor m.

*

Teres major m.

Post. humeral circumflex a.

Deltoid m.

Radial n., post. brachial cutaneous n.

Deep brachial a., deltoid br.

Brachial a.

Triceps brachii m., long head

Radial n.

Deep brachial a.

Triceps brachii m., lat. head

Inf. lat. brachial cutaneous n.

Biceps brachii m.

Triceps brachii m., lat. head

Radial collateral a., ant. br.

Brachialis m.

Middle collateral a.

Radial n., post. antebrachial cutaneous n.

Triceps brachii m., med. head

Lat. antebrachial cutaneous n. of musculocutaneous n.

Inf. ulnar collateral a.

Ulnar n.

Lat. epicondyle

Cubital arterial network

Ulnar recurrent a.

Brachioradialis m.; Extensor carpi radialis longus and brevis mm.

Anconeus m.

Fig. 403   Arteries and nerves of the posterior aspect of the left arm (45%).

* Quadrangular space

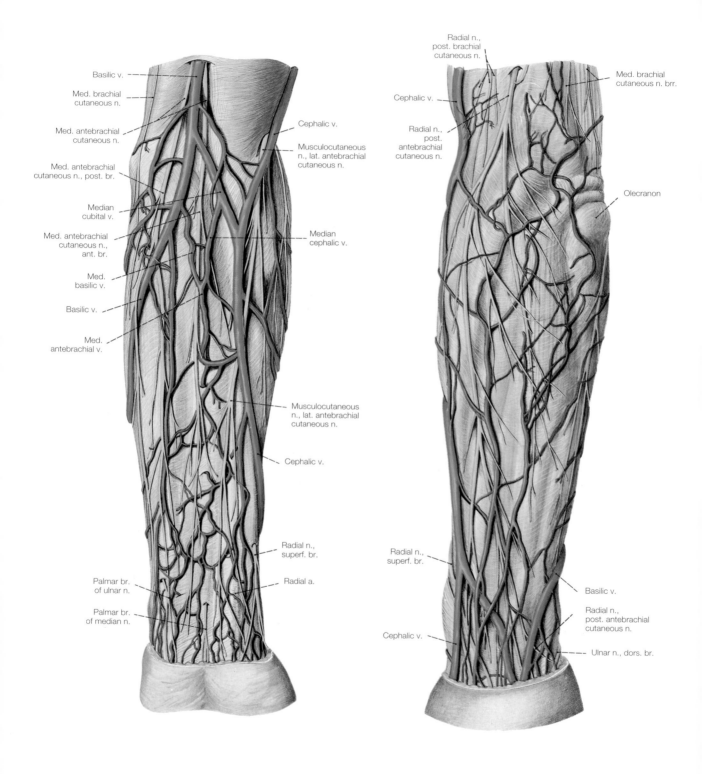

Basilic v.

Med. brachial
cutaneous n.

Med. antebrachial
cutaneous n.

Med. antebrachial
cutaneous n., post. br.

Median
cubital v.

Med. antebrachial
cutaneous n.,
ant. br.

Med.
basilic v.

Basilic v.

Med.
antebrachial v.

Cephalic v.

Musculocutaneous
n., lat. antebrachial
cutaneous n.

Median
cephalic v.

Musculocutaneous
n., lat. antebrachial
cutaneous n.

Cephalic v.

Radial n.,
superf. br.

Radial a.

Palmar br.
of ulnar n.

Palmar br.
of median n.

Radial n.,
post. brachial
cutaneous n.

Cephalic v.

Radial n.,
post.
antebrachial
cutaneous n.

Med. brachial
cutaneous n. brr.

Olecranon

Radial n.,
superf. br.

Cephalic v.

Basilic v.

Radial n.,
post. antebrachial
cutaneous n.

Ulnar n., dors. br.

Fig. 404 Superficial veins and nerves of the anterior
aspect of the left forearm (45%).

Fig. 405 Superficial veins and nerves of the posterior
aspect of the left forearm (45%).

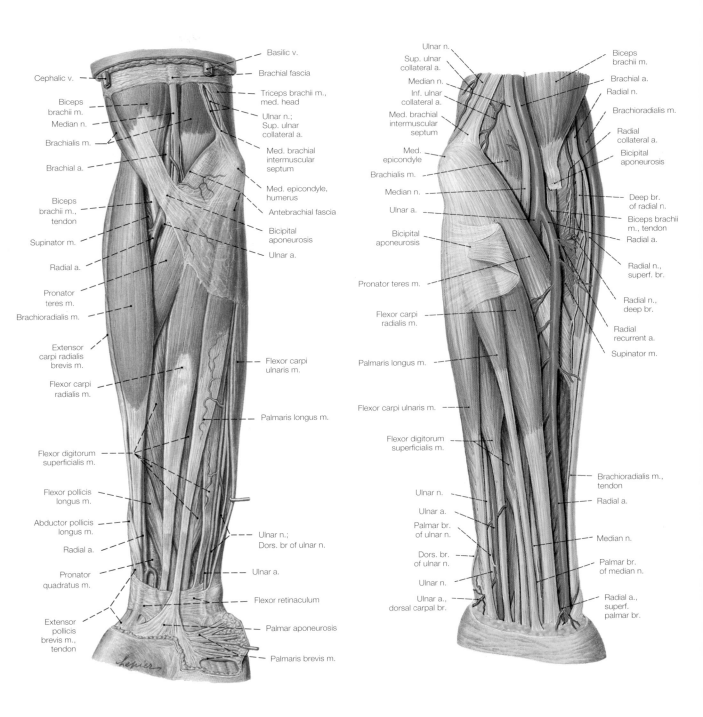

Fig. 406 Arteries and nerves of the anterior aspect of the right forearm (45%).

Fig. 407 Arteries and nerves of the anterior aspect of the left forearm (45%).

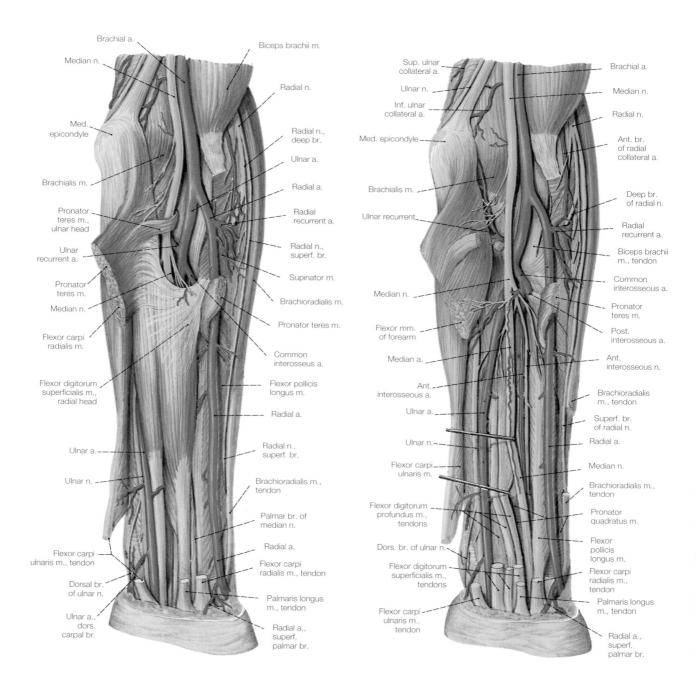

Brachial a.

Median n.

Med. epicondyle

Brachialis m.

Pronator teres m., ulnar head

Ulnar recurrent a.

Pronator teres m.

Median n.

Flexor carpi radialis m.

Flexor digitorum superficialis m., radial head

Ulnar a.

Ulnar n.

Flexor carpi ulnaris m., tendon

Dorsal br. of ulnar n.

Ulnar a., dors. carpal br.

Biceps brachii m.

Radial n.

Radial n., deep br.

Ulnar a.

Radial a.

Radial recurrent a.

Radial n., superf. br.

Supinator m.

Brachioradialis m.

Pronator teres m.

Common interosseus a.

Flexor pollicis longus m.

Radial a.

Radial n., superf. br.

Brachioradialis m., tendon

Palmar br. of median n.

Radial a.

Flexor carpi radialis m., tendon

Palmaris longus m., tendon

Radial a., superf. palmar br.

Sup. ulnar collateral a.

Ulnar n.

Inf. ulnar collateral a.

Med. epicondyle

Brachialis m.

Ulnar recurrent

Median n.

Flexor mm. of forearm

Median a.

Ant. interosseous a.

Ulnar a.

Ulnar n.

Flexor carpi ulnaris m.

Flexor digitorum profundus m., tendons

Dors. br. of ulnar n.

Flexor digitorum superficialis m., tendons

Flexor carpi ulnaris m., tendon

Brachial a.

Median n.

Radial n.

Ant. br. of radial collateral a.

Deep br. of radial n.

Radial recurrent a.

Biceps brachii m., tendon

Common interosseous a.

Pronator teres m.

Post. interosseous a.

Ant. interosseous n.

Brachioradialis m., tendon

Superf. br. of radial n.

Radial a.

Median n.

Brachioradialis m., tendon

Pronator quadratus m.

Flexor pollicis longus m.

Flexor carpi radialis m., tendon

Palmaris longus m., tendon

Radial a., superf. palmar br.

Fig. 408 Arteries and nerves of the anterior aspect of the left forearm, deep layer (45%).

Fig. 409 Arteries and nerves of the anterior aspect of the left forearm (45%). The deep layer after partial removal of the flexor digitorum superficialis muscle.

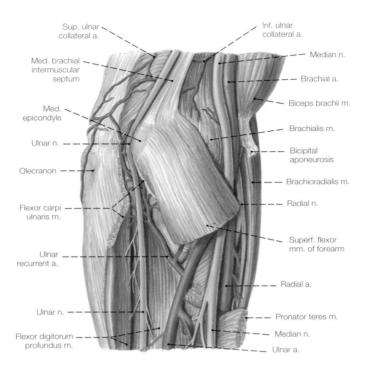

Sup. ulnar collateral a.

Med. brachial intermuscular septum

Med. epicondyle

Ulnar n.

Olecranon

Flexor carpi ulnaris m.

Ulnar recurrent a.

Ulnar n.

Flexor digitorum profundus m.

Inf. ulnar collateral a.

Median n.

Brachial a.

Biceps brachii m.

Brachialis m.

Bicipital aponeurosis

Brachioradialis m.

Radial n.

Superf. flexor mm. of forearm

Radial a.

Pronator teres m.

Median n.

Ulnar a.

Fig. 410 Arteries and nerves of the medial (ulnar) aspect of the left anterior cubital region (60%). The flexors of the forearm have been partially removed.

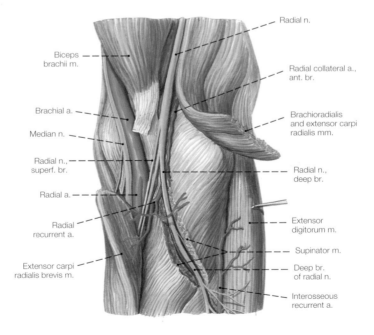

Biceps brachii m.

Brachial a.

Median n.

Radial n., superf. br.

Radial a.

Radial recurrent a.

Extensor carpi radialis brevis m.

Radial n.

Radial collateral a., ant. br.

Brachioradialis and extensor carpi radialis mm.

Radial n., deep br.

Extensor digitorum m.

Supinator m.

Deep br. of radial n.

Interosseous recurrent a.

Fig. 411 Arteries and nerves of the lateral (radial) aspect of the left anterior cubital region (60%). The radial group of muscles of the forearm has been sectioned.

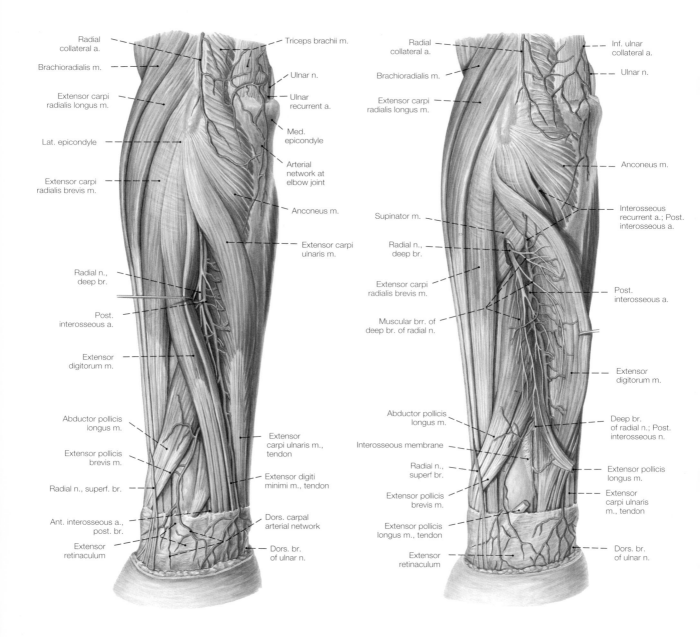

Radial collateral a.

Brachioradialis m.

Extensor carpi radialis longus m.

Lat. epicondyle

Extensor carpi radialis brevis m.

Radial n., deep br.

Post. interosseous a.

Extensor digitorum m.

Abductor pollicis longus m.

Extensor pollicis brevis m.

Radial n., superf. br.

Ant. interosseous a., post. br.

Extensor retinaculum

Triceps brachii m.

Ulnar n.

Ulnar recurrent a.

Med. epicondyle

Arterial network at elbow joint

Anconeus m.

Extensor carpi ulnaris m.

Extensor carpi ulnaris m., tendon

Extensor digiti minimi m., tendon

Dors. carpal arterial network

Dors. br. of ulnar n.

Radial collateral a.

Brachioradialis m.

Extensor carpi radialis longus m.

Supinator m.

Radial n., deep br.

Extensor carpi radialis brevis m.

Muscular brr. of deep br. of radial n.

Abductor pollicis longus m.

Interosseous membrane

Radial n., superf. br.

Extensor pollicis brevis m.

Extensor pollicis longus m., tendon

Extensor retinaculum

Inf. ulnar collateral a.

Ulnar n.

Anconeus m.

Interosseous recurrent a.; Post. interosseous a.

Post. interosseous a.

Extensor digitorum m.

Deep br. of radial n.; Post. interosseous n.

Extensor pollicis longus m.

Extensor carpi ulnaris m., tendon

Dors. br. of ulnar n.

Fig. 412 Arteries and nerves of the posterior aspect of the left forearm (45%).

Fig. 413 Arteries and nerves of the posterior aspect of the left forearm, deep layer (45%).

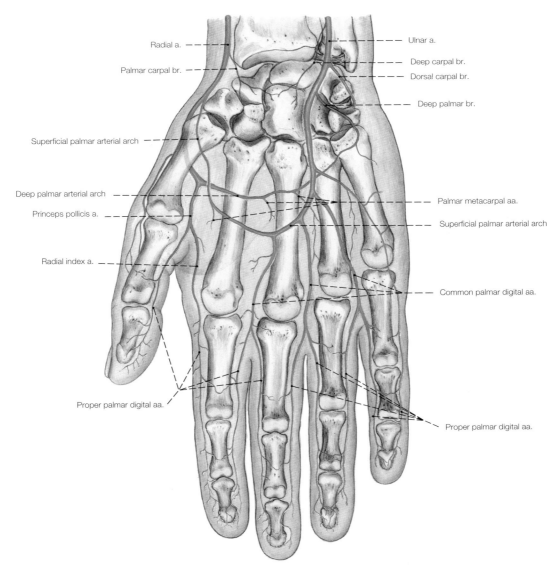

Radial a.

Palmar carpal br.

Ulnar a.

Deep carpal br.

Dorsal carpal br.

Deep palmar br.

Superficial palmar arterial arch

Deep palmar arterial arch

Princeps pollicis a.

Palmar metacarpal aa.

Superficial palmar arterial arch

Radial index a.

Common palmar digital aa.

Proper palmar digital aa.

Proper palmar digital aa.

Fig. 414 Arteries of the right hand, palmar aspect, overview (70%).

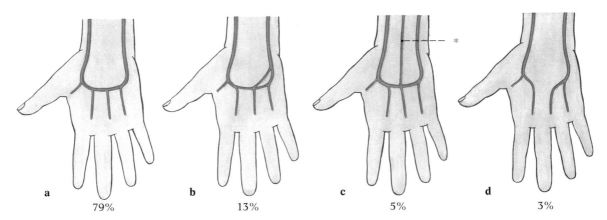

a 79%

b 13%

c 5%

d 3%

Fig. 415 a–d Variations of the deep palmar arterial arch. Percentages indicate the frequency of occurrence.

* Occasionally the anterior interosseous artery unites with the deep palmar arterial arch.

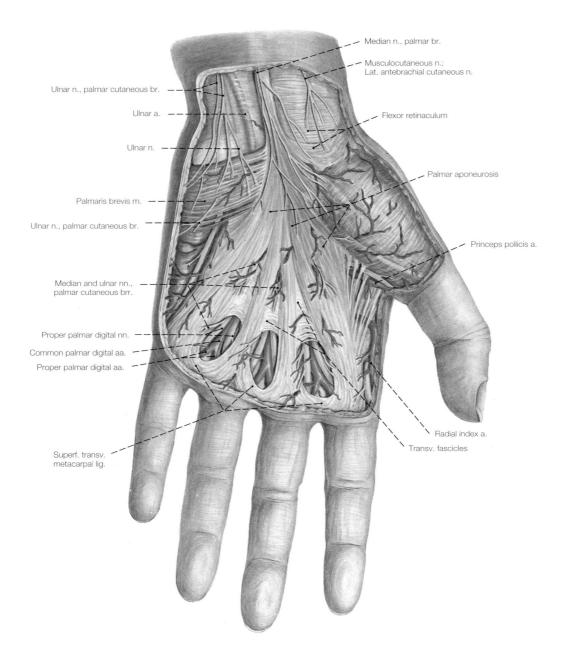

Median n., palmar br.

Musculocutaneous n.;
Lat. antebrachial cutaneous n.

Ulnar n., palmar cutaneous br.

Ulnar a.

Flexor retinaculum

Ulnar n.

Palmar aponeurosis

Palmaris brevis m.

Ulnar n., palmar cutaneous br.

Princeps pollicis a.

Median and ulnar nn.,
palmar cutaneous brr.

Proper palmar digital nn.

Common palmar digital aa.

Proper palmar digital aa.

Radial index a.

Transv. fascicles

Superf. transv.
metacarpal lig.

Fig. 416 Arteries and nerves of the palm of the left
hand, palmar aspect (70%).

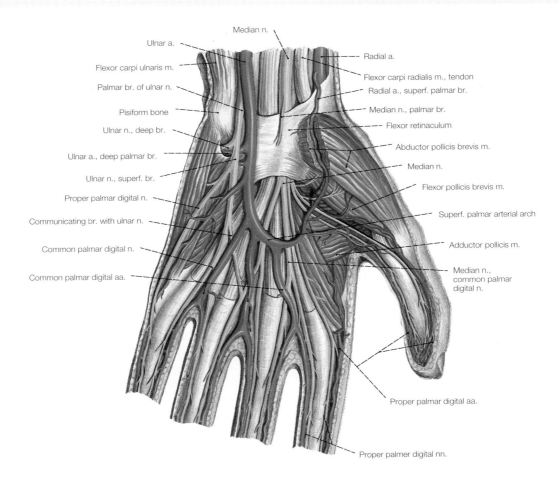

Median n.

Ulnar a.

Flexor carpi ulnaris m.

Palmar br. of ulnar n.

Pisiform bone

Ulnar n., deep br.

Ulnar a., deep palmar br.

Ulnar n., superf. br.

Proper palmar digital n.

Communicating br. with ulnar n.

Common palmar digital n.

Common palmar digital aa.

Radial a.

Flexor carpi radialis m., tendon

Radial a., superf. palmar br.

Median n., palmar br.

Flexor retinaculum

Abductor pollicis brevis m.

Median n.

Flexor pollicis brevis m.

Superf. palmar arterial arch

Adductor pollicis m.

Median n., common palmar digital n.

Proper palmar digital aa.

Proper palmer digital nn.

Fig. 417 Arteries and nerves of the palm of the left hand, palmar aspect (70%). The deep layer after removal of the palmar aponeurosis.

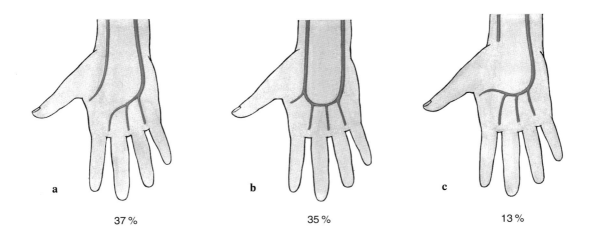

a

37 %

b

35 %

c

13 %

Fig. 418 a–c Variations of the superficial palmar arterial arch. Percentages indicate the frequency of occurrence.

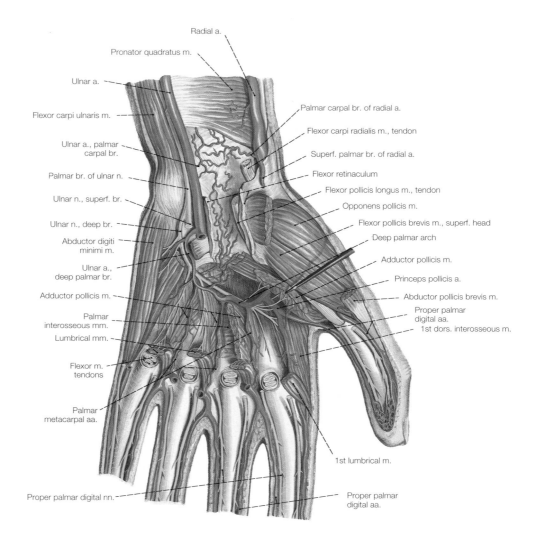

Radial a.

Pronator quadratus m.

Ulnar a.

Flexor carpi ulnaris m.

Ulnar a., palmar carpal br.

Palmar br. of ulnar n.

Ulnar n., superf. br.

Ulnar n., deep br.

Abductor digiti minimi m.

Ulnar a., deep palmar br.

Adductor pollicis m.

Palmar interosseous mm.

Lumbrical mm.

Flexor m. tendons

Palmar metacarpal aa.

Proper palmar digital nn.

Palmar carpal br. of radial a.

Flexor carpi radialis m., tendon

Superf. palmar br. of radial a.

Flexor retinaculum

Flexor pollicis longus m., tendon

Opponens pollicis m.

Flexor pollicis brevis m., superf. head

Deep palmar arch

Adductor pollicis m.

Princeps pollicis a.

Abductor pollicis brevis m.

Proper palmar digital aa.

1st dors. interosseous m.

1st lumbrical m.

Proper palmar digital aa.

Fig. 419 Arteries and nerves of the palm of the left hand, palmar aspect (75%). The deep layer with the transverse head of the adductor pollicis muscle sectioned.

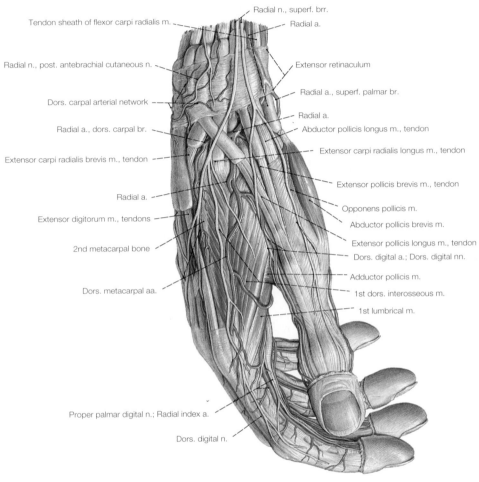

Tendon sheath of flexor carpi radialis m.

Radial n., post. antebrachial cutaneous n.

Dors. carpal arterial network

Radial a., dors. carpal br.

Extensor carpi radialis brevis m., tendon

Radial a.

Extensor digitorum m., tendons

2nd metacarpal bone

Dors. metacarpal aa.

Proper palmar digital n.; Radial index a.

Dors. digital n.

Radial n., superf. brr.

Radial a.

Extensor retinaculum

Radial a., superf. palmar br.

Radial a.

Abductor pollicis longus m., tendon

Extensor carpi radialis longus m., tendon

Extensor pollicis brevis m., tendon

Opponens pollicis m.

Abductor pollicis brevis m.

Extensor pollicis longus m., tendon

Dors. digital a.; Dors. digital nn.

Adductor pollicis m.

1st dors. interosseous m.

1st lumbrical m.

I–IV Tendon sheaths of extensor muscles:
I   Tendon sheath of abductor pollicis longus and extensor pollicis
      brevis muscles
II   Tendon sheath of extensor carpi radialis muscle
III   Tendon sheath of extensor pollicis longus muscle
IV   Tendon sheath of extensor digitorum and extensor indicis muscles

Fig. 420 Arteries and nerves of the right hand,
lateral (radial) aspect (65%).

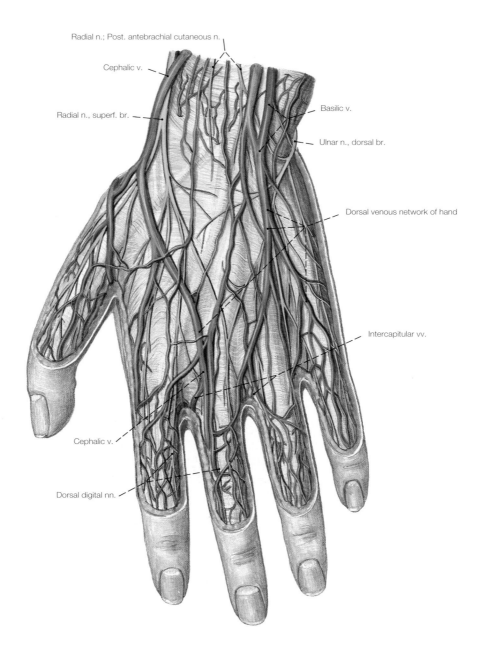

Radial n.; Post. antebrachial cutaneous n.

Cephalic v.

Radial n., superf. br.

Basilic v.

Ulnar n., dorsal br.

Dorsal venous network of hand

Intercapitular vv.

Cephalic v.

Dorsal digital nn.

Fig. 421 Blood vessels and nerves of the dorsum of the left hand, dorsal view (70%).

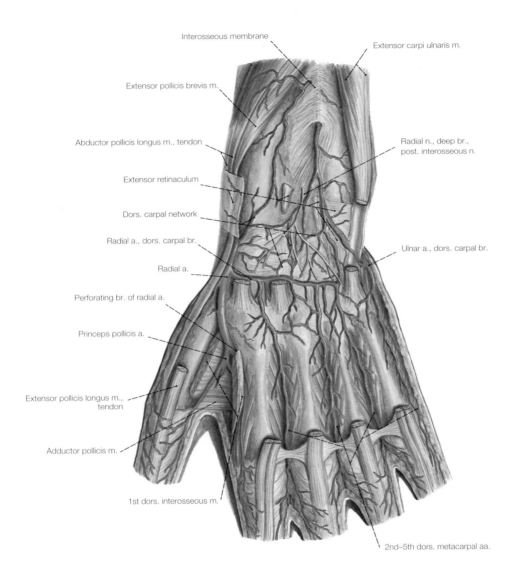

Interosseous membrane

Extensor carpi ulnaris m.

Extensor pollicis brevis m.

Abductor pollicis longus m., tendon

Radial n., deep br.,
post. interosseous n.

Extensor retinaculum

Dors. carpal network

Radial a., dors. carpal br.

Radial a.

Ulnar a., dors. carpal br.

Perforating br. of radial a.

Princeps pollicis a.

Extensor pollicis longus m.,
tendon

Adductor pollicis m.

1st dors. interosseous m.

2nd–5th dors. metacarpal aa.

Fig. 422 Arteries and nerves of the dorsum of
the left hand, deep layer, dorsal view (70%).

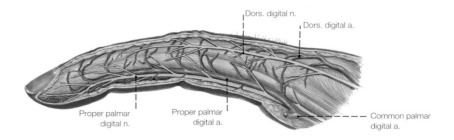

Fig. 423   Arteries and nerves of the right index finger, lateral (radial) aspect (80%).

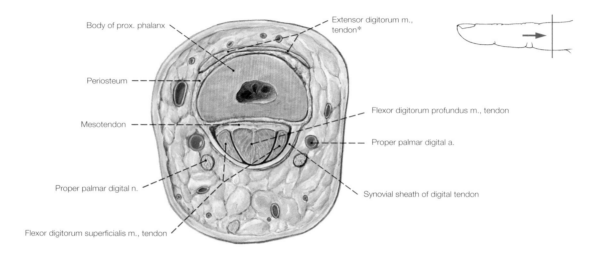

Fig. 424   The middle finger, the 3rd digit. Cross section through the shaft of the proximal phalanx, distal aspect.

* The extensor hood, i.e., aponeurosis of the tendons of the extensor digitorum muscle covering the dorsal surface of the phalanx, is reinforced by the tendons of the interosseous and lumbrical muscles.

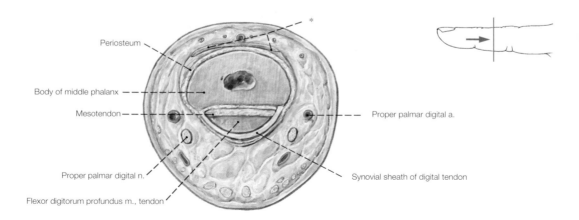

Fig. 425   The middle finger, the 3rd digit. Cross section through the shaft of the middle phalanx, distal aspect.

* Extensor hood (dorsal aponeurosis).
The location of the arteries and nerves of the finger is generally constant, making them easily accessible for anesthesia and hemostasis.

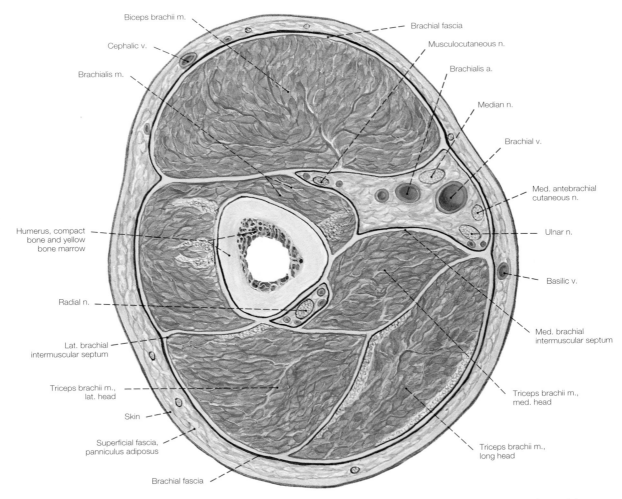

Biceps brachii m.

Cephalic v.

Brachialis m.

Humerus, compact bone and yellow bone marrow

Radial n.

Lat. brachial intermuscular septum

Triceps brachii m., lat. head

Skin

Superficial fascia, panniculus adiposus

Brachial fascia

Brachial fascia

Musculocutaneous n.

Brachialis a.

Median n.

Brachial v.

Med. antebrachial cutaneous n.

Ulnar n.

Basilic v.

Med. brachial intermuscular septum

Triceps brachii m., med. head

Triceps brachii m., long head

Fig. 426 The arm. Cross section at the level of the middle of the right arm, distal aspect (120%).

In fractures of the arm, the radial nerve is at risk due to its proximity to the shaft of the humerus as it courses in the sulcus of the radial nerve.

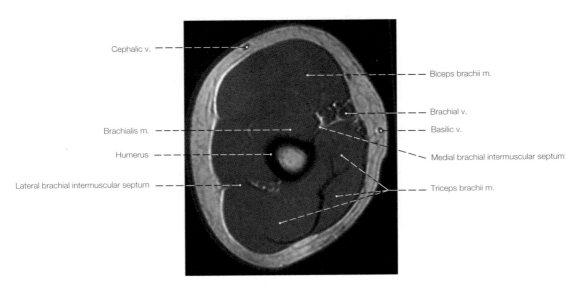

Cephalic v.

Brachialis m.

Humerus

Lateral brachial intermuscular septum

Biceps brachii m.

Brachial v.

Basilic v.

Medial brachial intermuscular septum

Triceps brachii m.

Fig. 427 The arm. Magnetic resonance image (MRI) cross section at the level of the middle of the right arm, distal aspect.

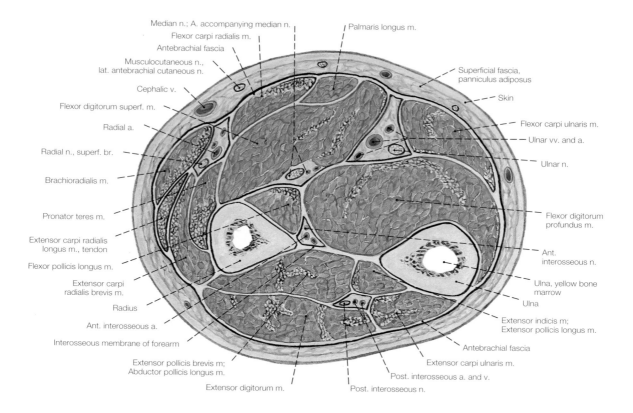

Median n.; A. accompanying median n.
Flexor carpi radialis m.
Antebrachial fascia
Musculocutaneous n.,
lat. antebrachial cutaneous n.
Cephalic v.
Flexor digitorum superf. m.
Radial a.
Radial n., superf. br.
Brachioradialis m.
Pronator teres m.
Extensor carpi radialis
longus m., tendon
Flexor pollicis longus m.
Extensor carpi
radialis brevis m.
Radius
Ant. interosseous a.
Interosseous membrane of forearm
Extensor pollicis brevis m;
Abductor pollicis longus m.
Extensor digitorum m.

Palmaris longus m.
Superficial fascia,
panniculus adiposus
Skin
Flexor carpi ulnaris m.
Ulnar vv. and a.
Ulnar n.
Flexor digitorum
profundus m.
Ant.
interosseous n.
Ulna, yellow bone
marrow
Ulna
Extensor indicis m;
Extensor pollicis longus m.
Antebrachial fascia
Extensor carpi ulnaris m.
Post. interosseous a. and v.
Post. interosseous n.

Fig. 428 The forearm. Cross section at the level of the middle of the right forearm, distal aspect (120%).

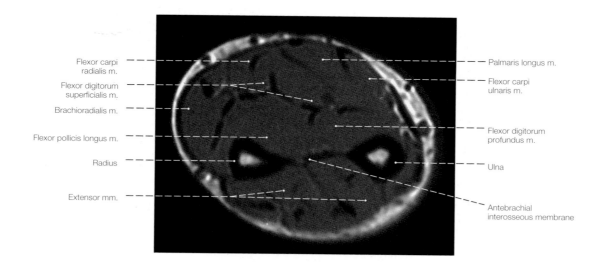

Flexor carpi
radialis m.
Flexor digitorum
superficialis m.
Brachioradialis m.
Flexor pollicis longus m.
Radius
Extensor mm.

Palmaris longus m.
Flexor carpi
ulnaris m.
Flexor digitorum
profundus m.
Ulna
Antebrachial
interosseous membrane

Fig. 429 The forearm. Magnetic resonance image (MRI) cross section at the level of the middle of the right forearm, distal aspect.

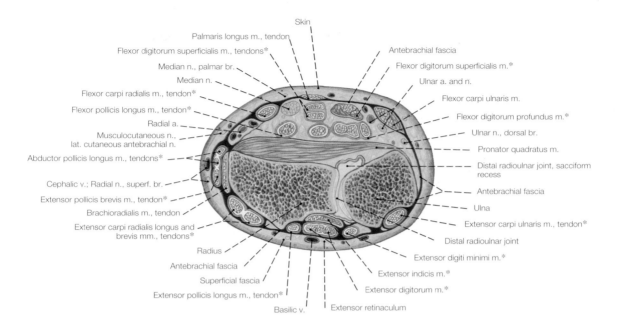

Skin
Palmaris longus m., tendon
Flexor digitorum superficialis m., tendons*
Median n., palmar br.
Median n.
Flexor carpi radialis m., tendon*
Flexor pollicis longus m., tendon*
Radial a.
Musculocutaneous n., lat. cutaneous antebrachial n.
Abductor pollicis longus m., tendons*
Cephalic v.; Radial n., superf. br.
Extensor pollicis brevis m., tendon*
Brachioradialis m., tendon
Extensor carpi radialis longus and brevis mm., tendons*
Radius
Antebrachial fascia
Superficial fascia
Extensor pollicis longus m., tendon*
Basilic v.

Antebrachial fascia
Flexor digitorum superficialis m.*
Ulnar a. and n.
Flexor carpi ulnaris m.
Flexor digitorum profundus m.*
Ulnar n., dorsal br.
Pronator quadratus m.
Distal radioulnar joint, sacciform recess
Antebrachial fascia
Ulna
Extensor carpi ulnaris m., tendon*
Distal radioulnar joint
Extensor digiti minimi m.*
Extensor indicis m.*
Extensor digitorum m.*
Extensor retinaculum

Fig. 430   The forearm. Cross section at the level of the right distal radioulnar joint, distal aspect (90%). At this level, the muscle tendons marked with an asterisk (*) are within the tendon sheaths.

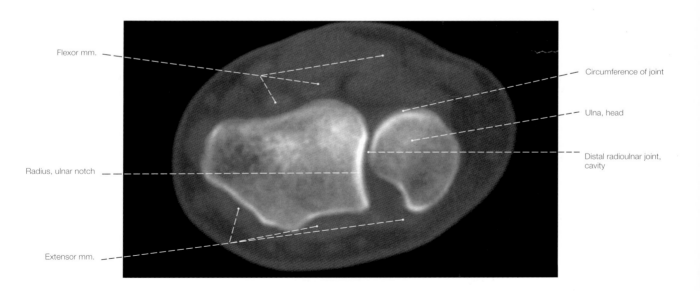

Flexor mm.
Radius, ulnar notch
Extensor mm.

Circumference of joint
Ulna, head
Distal radioulnar joint, cavity

Fig. 431   The forearm. Computed tomography (CT) cross section at the level of the right distal radioulnar joint, distal aspect.

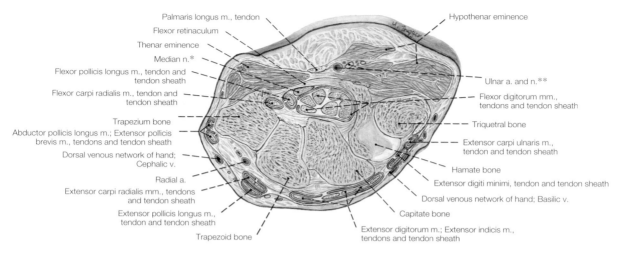

Palmaris longus m., tendon
Flexor retinaculum
Thenar eminence
Median n.*
Flexor pollicis longus m., tendon and tendon sheath
Flexor carpi radialis m., tendon and tendon sheath
Trapezium bone
Abductor pollicis longus m.; Extensor pollicis brevis m., tendons and tendon sheath
Dorsal venous network of hand; Cephalic v.
Radial a.
Extensor carpi radialis mm., tendons and tendon sheath
Extensor pollicis longus m., tendon and tendon sheath
Trapezoid bone

Hypothenar eminence
Ulnar a. and n.**
Flexor digitorum mm., tendons and tendon sheath
Triquetral bone
Extensor carpi ulnaris m., tendon and tendon sheath
Hamate bone
Extensor digiti minimi, tendon and tendon sheath
Dorsal venous network of hand; Basilic v.
Capitate bone
Extensor digitorum m.; Extensor indicis m., tendons and tendon sheath

Fig. 432 The right wrist. Cross section at the level of the hamulus of the hamate bone, distal aspect (100%). Carpal tunnel syndrome: Compression of the median nerve in the carpal tunnel (*); ulnar tunnel syndrome: compression of the ulnar nerve in the ulnar tunnel (GYON's box**)

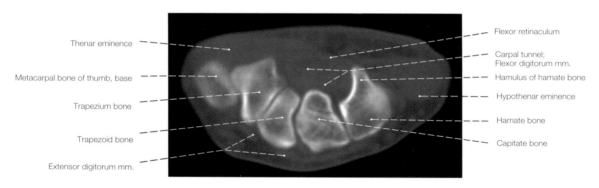

Thenar eminence
Metacarpal bone of thumb, base
Trapezium bone
Trapezoid bone
Extensor digitorum mm.

Flexor retinaculum
Carpal tunnel; Flexor digitorum mm.
Hamulus of hamate bone
Hypothenar eminence
Hamate bone
Capitate bone

Fig. 433 The right wrist. Computed tomography (CT) cross section at the level of the hamulus of the hamate bone, distal aspect.

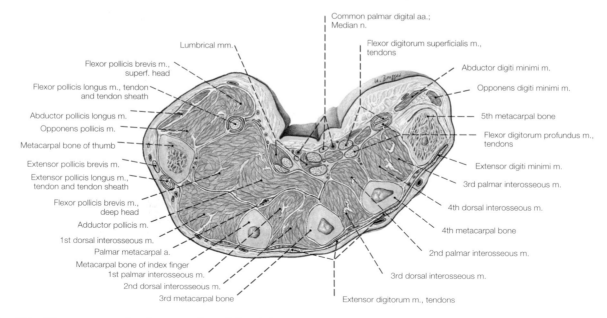

Common palmar digital aa.; Median n.
Flexor digitorum superficialis m., tendons
Lumbrical mm.
Flexor pollicis brevis m., superf. head
Flexor pollicis longus m., tendon and tendon sheath
Abductor pollicis longus m.
Opponens pollicis m.
Metacarpal bone of thumb
Extensor pollicis brevis m.
Extensor pollicis longus m., tendon and tendon sheath
Flexor pollicis brevis m., deep head
Adductor pollicis m.
1st dorsal interosseous m.
Palmar metacarpal a.
Metacarpal bone of index finger
1st palmar interosseous m.
2nd dorsal interosseous m.
3rd metacarpal bone

Abductor digiti minimi m.
Opponens digiti minimi m.
5th metacarpal bone
Flexor digitorum profundus m., tendons
Extensor digiti minimi m.
3rd palmar interosseous m.
4th dorsal interosseous m.
4th metacarpal bone
2nd palmar interosseous m.
3rd dorsal interosseous m.
Extensor digitorum m., tendons

Fig. 434 The metacarpals. Cross section of the right hand at the level of the middle of the 3rd metacarpal bone, distal aspect (95%).

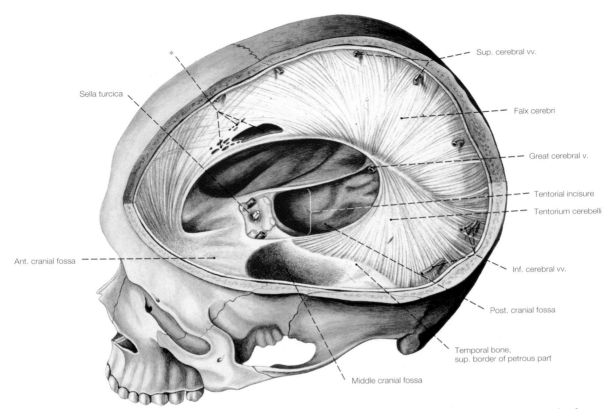

Sup. cerebral vv.

Sella turcica

Falx cerebri

Great cerebral v.

Tentorial incisure

Tentorium cerebelli

Ant. cranial fossa

Inf. cerebral vv.

Post. cranial fossa

Temporal bone,
sup. border of petrous part

Middle cranial fossa

Fig. 435 The cranial dura mater, viewed from the left in the skull opened laterally. The falx cerebri and the tentorium cerebelli divide the cranial cavity into three chambers that are incompletely separated from one another and which contain the two cerebral hemispheres and the cerebellum. The tentorial incisure surrounds the midbrain.

* Gaps in the falx cerebri

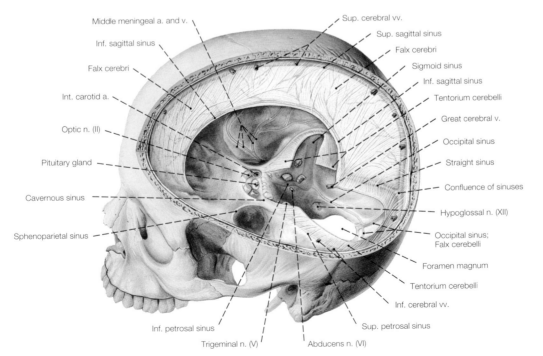

Middle meningeal a. and v.

Inf. sagittal sinus

Falx cerebri

Int. carotid a.

Optic n. (II)

Pituitary gland

Cavernous sinus

Sphenoparietal sinus

Sup. cerebral vv.

Sup. sagittal sinus

Falx cerebri

Sigmoid sinus

Inf. sagittal sinus

Tentorium cerebelli

Great cerebral v.

Occipital sinus

Straight sinus

Confluence of sinuses

Hypoglossal n. (XII)

Occipital sinus;
Falx cerebelli

Foramen magnum

Tentorium cerebelli

Inf. cerebral vv.

Sup. petrosal sinus

Inf. petrosal sinus

Trigeminal n. (V)

Abducens n. (VI)

Fig. 436 The cranial dura mater and the dural sinuses, viewed from the left. The skull has been opened laterally and the tentorium cerebelli partially removed.

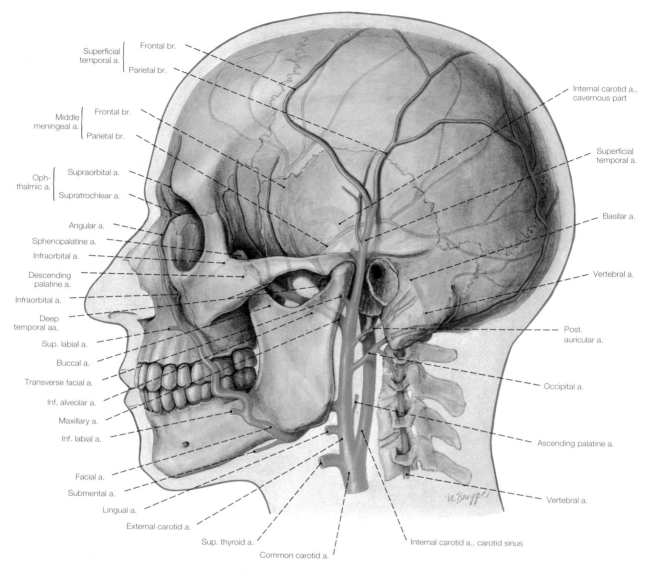

Fig. 437 Arteries of the head, viewed from the left.

The **internal carotid artery** is divided into four parts.

The **cervical part** begins at the bifurcation of the common carotid artery and runs through the carotid triangle to the base of the skull.

Within the petrous bone, the **petrous part** enters the carotid canal together with the (sympathetic) internal carotid plexus and the internal carotid venous plexus. Upon leaving the canal at the anterior edge of the apex of the petrous portion of the temporal bone, it is separated only by a thin bony or fibrous septum from the laterally positioned trigeminal ganglion.

The **cavernous part** traverses the cavernous sinus making a double curvature like the letter S, the "carotid siphon." As the artery curves forward, it lies lateral to the body of the sphenoid bone in a shallow groove that ascends in the caroticoclinoid canal on the medial aspect of the anterior clinoid process. In the cavernous sinus, it gives off a series of small arteries to the surrounding structures.

With an additional sharp bend, known as the "carotid genu," it perforates the inner layer of the cranial dura mater, gives off the ophthalmic artery and becomes the **cerebral part**. It then lies in the subarachnoid space and within the chiasmatic cistern divides into the anterior and middle cerebral arteries. Posteriorly the posterior communicating artery connects with the posterior cerebral artery.

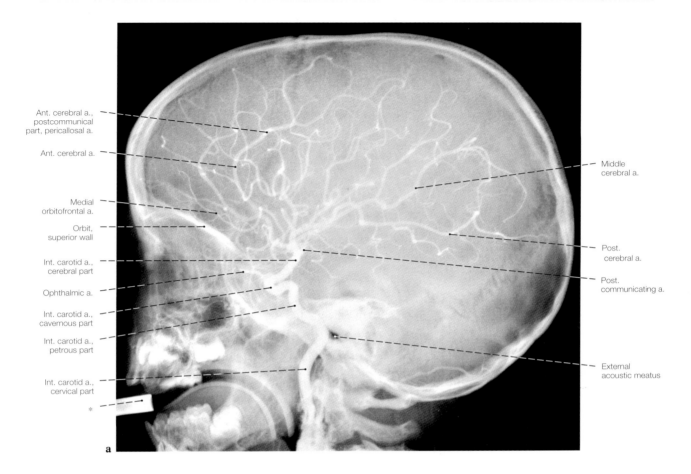

Ant. cerebral a., postcommunical part, pericallosal a.

Ant. cerebral a.

Medial orbitofrontal a.

Orbit, superior wall

Int. carotid a., cerebral part

Ophthalmic a.

Int. carotid a., cavernous part

Int. carotid a., petrous part

Int. carotid a., cervical part

*

Middle cerebral a.

Post. cerebral a.

Post. communicating a.

External acoustic meatus

a

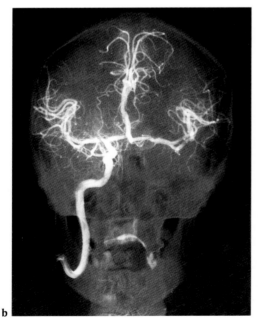

b

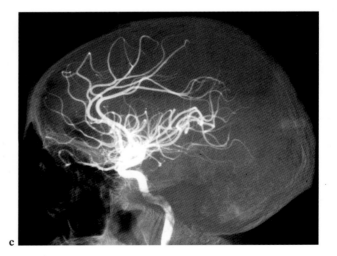

c

Fig. 438 a–c   The internal carotid artery. Radiographs (angiograms) after injection of contrast medium.
* Respiratory tube

a Conventional lateral radiograph, initial filling phase
b AP radiograph, digital subtraction angiography (DSA)
c Lateral radiograph, digital subtraction angiography (DSA)

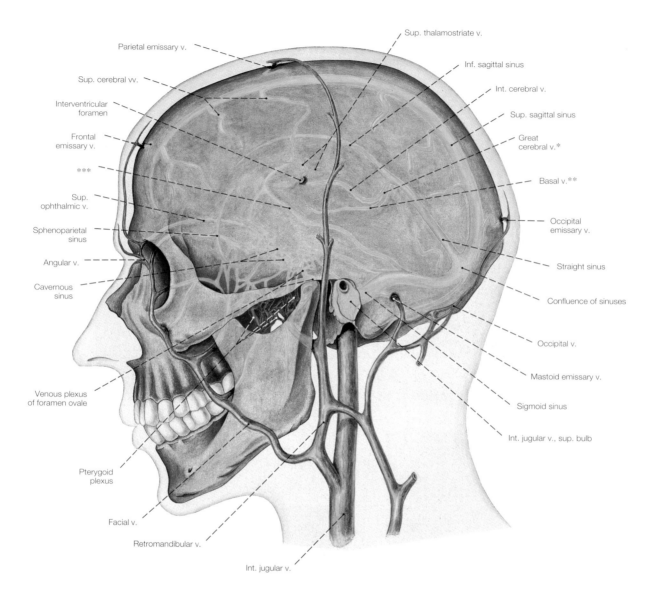

Parietal emissary v.

Sup. cerebral vv.

Interventricular foramen

Frontal emissary v.

***

Sup. ophthalmic v.

Sphenoparietal sinus

Angular v.

Cavernous sinus

Venous plexus of foramen ovale

Pterygoid plexus

Facial v.

Retromandibular v.

Int. jugular v.

Sup. thalamostriate v.

Inf. sagittal sinus

Int. cerebral v.

Sup. sagittal sinus

Great cerebral v.*

Basal v.**

Occipital emissary v.

Straight sinus

Confluence of sinuses

Occipital v.

Mastoid emissary v.

Sigmoid sinus

Int. jugular v., sup. bulb

Fig. 439 The veins of the head, viewed from the left.

*   Vein of GALEN
**   ROSENTHAL's vein
*** LABBÉ's anastomosis

Emissary veins — Sites of Passage Through the Skull

Parietal emissary v.—Parietal foramen
Mastoid emissary v.—Mastoid foramen
Occipital emissary v.—Opening in the region of the external occipital protuberance
Condylar emissary v.—Condylar canal

Venous plexus of hypoglossal canal—Hypoglossal canal
Venous plexus of foramen ovale—Foramen ovale
Venous plexus of the internal carotid—Carotid canal

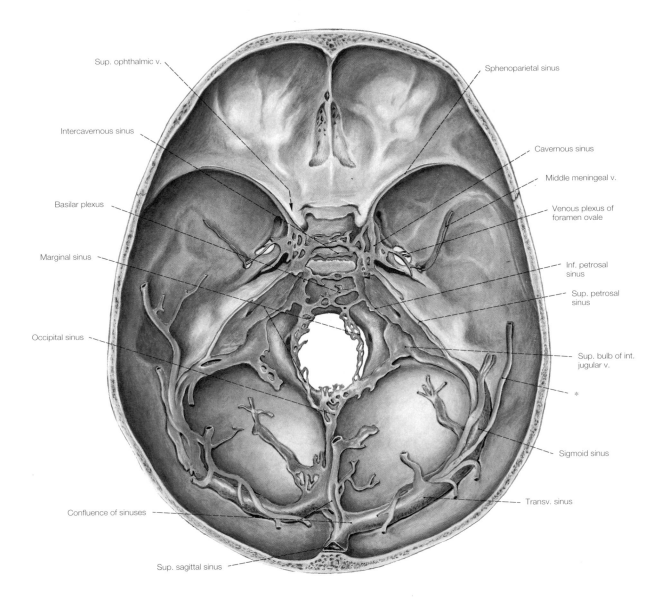

Sup. ophthalmic v.

Intercavernous sinus

Basilar plexus

Marginal sinus

Occipital sinus

Confluence of sinuses

Sup. sagittal sinus

Sphenoparietal sinus

Cavernous sinus

Middle meningeal v.

Venous plexus of foramen ovale

Inf. petrosal sinus

Sup. petrosal sinus

Sup. bulb of int. jugular v.

*

Sigmoid sinus

Transv. sinus

Fig. 440 Sinuses of the dura mater, viewed from above after removal of the calvaria. The venous sinuses have been injected with a plastic.

* LABBÉ's anastomosis with the superficial middle cerebral veins

The **sinuses of the dura mater** are venous channels, draining blood from the brain and from the bones that form the cranial cavity and carrying it into the internal jugular vein. The sinuses are situated between the two layers of the dura mater and are devoid of valves.

The main drainage from within the skull is through the sigmoid sinus into the internal jugular veins.

Additionally, the superior ophthalmic veins and the highly variable emissary veins form a series of smaller, likewise valveless, venous connections between the intra- and extracranial regions. The two cavernous sinuses assume a central position, being situated in the middle cranial fossa to the right and left of the sella turcica. They communicate with each other through the intercavernous sinus and either directly or indirectly with most other sinuses and with the veins of

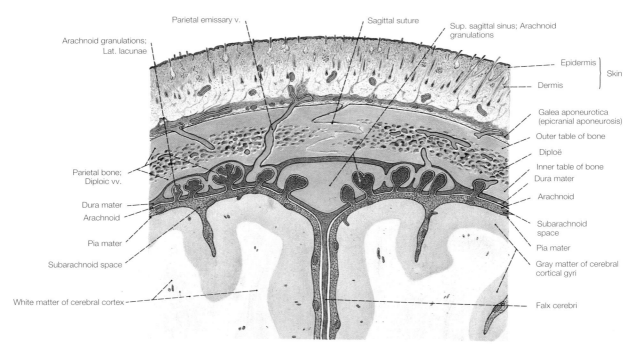

Parietal emissary v.

Sagittal suture

Sup. sagittal sinus; Arachnoid granulations

Arachnoid granulations; Lat. lacunae

Epidermis

Dermis

Skin

Galea aponeurotica (epicranial aponeurosis)

Outer table of bone

Diploë

Inner table of bone

Dura mater

Arachnoid

Parietal bone; Diploic vv.

Dura mater

Arachnoid

Subarachnoid space

Pia mater

Pia mater

Subarachnoid space

Gray matter of cerebral cortical gyri

White matter of cerebral cortex

Falx cerebri

Fig. 441 Calvaria (also called skullcap) and meninges. Frontal section through the cranium and upper cerebrum at the level of the crown of the head.

In the adult, cerebrospinal fluid is reabsorbed into the venous system mainly through the arachnoid granulations. Additionally, reabsorption occurs through the lymphatic sheaths of the small vessels of the pia mater and through the perineural sheaths of the cranial and spinal nerves.

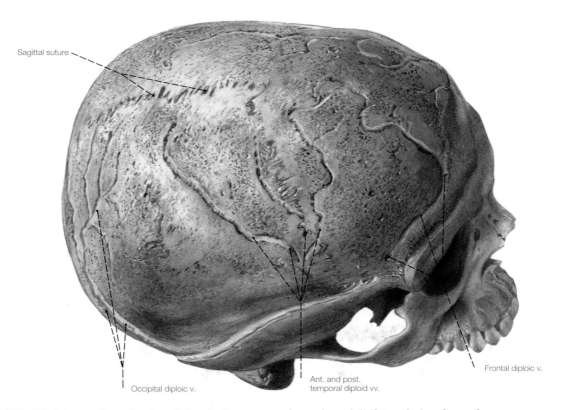

Sagittal suture

Occipital diploic v.

Ant. and post. temporal diploid vv.

Frontal diploic v.

Fig. 442 Diploic canals and veins of the skull exposed by removal of the outer table of compact bone, in a right lateral view from above.

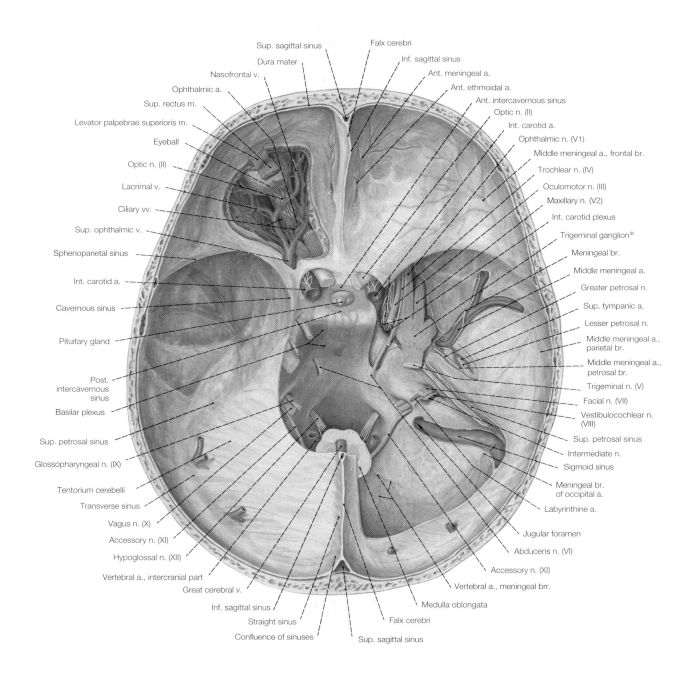

Sup. sagittal sinus
Dura mater
Nasofrontal v.
Ophthalmic a.
Sup. rectus m.
Levator palpebrae superioris m.
Eyeball
Optic n. (II)
Lacrimal v.
Ciliary vv.
Sup. ophthalmic v.
Sphenoparietal sinus
Int. carotid a.
Cavernous sinus
Pituitary gland
Post. intercavernous sinus
Basilar plexus
Sup. petrosal sinus
Glossopharyngeal n. (IX)
Tentorium cerebelli
Transverse sinus
Vagus n. (X)
Accessory n. (XI)
Hypoglossal n. (XII)
Vertebral a., intercranial part
Great cerebral v.
Inf. sagittal sinus
Straight sinus
Confluence of sinuses

Falx cerebri
Inf. sagittal sinus
Ant. meningeal a.
Ant. ethmoidal a.
Ant. intercavernous sinus
Optic n. (II)
Int. carotid a.
Ophthalmic n. (V1)
Middle meningeal a., frontal br.
Trochlear n. (IV)
Oculomotor n. (III)
Maxillary n. (V2)
Int. carotid plexus
Trigeminal ganglion*
Meningeal br.
Middle meningeal a.
Greater petrosal n.
Sup. tympanic a.
Lesser petrosal n.
Middle meningeal a., parietal br.
Middle meningeal a., petrosal br.
Trigeminal n. (V)
Facial n. (VII)
Vestibulocochlear n. (VIII)
Sup. petrosal sinus
Intermediate n.
Sigmoid sinus
Meningeal br. of occipital a.
Labyrinthine a.
Jugular foramen
Abducens n. (VI)
Accessory n. (XI)
Vertebral a., meningeal brr.
Medulla oblongata
Falx cerebri
Sup. sagittal sinus

Fig. 443 Internal surface of the base of the skull showing the cranial dura mater, venous sinuses, and cranial nerves, viewed from above. The roof of the left orbit and the falx cerebri with the right part of the tentorium cerebelli have been removed.

* Clinical: Semilunar or GASSERian ganglion

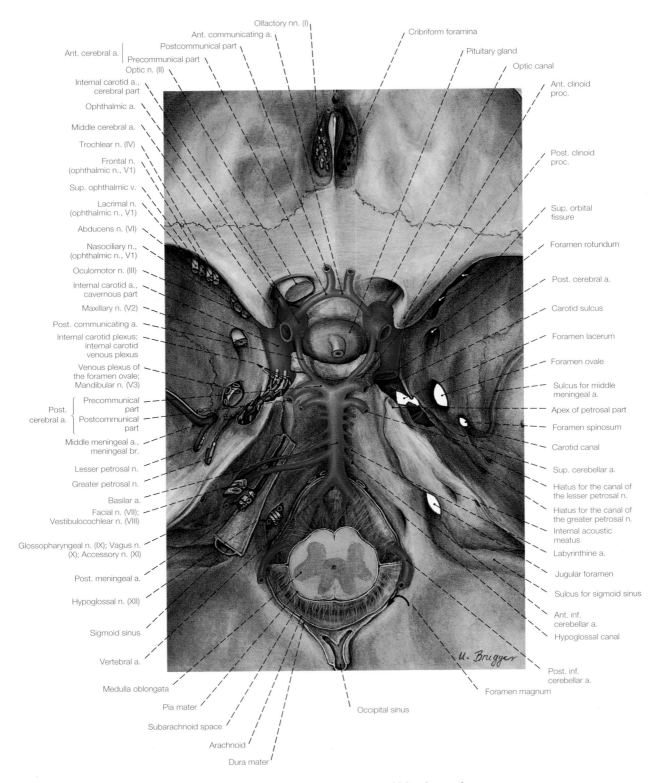

Ant. cerebral a.
Precommunical part
Postcommunical part
Optic n. (II)
Internal carotid a., cerebral part
Ophthalmic a.
Middle cerebral a.
Trochlear n. (IV)
Frontal n. (ophthalmic n., V1)
Sup. ophthalmic v.
Lacrimal n. (ophthalmic n., V1)
Abducens n. (VI)
Nasociliary n., (ophthalmic n., V1)
Oculomotor n. (III)
Internal carotid a., cavernous part
Maxillary n. (V2)
Post. communicating a.
Internal carotid plexus; internal carotid venous plexus
Venous plexus of the foramen ovale; Mandibular. n. (V3)
Post. cerebral a. { Precommunical part / Postcommunical part }
Middle meningeal a., meningeal br.
Lesser petrosal n.
Greater petrosal n.
Basilar a.
Facial n. (VII); Vestibulocochlear n. (VIII)
Glossopharyngeal n. (IX); Vagus n. (X); Accessory n. (XI)
Post. meningeal a.
Hypoglossal n. (XII)
Sigmoid sinus
Vertebral a.
Medulla oblongata
Pia mater
Subarachnoid space
Arachnoid
Dura mater

Olfactory nn. (I)
Ant. communicating a.
Cribriform foramina
Pituitary gland
Optic canal
Ant. clinoid proc.
Post. clinoid proc.
Sup. orbital fissure
Foramen rotundum
Post. cerebral a.
Carotid sulcus
Foramen lacerum
Foramen ovale
Sulcus for middle meningeal a.
Apex of petrosal part
Foramen spinosum
Carotid canal
Sup. cerebellar a.
Hiatus for the canal of the lesser petrosal n.
Hiatus for the canal of the greater petrosal n.
Internal acoustic meatus
Labyrinthine a.
Jugular foramen
Sulcus for sigmoid sinus
Ant. inf. cerebellar a.
Hypoglossal canal
Post. inf. cerebellar a.
Foramen magnum
Occipital sinus

U. Brügger

Fig. 444 Foramina for the passage of blood vessels and nerves through the base of the skull and the arterial circle (of WILLIS), internal aspect.

Contents of the Foramina of the Base of the Skull

Cribriform plate
Olfactory nn. (I)
Ant. ethmoidal a.

Optic canal
Optic n. (II)
Ophthalmic a.
Meninges; Sheath of the optic n.

Superior orbital fissure
Medial part:
Nasociliary n. (opthalmic n., V1)
Oculomotor n. (III)
Abducens n. (VI)

Lateral part:
Trochlear n. (IV)
Frontal n. (ophthalmic n., V1)
Lacrimal n. (ophthalmic n., V1)
Orbital br. (middle meningeal a.)
Sup. ophthalmic v.

Foramen rotundum
Maxillary n. (V2)

Foramen ovale
Mandibular n. (V3)
Venous plexus of the foramen ovale

Foramen spinosum
Meningeal br. (mandibular n., V3)
Middle meningeal a.

Foramen lacerum
Lesser petrosal n. (glossopharyngeal n., IX)

Sphenopetrosal fissure
Greater petrosal n. (facial n., VII)

Carotid canal
Internal carotid plexus (sympathetic trunk, sup. cervical ganglion)
Internal carotid venous plexus
Internal carotid a., petrous part

Internal acoustic meatus
Facial n. (VII)
Vestibulocochlear n. (VIII)
Labyrinthine a.
Labyrinthine vv.

Jugular foramen
Anterior part:
Glossopharyngeal n. (IX)
Inf. petrosal sinus

Posterior part:
Vagus n. (X)
Accessory n. (XI)
Sigmoid sinus; Sup. bulb of jugular vein
Post. meningeal a. (ascending pharyngeal a.)

Hypoglossal canal
Hypoglossal n. (XII)
Venous plexus of the hypoglossal canal

Condyloid canal
Condylar emissary v.

Foramen magnum
Medulla oblongata; Spinal medulla
Accessory n., spinal roots
Marginal sinus; Internal vertebral venous plexus
Vertebral a.
Ant. spinal a.
Meninges

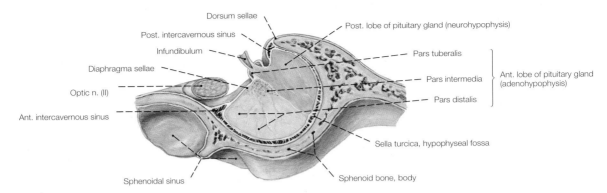

Dorsum sellae

Post. intercavernous sinus

Infundibulum

Diaphragma sellae

Optic n. (II)

Ant. intercavernous sinus

Sphenoidal sinus

Post. lobe of pituitary gland (neurohypophysis)

Pars tuberalis

Pars intermedia

Pars distalis

Ant. lobe of pituitary gland (adenohypophysis)

Sella turcica, hypophyseal fossa

Sphenoid bone, body

Fig. 445 The pituitary gland (hypophysis), median section, viewed from the left. The pituitary gland is imbedded in the venous sinus system of the cranial dura mater. The intercavernous sinuses (anterior and posterior) connect the right and left cavernous sinuses.

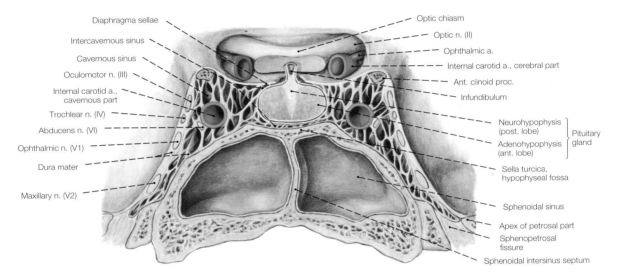

Diaphragma sellae

Intercavernous sinus

Cavernous sinus

Oculomotor n. (III)

Internal carotid a., cavernous part

Trochlear n. (IV)

Abducens n. (VI)

Ophthalmic n. (V1)

Dura mater

Maxillary n. (V2)

Optic chiasm

Optic n. (II)

Ophthalmic a.

Internal carotid a., cerebral part

Ant. clinoid proc.

Infundibulum

Neurohypophysis (post. lobe)

Adenohypophysis (ant. lobe)

Pituitary gland

Sella turcica, hypophyseal fossa

Sphenoidal sinus

Apex of petrosal part

Sphenopetrosal fissure

Sphenoidal intersinus septum

Fig. 446 The pituitary gland (hypophysis) and the cavernous sinus, frontal section, posterior view. The two sphenoidal sinuses are generally of unequal size, their septum being somewhat tortuous.

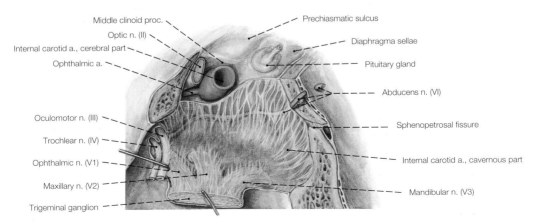

Middle clinoid proc.

Optic n. (II)

Internal carotid a., cerebral part

Ophthalmic a.

Oculomotor n. (III)

Trochlear n. (IV)

Ophthalmic n. (V1)

Maxillary n. (V2)

Trigeminal ganglion

Prechiasmatic sulcus

Diaphragma sellae

Pituitary gland

Abducens n. (VI)

Sphenopetrosal fissure

Internal carotid a., cavernous part

Mandibular n. (V3)

Fig. 447 The cavernous sinus, viewed from the left. The lateral part of the dura mater forming its wall has been removed, and the trigeminal ganglion has been retracted laterally.

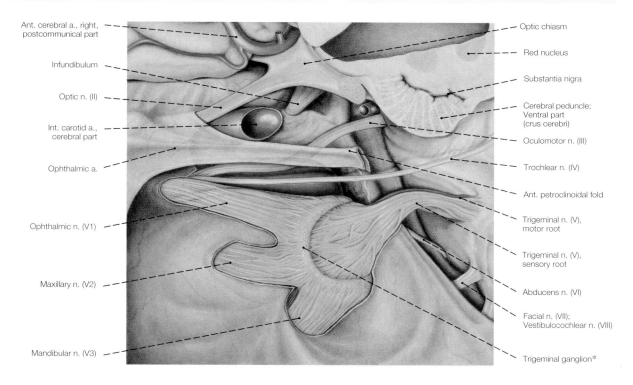

Ant. cerebral a., right, postcommunical part

Infundibulum

Optic n. (II)

Int. carotid a., cerebral part

Ophthalmic a.

Ophthalmic n. (V1)

Maxillary n. (V2)

Mandibular n. (V3)

Optic chiasm

Red nucleus

Substantia nigra

Cerebral peduncle; Ventral part (crus cerebri)

Oculomotor n. (III)

Trochlear n. (IV)

Ant. petroclinoidal fold

Trigeminal n. (V), motor root

Trigeminal n. (V), sensory root

Abducens n. (VI)

Facial n. (VII); Vestibulocochlear n. (VIII)

Trigeminal ganglion*

Fig. 448 Arteries and nerves in the region of the sella turcica and the cavernous sinus, lateral aspect viewed from above. The cranial dura mater has been partially removed.

* Clinical: Semilunar or GASSERian ganglion.

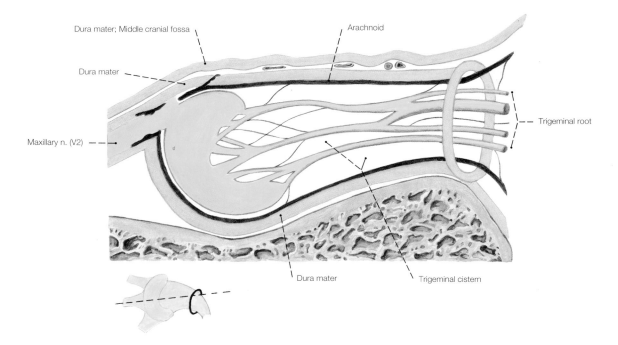

Dura mater; Middle cranial fossa

Arachnoid

Dura mater

Maxillary n. (V2)

Trigeminal root

Dura mater

Trigeminal cistern

Fig. 449 Trigeminal cistern and the trigeminal ganglion. Cross section at the level where the maxillary nerve joins the trigeminal ganglion.

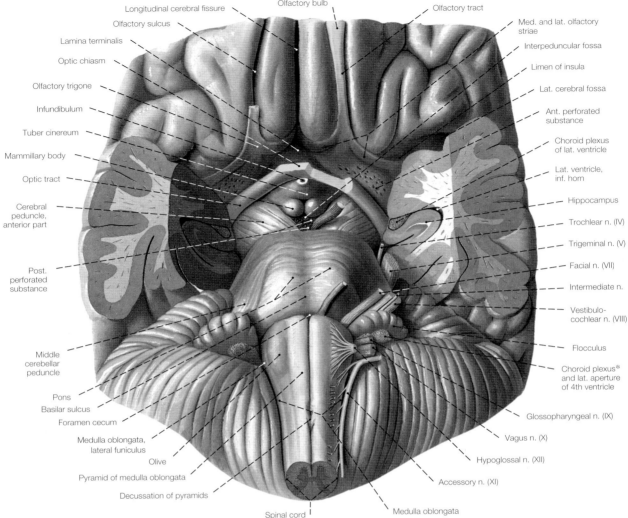

Olfactory bulb

Longitudinal cerebral fissure

Olfactory tract

Olfactory sulcus

Med. and lat. olfactory striae

Lamina terminalis

Interpeduncular fossa

Optic chiasm

Limen of insula

Olfactory trigone

Lat. cerebral fossa

Infundibulum

Ant. perforated substance

Tuber cinereum

Choroid plexus of lat. ventricle

Mammillary body

Lat. ventricle, inf. horn

Optic tract

Hippocampus

Cerebral peduncle, anterior part

Trochlear n. (IV)

Trigeminal n. (V)

Facial n. (VII)

Post. perforated substance

Intermediate n.

Vestibulo-cochlear n. (VIII)

Flocculus

Middle cerebellar peduncle

Choroid plexus* and lat. aperture of 4th ventricle

Pons

Basilar sulcus

Glossopharyngeal n. (IX)

Foramen cecum

Vagus n. (X)

Medulla oblongata, lateral funiculus

Hypoglossal n. (XII)

Olive

Accessory n. (XI)

Pyramid of medulla oblongata

Decussation of pyramids

Medulla oblongata

Spinal cord

Fig. 450 Origins of the cranial nerves, ventral view of the brain.

* Clinical: BOCHDALEK's flower basket

Cranial Nerves	Brain Exit or Entry	Functions of the Cranial Nerves (see also p. 290)
1. Olfactory nn. (I)	Olfactory bulb	(GSE) General somatic efferent: Motor fibers to the skeletal musculature of the body and the extremities (III, IV, VI, XII)
2. Optic n. (II)	Optic chiasm	
3. Oculomotor n. (III)	Cerebral peduncle, oculomotor sulcus	(GVE) General visceral efferent: Motor fibers to the visceral and vascular musculature (III, VII, IX, X)
4. Trochlear n. (IV)	Midbrain tectum, dorsal part	(SVE) Special visceral efferent: Motor fibers to the muscles of facial expression, muscles of mastication, pharynx, parts of the esophagus, sternocleidomastoid and trapezius muscles (V, VII, IX, X, XI)
5. Trigeminal n. (V)	Pons, lateral edge	
- Ophthalmic n. (V1)	Trigeminal ganglion	
- Maxillary n. (V2)	Trigeminal ganglion	
- Mandibular n. (V3)	Trigeminal ganglion	(GVA) General visceral afferent: Sensory fibers from the viscera and the blood vessels, etc. (IX, X)
6. Abducens n. (VI)	Between pons and pyramids of medulla oblongata	(SVA) Special visceral afferent: Smell, taste (I, VII, IX, X)
7. Facial n. (and intermediate n.) (VII)	Cerebellopontine angle	(GSA) General somatic afferent: Sensory fibers from exteroceptive receptors of the skin and proprioceptive receptors of skeletal muscles, tendons and joints (V, VII, IX, X)
8. Vestibulocochlear n. (VIII)	Cerebellopontine angle	
9. Glossopharyngeal n. (IX)	Medulla oblongata posterolateral sulcus (retro-olivary)	(SSA) Special somatic afferent: Vision, audition, equilibration (II, VIII)
10. Vagus n. (X)	(retro-olivary)	
11. Accessory n. (XI)	(retro-olivary)	
12. Hypoglossal n. (XII)	Medulla oblongata, anterolateral sulcus	

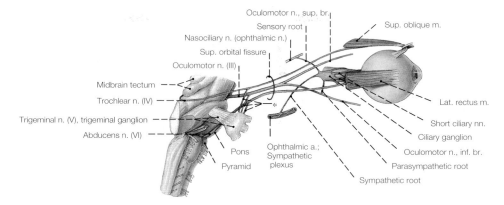

Oculomotor n., sup. br.
Sensory root
Nasociliary n. (ophthalmic n.)
Sup. orbital fissure
Oculomotor n. (III)
Midbrain tectum
Trochlear n. (IV)
Trigeminal n. (V), trigeminal ganglion
Abducens n. (VI)
Pons
Pyramid
Ophthalmic a.;
Sympathetic plexus
Sup. oblique m.
Lat. rectus m.
Short ciliary nn.
Ciliary ganglion
Oculomotor n., inf. br.
Parasympathetic root
Sympathetic root

Fig. 451 Oculomotor (III), trochlear (IV) and abducens (VI) nerves, lateral view of the right nerves.

* Connections with the trigeminal ganglion

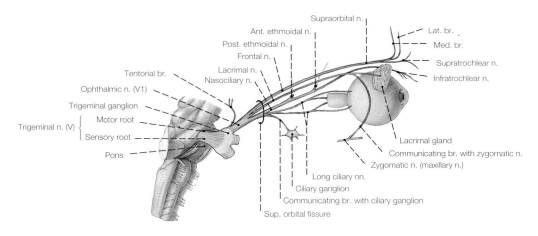

Supraorbital n.
Ant. ethmoidal n.
Post. ethmoidal n.
Frontal n.
Lacrimal n.
Nasociliary n.
Tentorial br.
Ophthalmic n. (V1)
Trigeminal ganglion
Trigeminal n. (V) { Motor root / Sensory root
Pons
Lat. br.
Med. br.
Supratrochlear n.
Infratrochlear n.
Lacrimal gland
Communicating br. with zygomatic n.
Zygomatic n. (maxillary n.)
Long ciliary nn.
Ciliary ganglion
Communicating br. with ciliary ganglion
Sup. orbital fissure

Fig. 452 Ophthalmic nerve (V1), lateral view of the right nerve.

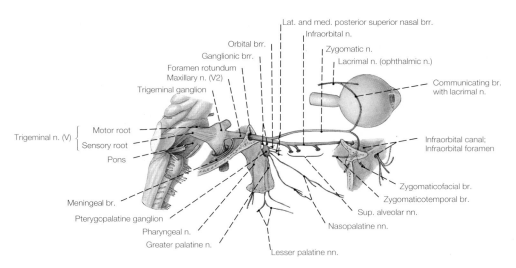

Lat. and med. posterior superior nasal brr.
Infraorbital n.
Orbital brr.
Ganglionic brr.
Foramen rotundum
Maxillary n. (V2)
Trigeminal ganglion
Zygomatic n.
Lacrimal n. (ophthalmic n.)
Trigeminal n. (V) { Motor root / Sensory root
Pons
Meningeal br.
Pterygopalatine ganglion
Pharyngeal n.
Greater palatine n.
Lesser palatine nn.
Nasopalatine nn.
Sup. alveolar nn.
Zygomaticotemporal br.
Zygomaticofacial br.
Infraorbital canal;
Infraorbital foramen
Communicating br. with lacrimal n.

Fig. 453 Maxillary nerve (V2), lateral view of the right nerve.

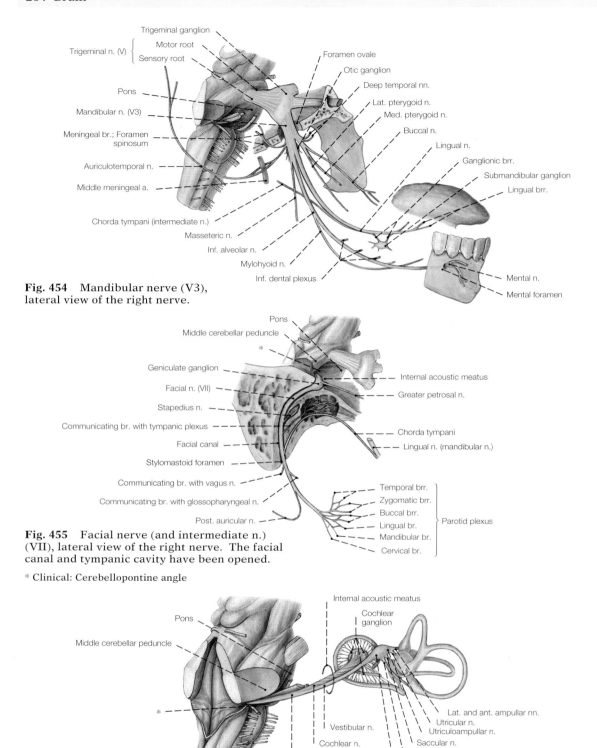

Fig. 454 Mandibular nerve (V3), lateral view of the right nerve.

Fig. 455 Facial nerve (and intermediate n.) (VII), lateral view of the right nerve. The facial canal and tympanic cavity have been opened.

* Clinical: Cerebellopontine angle

Fig. 456 Vestibulocochlear nerve (VIII), posterolateral view of the right nerve. The membranous labyrinth has been greatly enlarged.

* Clinical: Cerebellopontine angle

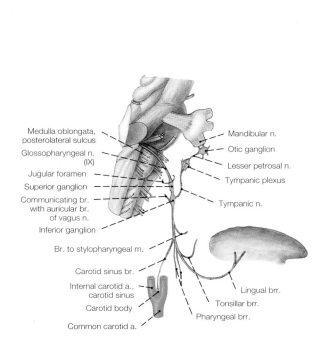

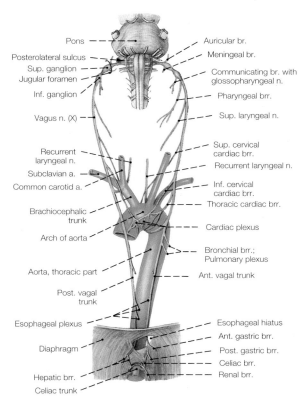

Fig. 457 Glossopharyngeal nerve (IX), lateral view of the right nerve.

Fig. 458 Vagus nerve (X), anterior view of both nerves.

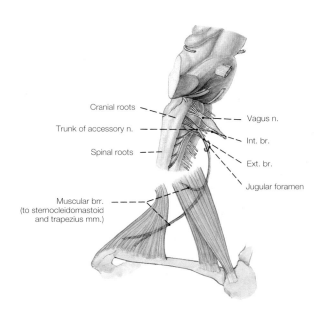

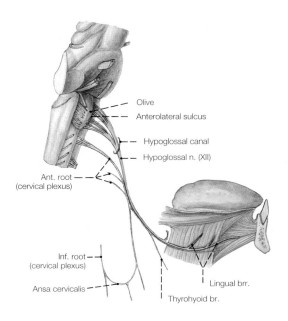

Fig. 459 Accessory nerve (XI), lateral view of the right nerve.

Fig. 460 Hypoglossal nerve (XII), lateral view of the right nerve.

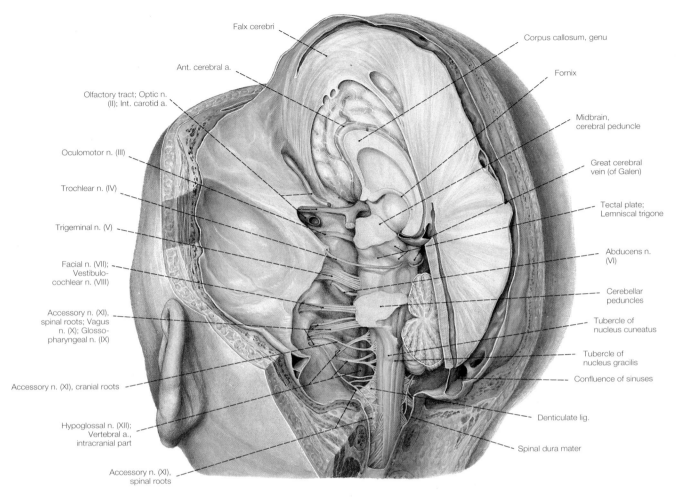

Falx cerebri

Ant. cerebral a.

Olfactory tract; Optic n.
(II); Int. carotid a.

Oculomotor n. (III)

Trochlear n. (IV)

Trigeminal n. (V)

Facial n. (VII);
Vestibulo-
cochlear n. (VIII)

Accessory n. (XI),
spinal roots; Vagus
n. (X); Glosso-
pharyngeal n. (IX)

Accessory n. (XI), cranial roots

Hypoglossal n. (XII);
Vertebral a.,
intracranial part

Accessory n. (XI),
spinal roots

Corpus callosum, genu

Fornix

Midbrain,
cerebral peduncle

Great cerebral
vein (of Galen)

Tectal plate;
Lemniscal trigone

Abducens n.
(VI)

Cerebellar
peduncles

Tubercle of
nucleus cuneatus

Tubercle of
nucleus gracilis

Confluence of sinuses

Denticulate lig.

Spinal dura mater

Fig. 461 Course of the cranial nerves in the subarachnoid space, viewed posteriorly from above.

The left half of the cerebrum and cerebellum and the tentorium cerebelli have been removed.

Cranial Parasympathetic Ganglia

These ganglia contain the perikarya of the postganglionic parasympathetic nerve cells. The preganglionic fibers from the accessory nucleus of the oculomotor nerve and the superior and inferior salivatory nuclei terminate in these ganglia.

The **ciliary ganglion** is the site of synapse of fibers from the accessory oculomotor nucleus, which reach the ganglion via the oculomotor nerve (parasympathetic root). Sensory fibers from the nasociliary nerve (sensory root) and sympathetic fibers from the internal carotid plexus (sympathetic root) traverse the ganglion without synapsing. Postganglionic parasympathetic fibers travel to the ciliary muscle (accommodation) and to the pupillary sphincter muscle (pupillary constriction) via the short ciliary nerves.

The **pterygopalatine ganglion** receives parasympathetic fibers from the superior salivatory nucleus traveling in the trunk of the facial nerve to the greater petrosal nerve and continuing in the nerve of the pterygoid canal to synapse in the ganglion. Sensory fibers from the maxillary nerve and sympathetic fibers from the superior cervical ganglion traverse the gan-

glion without synapsing. A series of small postganglionic parasympathetic branches supply secretory innervation to the lacrimal gland, the mucous membrane and glands of the paranasal sinuses, the nasal cavity, and the gingiva.

The **submandibular ganglion** contains the synapses of parasympathetic fibers from the chorda tympani of the facial nerve which join the lingual nerve, as well as those from the superior salivatory nucleus. Sympathetic roots emanating from the superior cervical ganglion traverse the submandibular ganglion. Postganglionic parasympathetic fibers travel to the submandibular and sublingual glands with the lingual nerve.

The **otic ganglion** contains the synapses of parasympathetic fibers from the inferior salivatory nucleus, which reach the ganglion via the trunk of the glossopharyngeal nerve and its tympanic nerve. Sympathetic roots arising from the superior cervical ganglion traverse the otic ganglion. Postganglionic parasympathetic fibers travel in the communicating branch to the auriculotemporal nerve and on to the parotid gland.

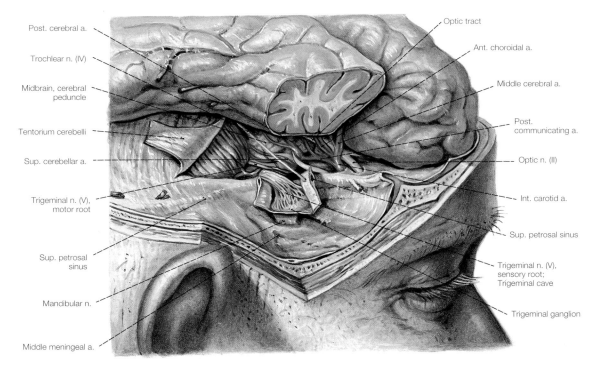

Post. cerebral a.

Trochlear n. (IV)

Midbrain, cerebral peduncle

Tentorium cerebelli

Sup. cerebellar a.

Trigeminal n. (V), motor root

Sup. petrosal sinus

Mandibular n.

Middle meningeal a.

Optic tract

Ant. choroidal a.

Middle cerebral a.

Post. communicating a.

Optic n. (II)

Int. carotid a.

Sup. petrosal sinus

Trigeminal n. (V), sensory root; Trigeminal cave

Trigeminal ganglion

Fig. 462   Course of the cranial nerves in the middle cranial fossa, lateral aspect. The temporal lobe has been partially removed and the remaining portion elevated.

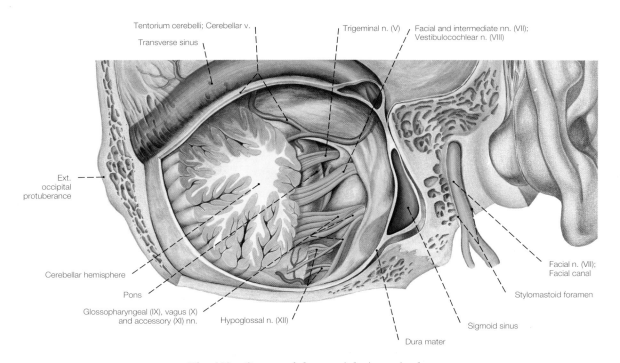

Tentorium cerebelli; Cerebellar v.

Transverse sinus

Trigeminal n. (V)

Facial and intermediate nn. (VII); Vestibulocochlear n. (VIII)

Ext. occipital protuberance

Cerebellar hemisphere

Pons

Glossopharyngeal (IX), vagus (X) and accessory (XI) nn.

Hypoglossal n. (XII)

Dura mater

Sigmoid sinus

Stylomastoid foramen

Facial n. (VII); Facial canal

Fig. 463   Course of the cranial nerves in the posterior cranial fossa, the right side viewed from posterior. The left cerebellar hemisphere and the tentorium cerebelli have been partially removed.

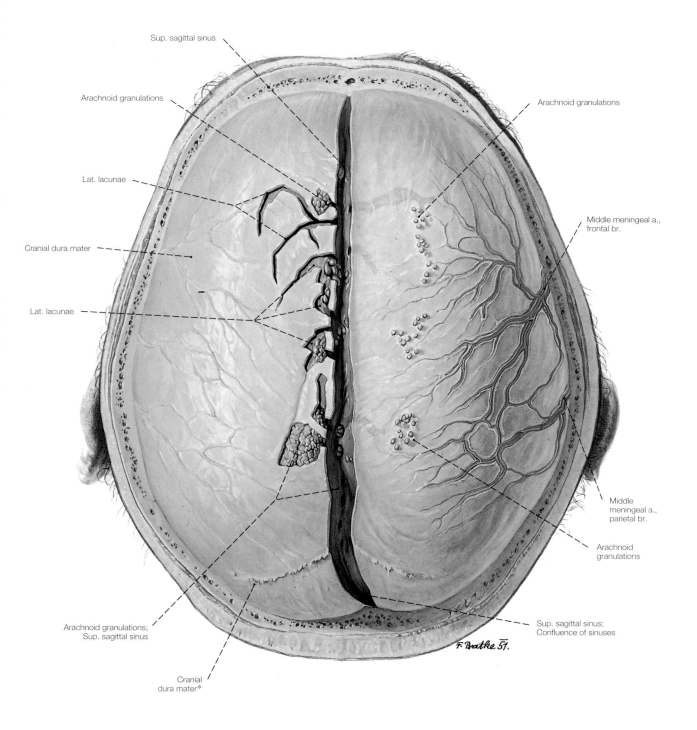

Sup. sagittal sinus

Arachnoid granulations

Lat. lacunae

Cranial dura mater

Lat. lacunae

Arachnoid granulations;
Sup. sagittal sinus

Cranial
dura mater*

Arachnoid granulations

Middle meningeal a.,
frontal br.

Middle
meningeal a.,
parietal br.

Arachnoid
granulations

Sup. sagittal sinus;
Confluence of sinuses

F. Bratke 51.

Fig. 464 The cranial dura mater, viewed from above. The calvaria has been removed and the superior sagittal sinus with its lateral lacunae has been opened.

* Sites where the dura mater is attached in the region of the lambdoidal suture

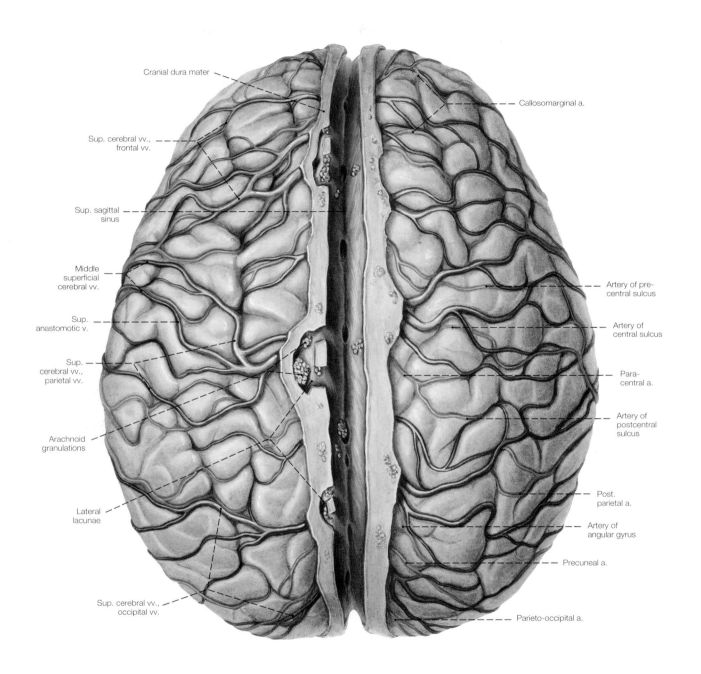

Cranial dura mater

Callosomarginal a.

Sup. cerebral vv.,
frontal vv.

Sup. sagittal
sinus

Middle
superficial
cerebral vv.

Sup.
anastomotic v.

Sup.
cerebral vv.,
parietal vv.

Arachnoid
granulations

Lateral
lacunae

Sup. cerebral vv.,
occipital vv.

Artery of pre-
central sulcus

Artery of
central sulcus

Para-
central a.

Artery of
postcentral
sulcus

Post.
parietal a.

Artery of
angular gyrus

Precuneal a.

Parieto-occipital a.

Fig. 465 Superficial arteries and veins of the brain,
viewed from above. The cranial dura mater has been
removed and the superior sagittal sinus opened. The
arachnoid granulations are the sites where
cerebrospinal fluid passes back into the venous
circulation.

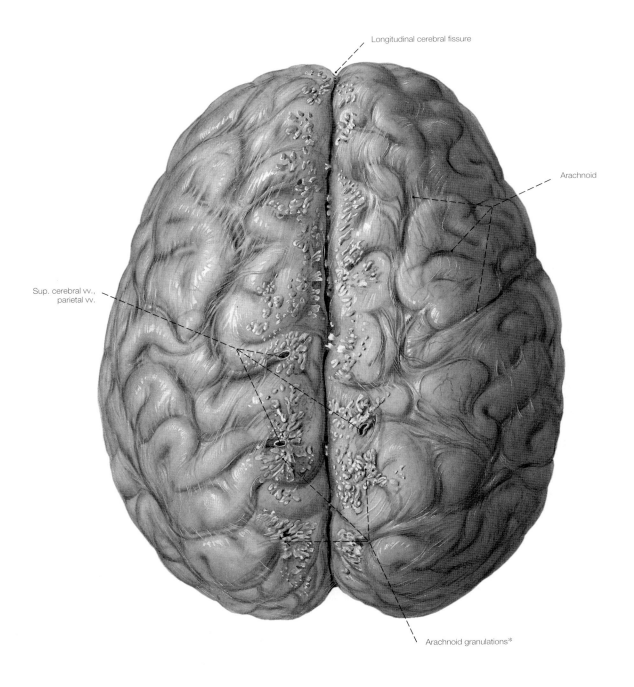

Longitudinal cerebral fissure

Arachnoid

Sup. cerebral vv.,
parietal vv.

Arachnoid granulations*

Fig. 466 The brain with the arachnoid, viewed from above.

* PACCHIONian bodies or arachnoid villi

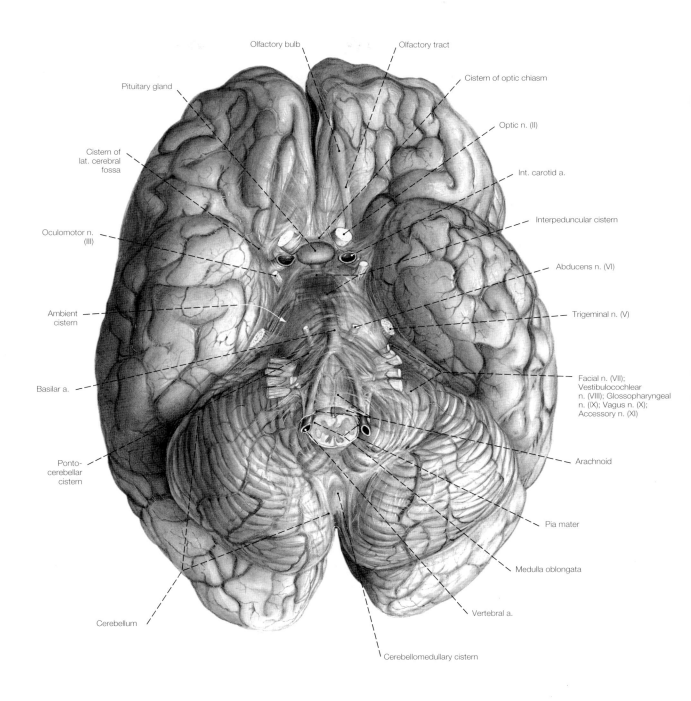

Olfactory bulb

Olfactory tract

Cistern of optic chiasm

Pituitary gland

Optic n. (II)

Cistern of lat. cerebral fossa

Int. carotid a.

Interpeduncular cistern

Oculomotor n. (III)

Abducens n. (VI)

Ambient cistern

Trigeminal n. (V)

Basilar a.

Facial n. (VII); Vestibulocochlear n. (VIII); Glossopharyngeal n. (IX); Vagus n. (X); Accessory n. (XI)

Ponto-cerebellar cistern

Arachnoid

Pia mater

Medulla oblongata

Cerebellum

Vertebral a.

Cerebellomedullary cistern

Fig. 467 The brain with the arachnoid, viewed from below.

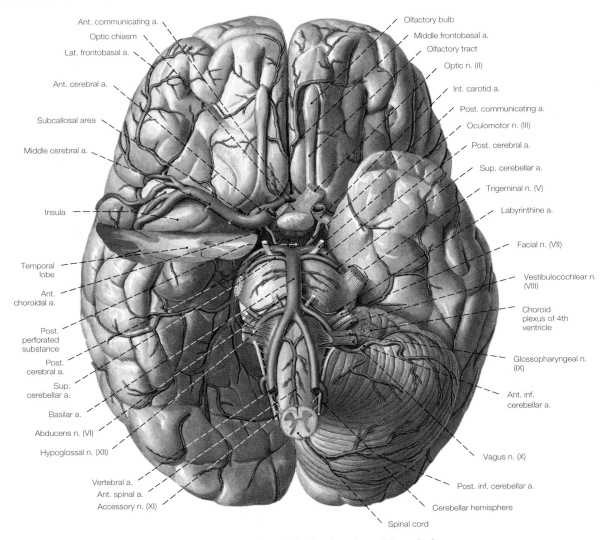

Ant. communicating a.
Optic chiasm
Lat. frontobasal a.
Ant. cerebral a.
Subcallosal area
Middle cerebral a.
Insula
Temporal lobe
Ant. choroidal a.
Post. perforated substance
Post. cerebral a.
Sup. cerebellar a.
Basilar a.
Abducens n. (VI)
Hypoglossal n. (XII)
Vertebral a.
Ant. spinal a.
Accessory n. (XI)
Spinal cord

Olfactory bulb
Middle frontobasal a.
Olfactory tract
Optic n. (II)
Int. carotid a.
Post. communicating a.
Oculomotor n. (III)
Post. cerebral a.
Sup. cerebellar a.
Trigeminal n. (V)
Labyrinthine a.
Facial n. (VII)
Vestibulocochlear n. (VIII)
Choroid plexus of 4th ventricle
Glossopharyngeal n. (IX)
Ant. inf. cerebellar a.
Vagus n. (X)
Post. inf. cerebellar a.
Cerebellar hemisphere

Fig. 468 Arteries of the brain, viewed from below.
The temporal lobe has been partially removed.

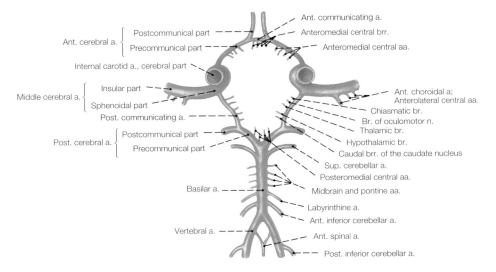

Ant. cerebral a.
  Postcommunical part
  Precommunical part
Internal carotid a., cerebral part
Middle cerebral a.
  Insular part
  Sphenoidal part
Post. communicating a.
Post. cerebral a.
  Postcommunical part
  Precommunical part
Basilar a.
Vertebral a.

Ant. communicating a.
Anteromedial central brr.
Anteromedial central aa.
Ant. choroidal a;
Anterolateral central aa.
Chiasmatic br.
Br. of oculomotor n.
Thalamic br.
Hypothalamic br.
Caudal brr. of the caudate nucleus
Sup. cerebellar a.
Posteromedial central aa.
Midbrain and pontine aa.
Labyrinthine a.
Ant. inferior cerebellar a.
Ant. spinal a.
Post. inferior cerebellar a.

Fig. 469 Arterial circle (of WILLIS).

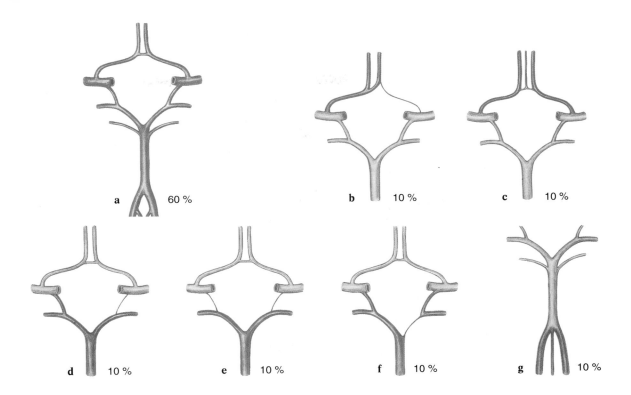

Fig. 470 a–g Variations in the arterial circle (of WILLIS).
Percentages indicate the frequency of occurrence.

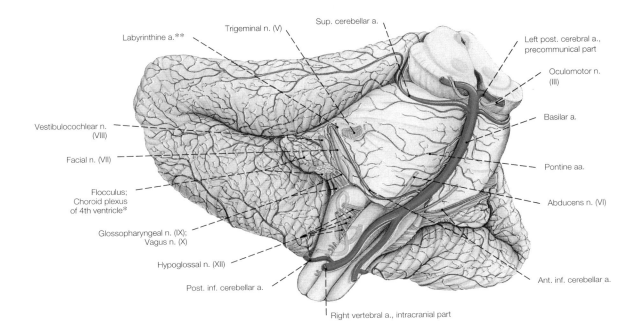

Labyrinthine a.**

Trigeminal n. (V)

Sup. cerebellar a.

Left post. cerebral a.,
precommunical part

Oculomotor n.
(III)

Vestibulocochlear n.
(VIII)

Basilar a.

Facial n. (VII)

Pontine aa.

Flocculus;
Choroid plexus
of 4th ventricle*

Abducens n. (VI)

Glossopharyngeal n. (IX);
Vagus n. (X)

Hypoglossal n. (XII)

Ant. inf. cerebellar a.

Post. inf. cerebellar a.

Right vertebral a., intracranial part

Fig. 471 Arteries of the hindbrain, viewed from the
right and below. The midbrain has been sectioned.
The inferior anterior cerebellar artery generally
courses over the abducens nerve (approx. 80% of

cases); however, on the left side of the figure, it
courses under the nerve.

* Clinical: BOCHDALEK's flower basket
** In approx. 15% of cases the labyrinthine artery originates
directly from the basilar artery.

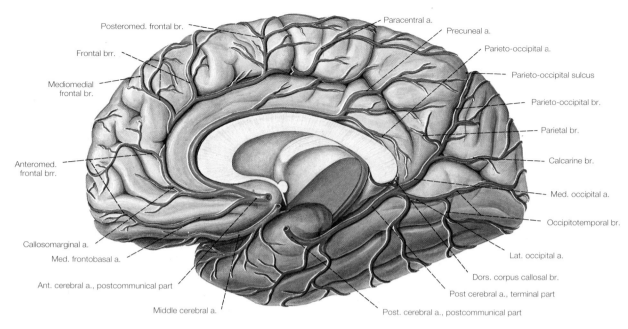

Posteromed. frontal br.

Frontal brr.

Mediomedial frontal br.

Anteromed. frontal brr.

Callosomarginal a.

Med. frontobasal a.

Ant. cerebral a., postcommunical part

Middle cerebral a.

Paracentral a.

Precuneal a.

Parieto-occipital a.

Parieto-occipital sulcus

Parieto-occipital br.

Parietal br.

Calcarine br.

Med. occipital a.

Occipitotemporal br.

Lat. occipital a.

Dors. corpus callosal br.

Post cerebral a., terminal part

Post. cerebral a., postcommunical part

Fig. 472 The arteries of the medial and inferior surfaces of the right cerebral hemisphere, medial aspect.

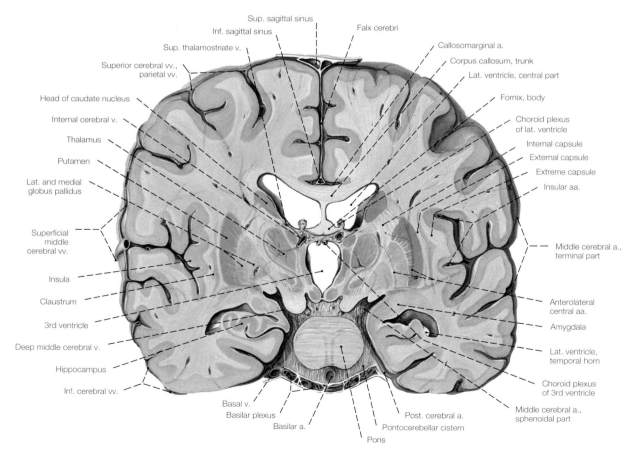

Sup. sagittal sinus

Inf. sagittal sinus

Sup. thalamostriate v.

Superior cerebral vv., parietal vv.

Head of caudate nucleus

Internal cerebral v.

Thalamus

Putamen

Lat. and medial globus pallidus

Superficial middle cerebral vv.

Insula

Claustrum

3rd ventricle

Deep middle cerebral v.

Hippocampus

Inf. cerebral vv.

Basal v.

Basilar plexus

Basilar a.

Pons

Falx cerebri

Callosomarginal a.

Corpus callosum, trunk

Lat. ventricle, central part

Fornix, body

Choroid plexus of lat. ventricle

Internal capsule

External capsule

Extreme capsule

Insular aa.

Middle cerebral a., terminal part

Anterolateral central aa.

Amygdala

Lat. ventricle, temporal horn

Choroid plexus of 3rd ventricle

Middle cerebral a., sphenoidal part

Post. cerebral a.

Pontocerebellar cistern

Fig. 473 Arteries and veins of the brain. Frontal section, posterior aspect, with arteries shown on the right and veins on the left.

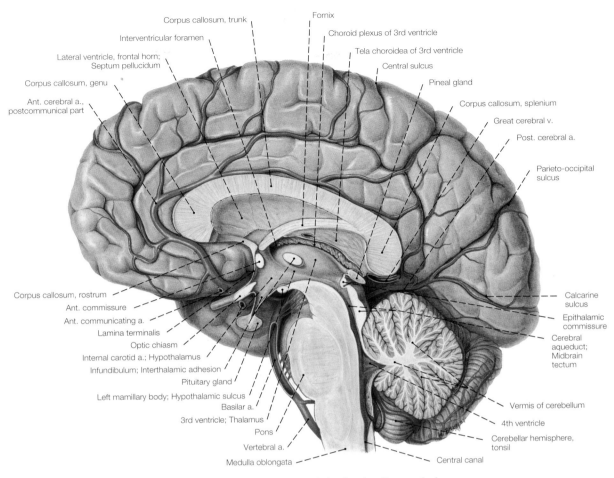

Corpus callosum, trunk

Interventricular foramen

Lateral ventricle, frontal horn;
Septum pellucidum

Corpus callosum, genu

Ant. cerebral a.,
postcommunical part

Fornix

Choroid plexus of 3rd ventricle

Tela choroidea of 3rd ventricle

Central sulcus

Pineal gland

Corpus callosum, splenium

Great cerebral v.

Post. cerebral a.

Parieto-occipital
sulcus

Corpus callosum, rostrum

Ant. commissure

Ant. communicating a.

Lamina terminalis

Optic chiasm

Internal carotid a.; Hypothalamus

Infundibulum; Interthalamic adhesion

Pituitary gland

Left mamillary body; Hypothalamic sulcus

Basilar a.

3rd ventricle; Thalamus

Pons

Vertebral a.

Medulla oblongata

Calcarine
sulcus

Epithalamic
commissure

Cerebral
aqueduct;
Midbrain
tectum

Vermis of cerebellum

4th ventricle

Cerebellar hemisphere,
tonsil

Central canal

Fig. 474 Medial surface of the brain, diencephalon,
and brainstem, viewed from the left. Sectioning in
the median plane has been staggered anteriorly.

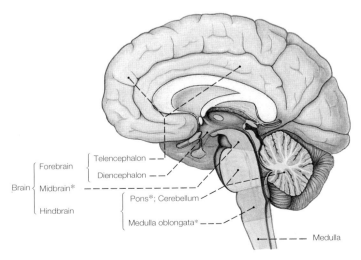

Brain

Forebrain

Midbrain*

Hindbrain

Telencephalon

Diencephalon

Pons*; Cerebellum

Medulla oblongata*

Medulla

Fig. 475 Diagram of the regions of the central
nervous system, median section.

The regions of the brain marked with an asterisk (*)
together form the brainstem.

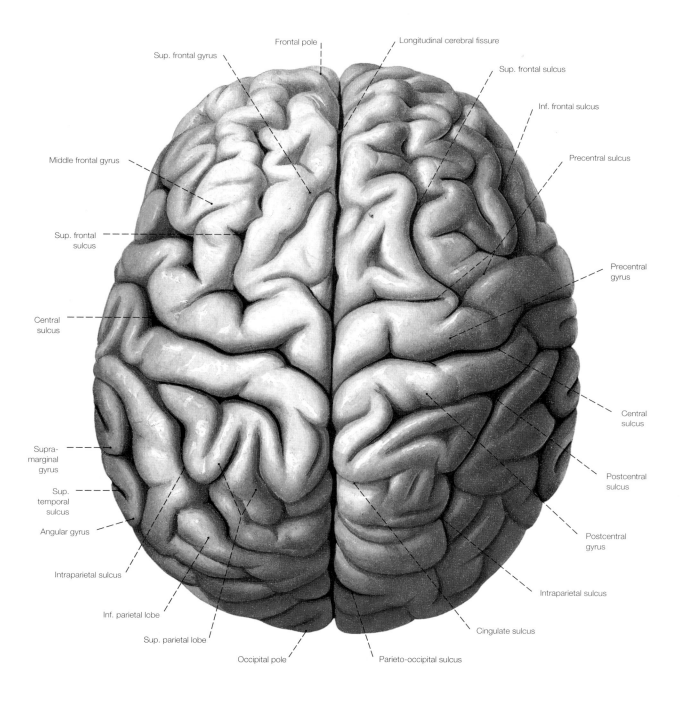

Frontal pole

Longitudinal cerebral fissure

Sup. frontal gyrus

Sup. frontal sulcus

Inf. frontal sulcus

Middle frontal gyrus

Precentral sulcus

Sup. frontal sulcus

Precentral gyrus

Central sulcus

Central sulcus

Supra-marginal gyrus

Postcentral sulcus

Sup. temporal sulcus

Postcentral gyrus

Angular gyrus

Intraparietal sulcus

Intraparietal sulcus

Cingulate sulcus

Inf. parietal lobe

Sup. parietal lobe

Occipital pole

Parieto-occipital sulcus

Fig. 476 The cerebrum, viewed from above. The leptomeninges (i.e., arachnoid and pia mater) have been removed.

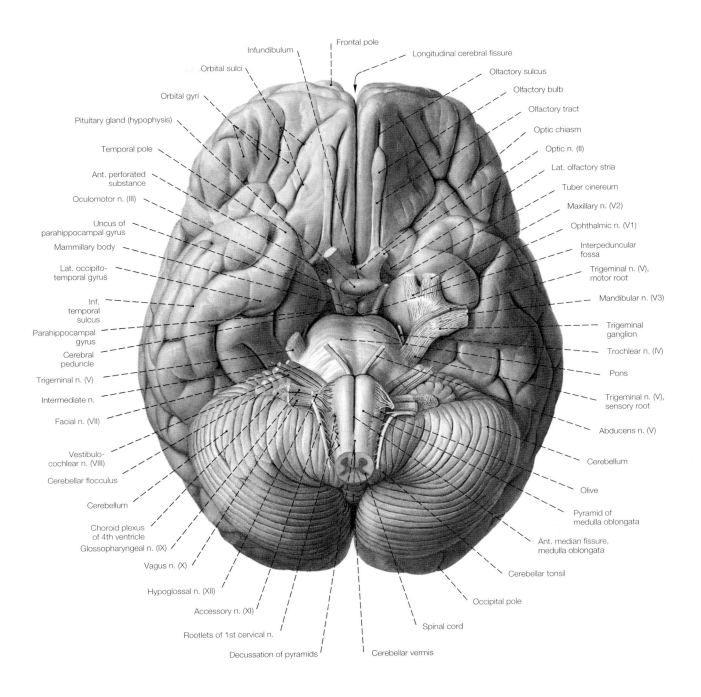

Infundibulum

Frontal pole

Orbital sulci

Longitudinal cerebral fissure

Orbital gyri

Olfactory sulcus

Pituitary gland (hypophysis)

Olfactory bulb

Temporal pole

Olfactory tract

Ant. perforated substance

Optic chiasm

Oculomotor n. (III)

Optic n. (II)

Uncus of parahippocampal gyrus

Lat. olfactory stria

Mammillary body

Tuber cinereum

Lat. occipito-temporal gyrus

Maxillary n. (V2)

Inf. temporal sulcus

Ophthalmic n. (V1)

Parahippocampal gyrus

Interpeduncular fossa

Cerebral peduncle

Trigeminal n. (V), motor root

Trigeminal n. (V)

Mandibular n. (V3)

Intermediate n.

Trigeminal ganglion

Facial n. (VII)

Trochlear n. (IV)

Vestibulo-cochlear n. (VIII)

Pons

Cerebellar flocculus

Trigeminal n. (V), sensory root

Cerebellum

Abducens n. (V)

Choroid plexus of 4th ventricle

Cerebellum

Glossopharyngeal n. (IX)

Olive

Vagus n. (X)

Pyramid of medulla oblongata

Hypoglossal n. (XII)

Ant. median fissure, medulla oblongata

Accessory n. (XI)

Cerebellar tonsil

Rootlets of 1st cervical n.

Occipital pole

Decussation of pyramids

Spinal cord

Cerebellar vermis

Fig. 477 The cerebrum and brainstem with cerebellum and cranial nerves, viewed from below. The leptomeninges (i.e., arachnoid and pia mater) have been removed.

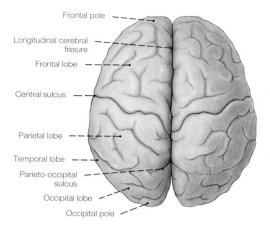

Fig. 478 The lobes of the cerebrum, viewed from above.

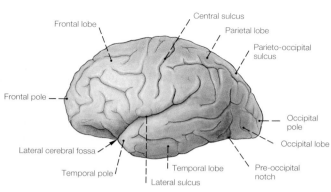

Fig. 479 The lobes of the cerebrum, lateral aspect.

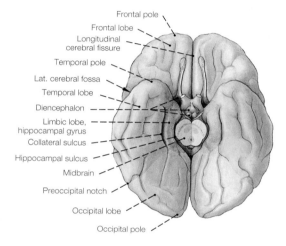

Fig. 480 The lobes of the cerebrum, viewed from below.

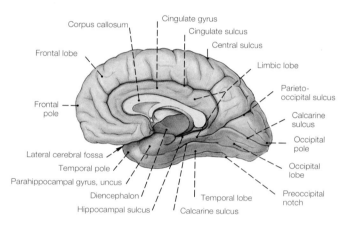

Fig. 481 The lobes of the cerebrum, medial aspect.

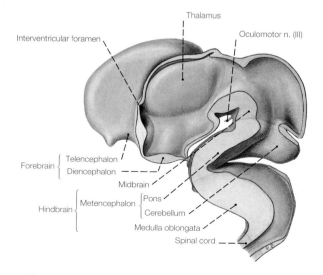

Fig. 482 Development of the brain. Median section of a model of the brain of a 2-month-old embryo. Compare Fig. 475.

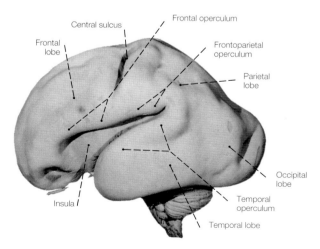

Fig. 483 Development of the brain. The brain of a 4-month-old fetus (crown-rump length, CRL, 20 cm), lateral aspect.

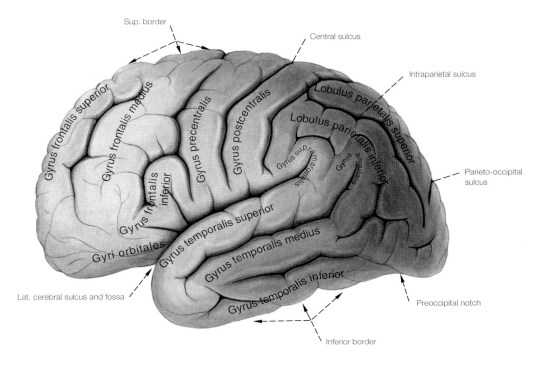

Fig. 484 Gyri of the left cerebral hemisphere, lateral aspect.

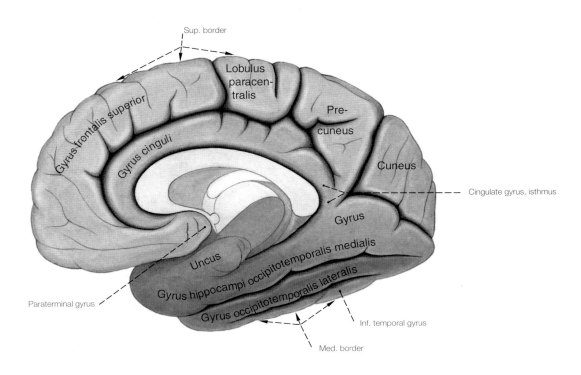

Fig. 485 Gyri of the right cerebral hemisphere, medial aspect.

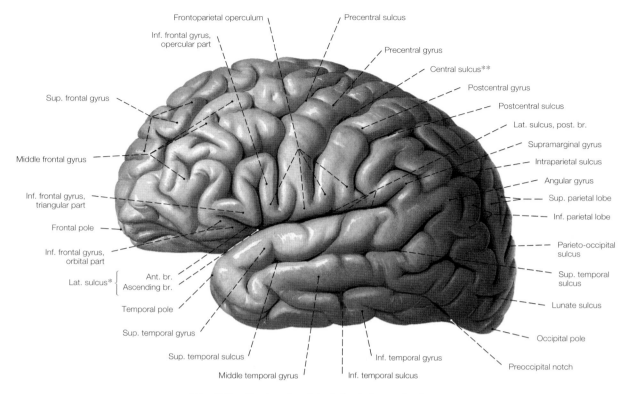

Frontoparietal operculum

Inf. frontal gyrus,
opercular part

Precentral sulcus

Precentral gyrus

Central sulcus**

Postcentral gyrus

Postcentral sulcus

Lat. sulcus, post. br.

Supramarginal gyrus

Intraparietal sulcus

Angular gyrus

Sup. parietal lobe

Inf. parietal lobe

Parieto-occipital sulcus

Sup. temporal sulcus

Lunate sulcus

Occipital pole

Preoccipital notch

Sup. frontal gyrus

Middle frontal gyrus

Inf. frontal gyrus,
triangular part

Frontal pole

Inf. frontal gyrus,
orbital part

Lat. sulcus* { Ant. br. Ascending br.

Temporal pole

Sup. temporal gyrus

Sup. temporal sulcus

Middle temporal gyrus

Inf. temporal sulcus

Inf. temporal gyrus

Fig. 486 Gyri and sulci of the left cerebral hemisphere, lateral aspect.

* SYLVIAN sulcus
** Sulcus of ROLANDO

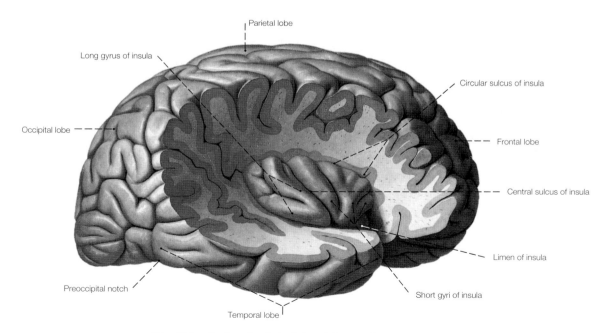

Parietal lobe

Long gyrus of insula

Occipital lobe

Circular sulcus of insula

Frontal lobe

Central sulcus of insula

Limen of insula

Short gyri of insula

Preoccipital notch

Temporal lobe

Fig. 487 Gyri and sulci of the right cerebral hemisphere, lateral aspect. The insula has been exposed by removing the frontal, frontoparietal and temporal opercula.

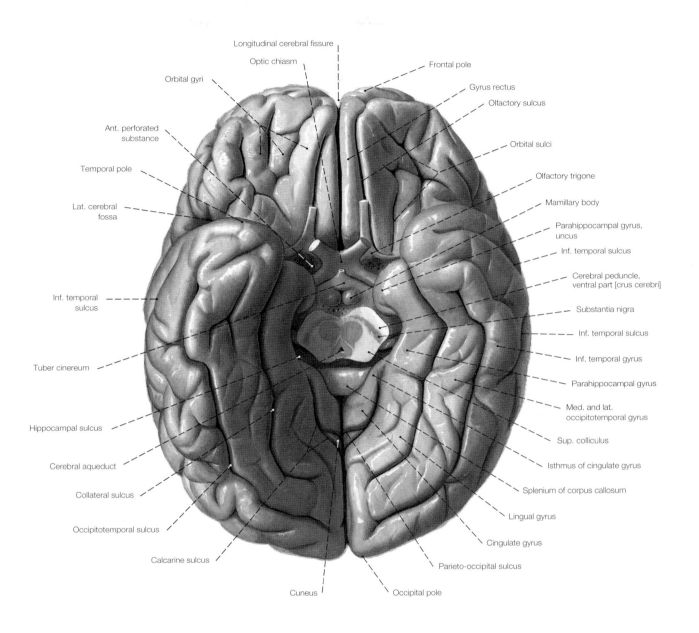

Longitudinal cerebral fissure

Optic chiasm

Orbital gyri

Ant. perforated substance

Temporal pole

Lat. cerebral fossa

Inf. temporal sulcus

Tuber cinereum

Hippocampal sulcus

Cerebral aqueduct

Collateral sulcus

Occipitotemporal sulcus

Calcarine sulcus

Cuneus

Frontal pole

Gyrus rectus

Olfactory sulcus

Orbital sulci

Olfactory trigone

Mamillary body

Parahippocampal gyrus, uncus

Inf. temporal sulcus

Cerebral peduncle, ventral part [crus cerebri]

Substantia nigra

Inf. temporal sulcus

Inf. temporal gyrus

Parahippocampal gyrus

Med. and lat. occipitotemporal gyrus

Sup. colliculus

Isthmus of cingulate gyrus

Splenium of corpus callosum

Lingual gyrus

Cingulate gyrus

Parieto-occipital sulcus

Occipital pole

Fig. 488 Gyri and sulci of the cerebral hemispheres, viewed from below. The midbrain has been sectioned.

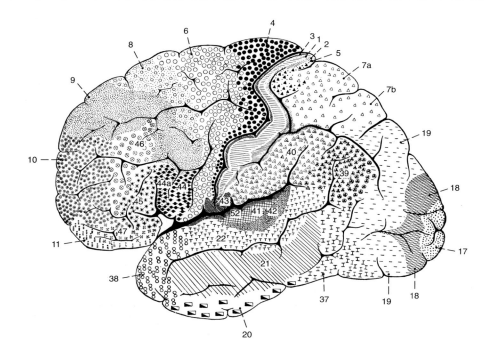

Fig. 489 Cytoarchitectonic cortical areas of the left cerebral hemisphere as described by BRODMANN, lateral aspect. The individual areas are numbered; the various symbols indicate different cell types.

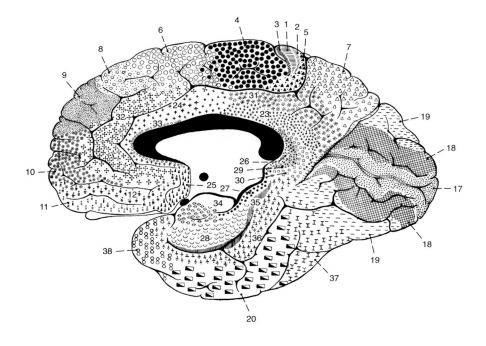

Fig. 490 Cytoarchitectonic cortical areas of the right cerebral hemisphere as described by BRODMANN, medial aspect. The individual areas are numbered; the various symbols indicate different cell types.

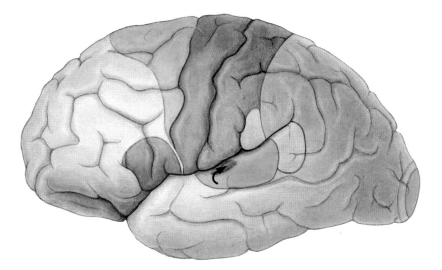

Fig. 491 Functional cortical areas of the cerebral hemispheres according to FOERSTER, lateral aspect.

The primary receiving area for auditory impulses (↰) extends over the upper edge of the temporal lobe onto its inner surface.

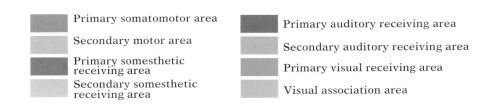

Primary somatomotor area

Secondary motor area

Primary somesthetic receiving area

Secondary somesthetic receiving area

Primary auditory receiving area

Secondary auditory receiving area

Primary visual receiving area

Visual association area

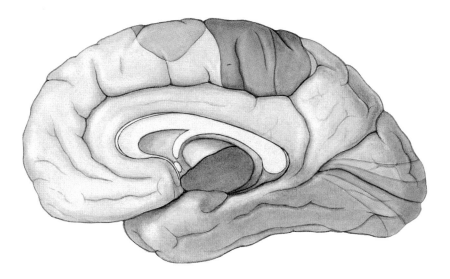

Fig. 492 Functional cortical areas of the cerebral hemispheres according to FOERSTER, medial aspect.

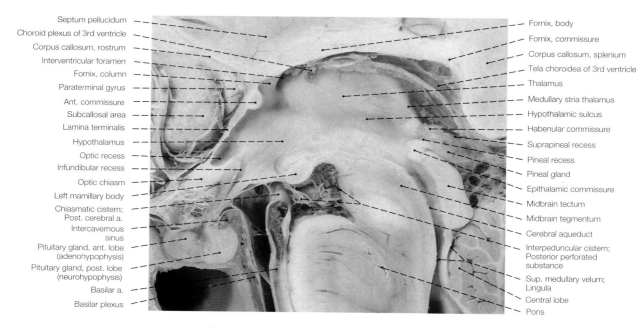

Septum pellucidum
Choroid plexus of 3rd ventricle
Corpus callosum, rostrum
Interventricular foramen
Fornix, column
Paraterminal gyrus
Ant. commissure
Subcallosal area
Lamina terminalis
Hypothalamus
Optic recess
Infundibular recess
Optic chiasm
Left mamillary body
Chiasmatic cistern;
Post. cerebral a.
Intercavernous
sinus
Pituitary gland, ant. lobe
(adenohypophysis)
Pituitary gland, post. lobe
(neurohypophysis)
Basilar a.
Basilar plexus

Fornix, body
Fornix, commissure
Corpus callosum, splenium
Tela choroidea of 3rd ventricle
Thalamus
Medullary stria thalamus
Hypothalamic sulcus
Habenular commissure
Suprapineal recess
Pineal recess
Pineal gland
Epithalamic commissure
Midbrain tectum
Midbrain tegmentum
Cerebral aqueduct
Interpeduncular cistern;
Posterior perforated
substance
Sup. medullary velum;
Lingula
Central lobe
Pons

Fig. 493 The third ventricle, median section, medial aspect.

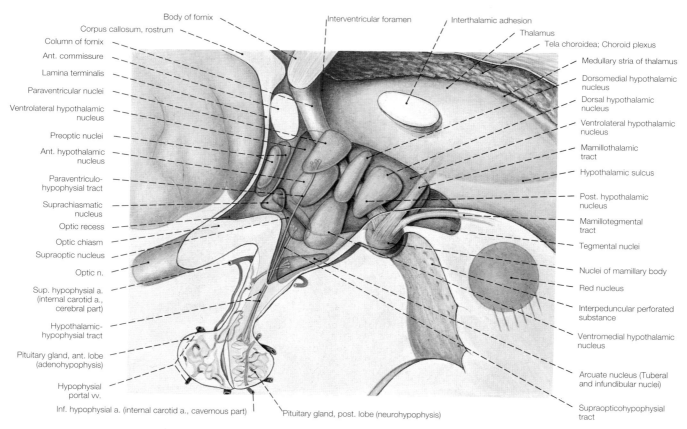

Body of fornix
Corpus callosum, rostrum
Column of fornix
Ant. commissure
Lamina terminalis
Paraventricular nuclei
Ventrolateral hypothalamic
nucleus
Preoptic nuclei
Ant. hypothalamic
nucleus
Paraventriculo-
hypophysial tract
Suprachiasmatic
nucleus
Optic recess
Optic chiasm
Supraoptic nucleus
Optic n.
Sup. hypophysial a.
(internal carotid a.,
cerebral part)
Hypothalamic-
hypophysial tract
Pituitary gland, ant. lobe
(adenohypophysis)
Hypophysial
portal vv.
Inf. hypophysial a. (internal carotid a., cavernous part)
Pituitary gland, post. lobe (neurohypophysis)

Interventricular foramen
Interthalamic adhesion
Thalamus
Tela choroidea; Choroid plexus
Medullary stria of thalamus
Dorsomedial hypothalamic
nucleus
Dorsal hypothalamic
nucleus
Ventrolateral hypothalamic
nucleus
Mamillothalamic
tract
Hypothalamic sulcus
Post. hypothalamic
nucleus
Mamillotegmental
tract
Tegmental nuclei
Nuclei of mamillary body
Red nucleus
Interpeduncular perforated
substance
Ventromedial hypothalamic
nucleus
Arcuate nucleus (Tuberal
and infundibular nuclei)
Supraopticohypophysial
tract

Fig. 494 The hypothalamus, overview, medial aspect. The nuclear regions are depicted as transparent.

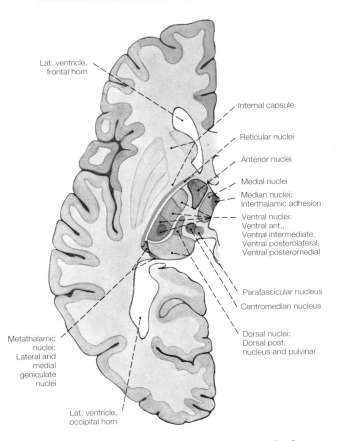

Lat. ventricle, frontal horn

Internal capsule

Reticular nuclei

Anterior nuclei

Medial nuclei

Median nuclei; Interthalamic adhesion

Ventral nuclei: Ventral ant., Ventral intermediate, Ventral posterolateral, Ventral posteromedial

Parafascicular nucleus

Centromedian nucleus

Dorsal nuclei: Dorsal post. nucleus and pulvinar

Metathalamic nuclei: Lateral and medial geniculate nuclei

Lat. ventricle, occipital horn

a Horizontal section through the left cerebral hemisphere, viewed from above.

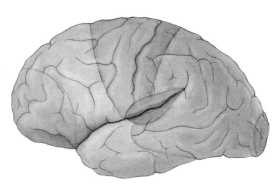

b The left cerebral hemisphere, lateral aspect.

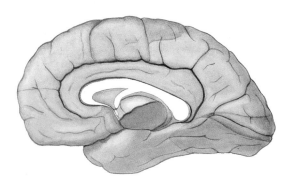

c The right cerebral hemisphere, medial aspect.

Fig. 495 a–c   Nuclei and cortical projections of the thalamus. Each color identifies a nucleus and its related cortical projection area.

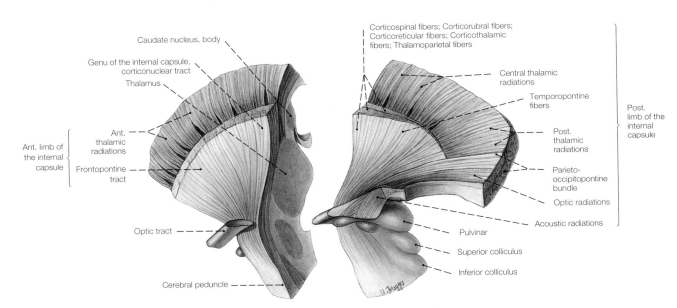

Caudate nucleus, body

Genu of the internal capsule, corticonuclear tract

Thalamus

Corticospinal fibers; Corticorubral fibers; Corticoreticular fibers; Corticothalamic fibers; Thalamoparietal fibers

Central thalamic radiations

Temporopontine fibers

Post. thalamic radiations

Parieto-occipitopontine bundle

Optic radiations

Acoustic radiations

Post. limb of the internal capsule

Ant. limb of the internal capsule

Ant. thalamic radiations

Frontopontine tract

Optic tract

Pulvinar

Superior colliculus

Inferior colliculus

Cerebral peduncle

Fig. 496   Thalamic radiations and the left internal capsule, divided in two by a frontal section, lateral aspect.

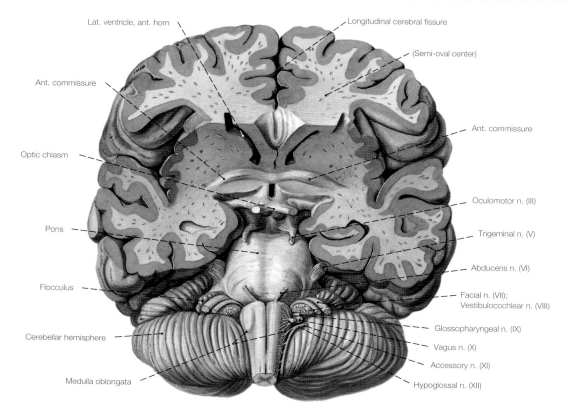

Lat. ventricle, ant. horn

Longitudinal cerebral fissure

Ant. commissure

(Semi-oval center)

Ant. commissure

Optic chiasm

Oculomotor n. (III)

Pons

Trigeminal n. (V)

Abducens n. (VI)

Flocculus

Facial n. (VII);
Vestibulocochlear n. (VIII)

Glossopharyngeal n. (IX)

Cerebellar hemisphere

Vagus n. (X)

Accessory n. (XI)

Medulla oblongata

Hypoglossal n. (XII)

Fig. 497 Anterior commissure and brainstem, viewed from below. Basal parts of the cerebral hemispheres have been partially removed.

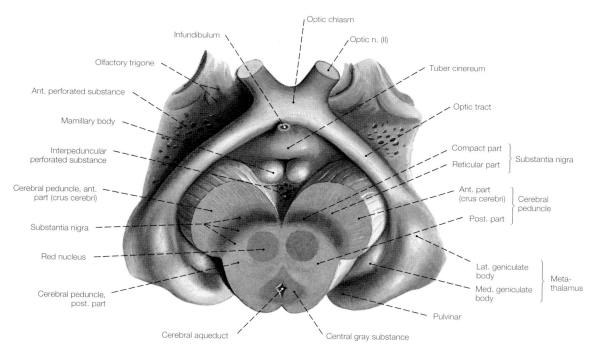

Infundibulum

Optic chiasm

Optic n. (II)

Olfactory trigone

Tuber cinereum

Ant. perforated substance

Optic tract

Mamillary body

Compact part

Reticular part

Substantia nigra

Interpeduncular perforated substance

Cerebral peduncle, ant. part (crus cerebri)

Ant. part (crus cerebri)

Post. part

Cerebral peduncle

Substantia nigra

Red nucleus

Lat. geniculate body

Med. geniculate body

Meta-thalamus

Cerebral peduncle, post. part

Pulvinar

Cerebral aqueduct

Central gray substance

Fig. 498 Midbrain and diencephalon, viewed from below. The midbrain has been cross-sectioned.

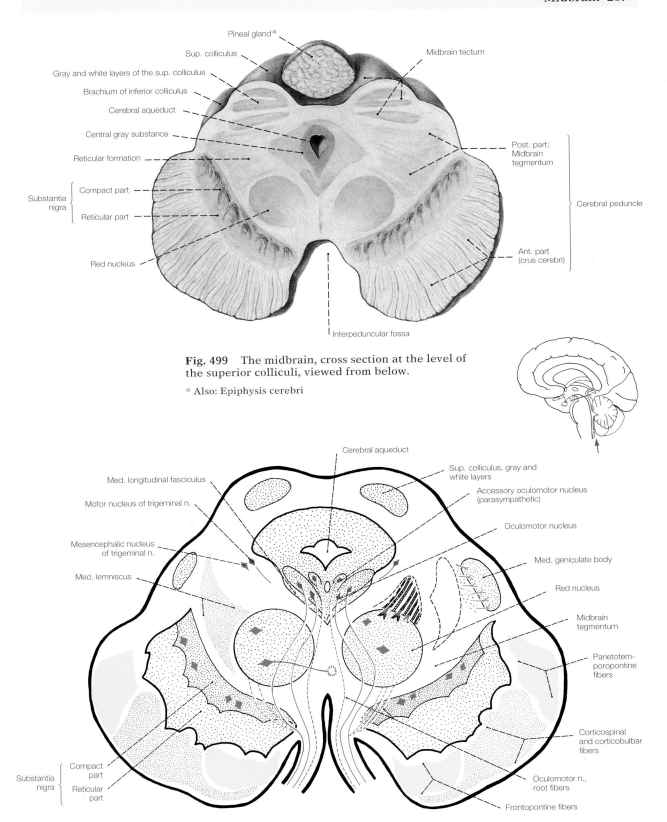

Pineal gland*

Sup. colliculus

Gray and white layers of the sup. colliculus

Brachium of inferior colliculus

Cerebral aqueduct

Central gray substance

Reticular formation

Substantia nigra { Compact part

Reticular part

Red nucleus

Midbrain tectum

Post. part; Midbrain tegmentum

Cerebral peduncle

Ant. part (crus cerebri)

Interpeduncular fossa

Fig. 499   The midbrain, cross section at the level of the superior colliculi, viewed from below.

* Also: Epiphysis cerebri

Cerebral aqueduct

Med. longitudinal fasciculus

Motor nucleus of trigeminal n.

Mesencephalic nucleus of trigeminal n.

Med. lemniscus

Substantia nigra { Compact part

Reticular part

Sup. colliculus, gray and white layers

Accessory oculomotor nucleus (parasympathetic)

Oculomotor nucleus

Med. geniculate body

Red nucleus

Midbrain tegmentum

Parietotem-poropontine fibers

Corticospinal and corticobulbar fibers

Oculomotor n., root fibers

Frontopontine fibers

Fig. 500   Nuclei and fiber tracts of the midbrain. Schematic cross section at the level of the superior colliculi.

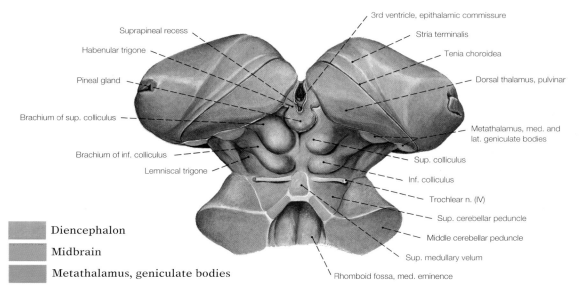

Suprapineal recess

Habenular trigone

Pineal gland

Brachium of sup. colliculus

Brachium of inf. colliculus

Lemniscal trigone

3rd ventricle, epithalamic commissure

Stria terminalis

Tenia choroidea

Dorsal thalamus, pulvinar

Metathalamus, med. and lat. geniculate bodies

Sup. colliculus

Inf. colliculus

Trochlear n. (IV)

Sup. cerebellar peduncle

Middle cerebellar peduncle

Sup. medullary velum

Rhomboid fossa, med. eminence

Diencephalon

Midbrain

Metathalamus, geniculate bodies

Fig. 501 The midbrain and pineal gland, viewed posteriorly from above.

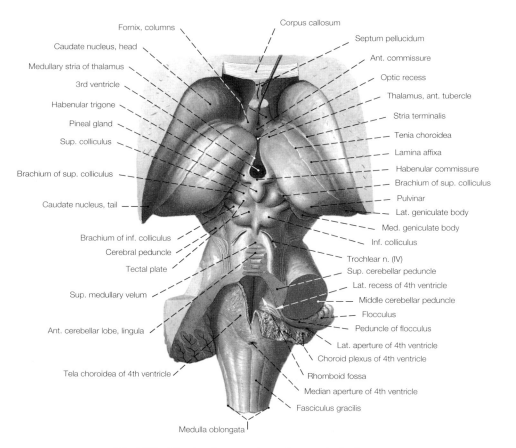

Fornix, columns

Caudate nucleus, head

Medullary stria of thalamus

3rd ventricle

Habenular trigone

Pineal gland

Sup. colliculus

Brachium of sup. colliculus

Caudate nucleus, tail

Brachium of inf. colliculus

Cerebral peduncle

Tectal plate

Sup. medullary velum

Ant. cerebellar lobe, lingula

Tela choroidea of 4th ventricle

Medulla oblongata

Corpus callosum

Septum pellucidum

Ant. commissure

Optic recess

Thalamus, ant. tubercle

Stria terminalis

Tenia choroidea

Lamina affixa

Habenular commissure

Brachium of sup. colliculus

Pulvinar

Lat. geniculate body

Med. geniculate body

Inf. colliculus

Trochlear n. (IV)

Sup. cerebellar peduncle

Lat. recess of 4th ventricle

Middle cerebellar peduncle

Flocculus

Peduncle of flocculus

Lat. aperture of 4th ventricle

Choroid plexus of 4th ventricle

Rhomboid fossa

Median aperture of 4th ventricle

Fasciculus gracilis

Fig. 502 The brainstem viewed posteriorly from above. The corpus callosum and most of the cerebellum have been removed. The tela choroidea of the 4th ventricle has been split in the midline and reflected to the right.

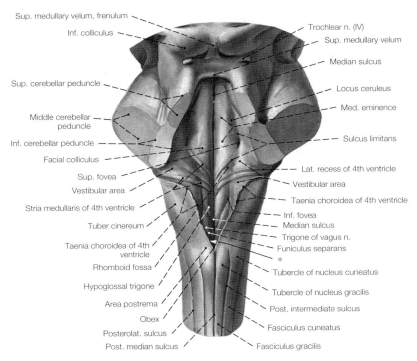

Fig. 503 Rhomboid fossa. Dorsal view of the floor of the fourth ventricle after sectioning the cerebellar peduncles.

* Formerly: Calamus scriptorius

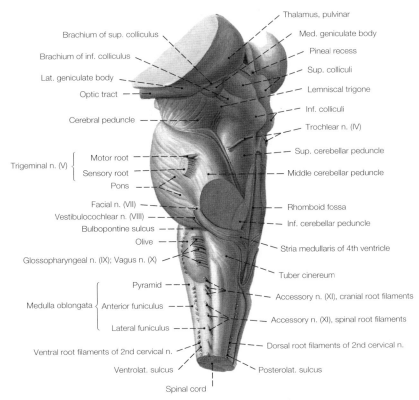

Fig. 504 Brainstem. Oblique lateral view of the floor of the fourth ventricle after sectioning the cerebellar peduncles.

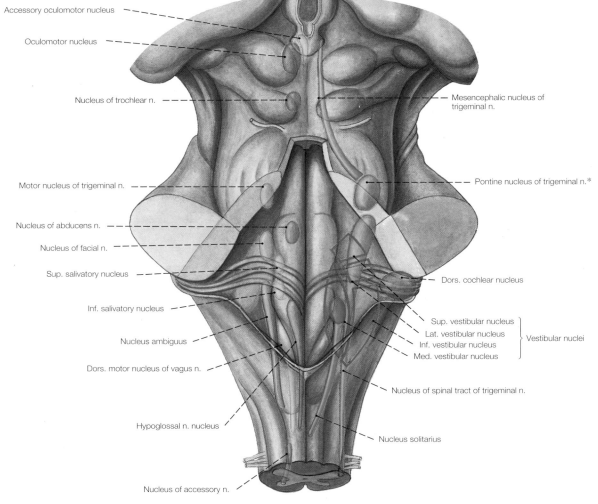

Accessory oculomotor nucleus

Oculomotor nucleus

Nucleus of trochlear n.

Mesencephalic nucleus of trigeminal n.

Motor nucleus of trigeminal n.

Pontine nucleus of trigeminal n.*

Nucleus of abducens n.

Nucleus of facial n.

Sup. salivatory nucleus

Dors. cochlear nucleus

Inf. salivatory nucleus

Sup. vestibular nucleus
Lat. vestibular nucleus
Inf. vestibular nucleus   Vestibular nuclei
Med. vestibular nucleus

Nucleus ambiguus

Dors. motor nucleus of vagus n.

Nucleus of spinal tract of trigeminal n.

Hypoglossal n. nucleus

Nucleus solitarius

Nucleus of accessory n.

Fig. 505 Nuclei of the cranial nerves projected schematically onto a dorsal view of the brainstem.

On the left are the motor nuclei and on the right, the sensory nuclei.

* Clinical: Principal sensory nucleus of trigeminal n.

General somatic efferent nuclei (GSE)

General visceral efferent nuclei (GVE)

Special visceral efferent nuclei (SVE)

General and special visceral afferent nuclei (G/SVA)

General somatic afferent nuclei (GSA)

Special somatic afferent nuclei (SSA)

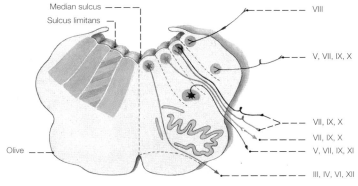

Median sulcus

Sulcus limitans

VIII

V, VII, IX, X

VII, IX, X

VII, IX, X

V, VII, IX, XI

Olive

III, IV, VI, XII

Fig. 506 Nuclei of the cranial nerves projected onto a diagram of a cross section of the brainstem

at the level of the rhomboid fossa. See table, page 262.

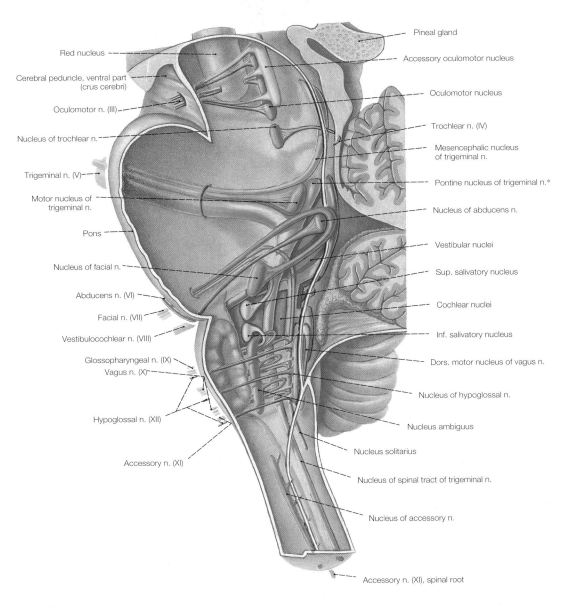

Red nucleus

Cerebral peduncle, ventral part (crus cerebri)

Oculomotor n. (III)

Nucleus of trochlear n.

Trigeminal n. (V)

Motor nucleus of trigeminal n.

Pons

Nucleus of facial n.

Abducens n. (VI)

Facial n. (VII)

Vestibulocochlear n. (VIII)

Glossopharyngeal n. (IX)

Vagus n. (X)

Hypoglossal n. (XII)

Accessory n. (XI)

Pineal gland

Accessory oculomotor nucleus

Oculomotor nucleus

Trochlear n. (IV)

Mesencephalic nucleus of trigeminal n.

Pontine nucleus of trigeminal n.*

Nucleus of abducens n.

Vestibular nuclei

Sup. salivatory nucleus

Cochlear nuclei

Inf. salivatory nucleus

Dors. motor nucleus of vagus n.

Nucleus of hypoglossal n.

Nucleus ambiguus

Nucleus solitarius

Nucleus of spinal tract of trigeminal n.

Nucleus of accessory n.

Accessory n. (XI), spinal root

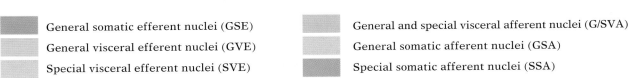

General somatic efferent nuclei (GSE)

General visceral efferent nuclei (GVE)

Special visceral efferent nuclei (SVE)

General and special visceral afferent nuclei (G/SVA)

General somatic afferent nuclei (GSA)

Special somatic afferent nuclei (SSA)

Fig. 507 The nuclei of the cranial nerves projected onto a spatial diagram of the median plane of the brainstem, medial aspect.

* Clinical: Principle sensory nucleus of trigeminal n.

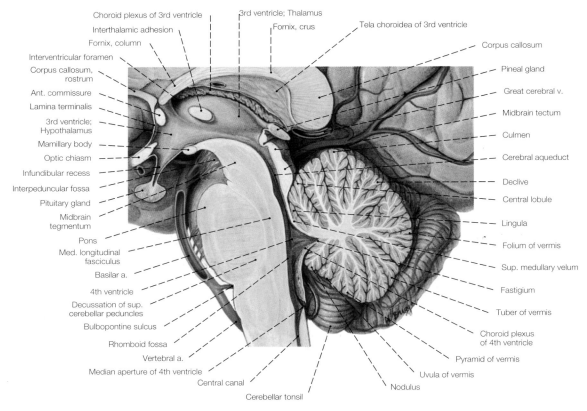

Choroid plexus of 3rd ventricle
Interthalamic adhesion
Fornix, column
Interventricular foramen
Corpus callosum, rostrum
Ant. commissure
Lamina terminalis
3rd ventricle; Hypothalamus
Mamillary body
Optic chiasm
Infundibular recess
Interpeduncular fossa
Pituitary gland
Midbrain tegmentum
Pons
Med. longitudinal fasciculus
Basilar a.
4th ventricle
Decussation of sup. cerebellar peduncles
Bulbopontine sulcus
Rhomboid fossa
Vertebral a.
Median aperture of 4th ventricle
Central canal
Cerebellar tonsil

3rd ventricle; Thalamus
Fornix, crus
Tela choroidea of 3rd ventricle

Corpus callosum
Pineal gland
Great cerebral v.
Midbrain tectum
Culmen
Cerebral aqueduct
Declive
Central lobule
Lingula
Folium of vermis
Sup. medullary velum
Fastigium
Tuber of vermis
Choroid plexus of 4th ventricle
Pyramid of vermis
Uvula of vermis
Nodulus

Fig. 508 The third and fourth ventricles. Median section through the brainstem, medial aspect.

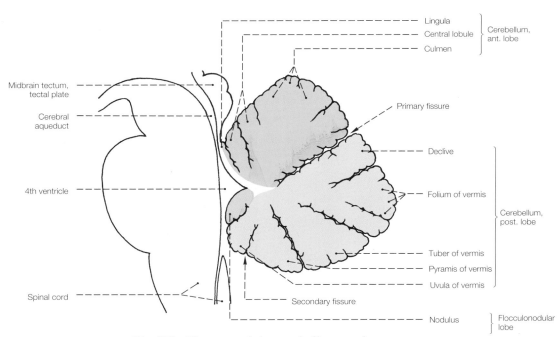

Lingula
Central lobule
Culmen
} Cerebellum, ant. lobe

Midbrain tectum, tectal plate
Cerebral aqueduct

Primary fissure

4th ventricle

Declive
Folium of vermis
} Cerebellum, post. lobe

Tuber of vermis
Pyramis of vermis
Uvula of vermis

Spinal cord

Secondary fissure

Nodulus } Flocculonodular lobe

Fig. 509 The parts of the cerebellar vermis. Diagram of a median section.

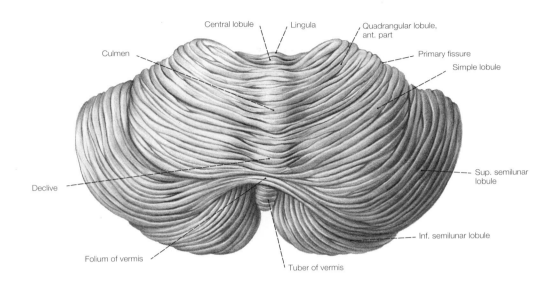

Fig. 510 Cerebellum, viewed posteriorly from above.

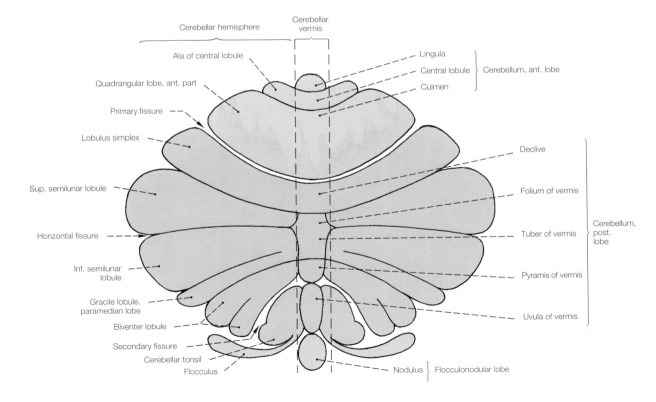

Fig. 511 Cerebellum. Diagram of the cerebellar lobes and their lobules.

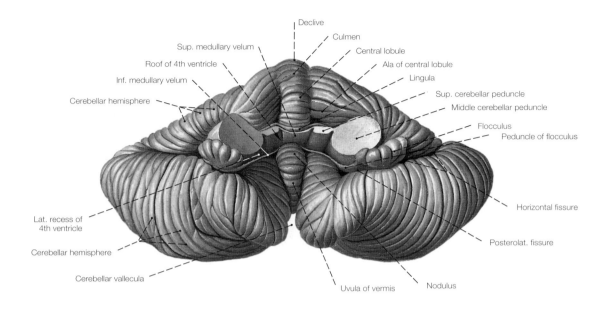

Fig. 512 Cerebellum, with the cerebellar peduncles sectioned, anterior view.

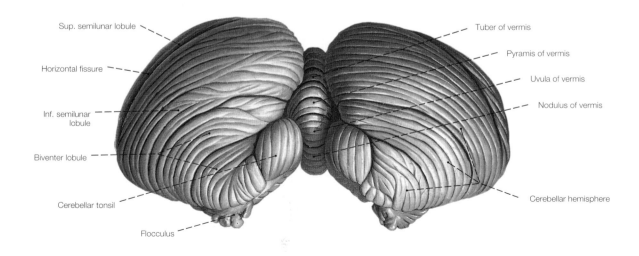

Fig. 513 Cerebellum, posterior view.

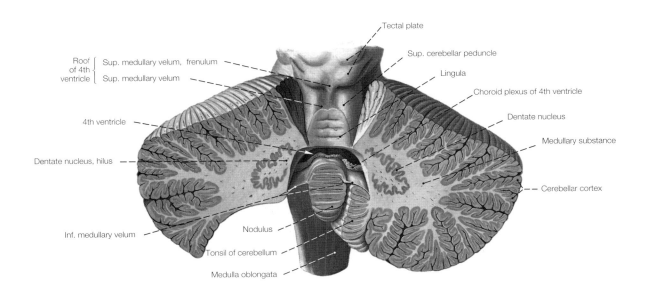

Tectal plate

Roof of 4th ventricle { Sup. medullary velum, frenulum

Sup. medullary velum

Sup. cerebellar peduncle

Lingula

Choroid plexus of 4th ventricle

4th ventricle

Dentate nucleus

Medullary substance

Dentate nucleus, hilus

Cerebellar cortex

Inf. medullary velum

Nodulus

Tonsil of cerebellum

Medulla oblongata

Fig. 514 Cerebellum. Frontal section, posterior view.

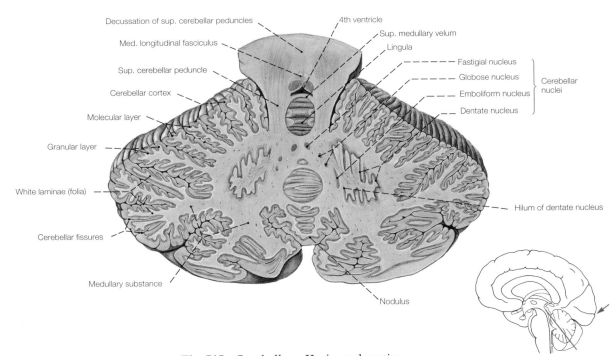

Decussation of sup. cerebellar peduncles

4th ventricle

Med. longitudinal fasciculus

Sup. medullary velum

Lingula

Sup. cerebellar peduncle

Fastigial nucleus

Globose nucleus

Cerebellar cortex

Emboliform nucleus

Molecular layer

Dentate nucleus

Granular layer

White laminae (folia)

Hilum of dentate nucleus

Cerebellar fissures

Medullary substance

Nodulus

Cerebellar nuclei

Fig. 515 Cerebellum. Horizontal section through the middle cerebellar peduncles, posterior view.

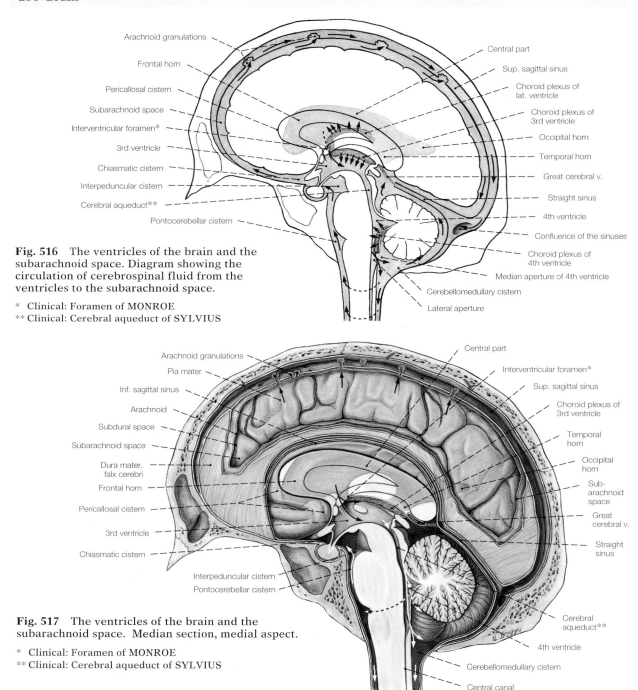

Fig. 516 The ventricles of the brain and the subarachnoid space. Diagram showing the circulation of cerebrospinal fluid from the ventricles to the subarachnoid space.

* Clinical: Foramen of MONROE
** Clinical: Cerebral aqueduct of SYLVIUS

Fig. 517 The ventricles of the brain and the subarachnoid space. Median section, medial aspect.

* Clinical: Foramen of MONROE
** Clinical: Cerebral aqueduct of SYLVIUS

The cerebrospinal fluid is formed by the ependyma lining the ventricles, especially by the choroid plexus. It circulates from its sites of formation in the lateral ventricles, through both interventricular foramina (of MONROE) into the third ventricle, and then through the cerebral aqueduct (of SYLVIUS) into the fourth ventricle and into the central canal of the medulla. It passes into the cerebromedullary cistern (great cistern) and the pontine cistern via the median aperture (of MAGENDI) and the lateral apertures (of LUSCHKA) of the fourth ventricle and thereby into the subarachnoid space.

Within the subarachnoid space the cerebrospinal fluid circulates around the surfaces of the cerebrum, cerebellum, and spinal cord. As it circulates, cerebrospinal fluid is interposed between the blood vessels with their penetrating branches, the connective tissue of the pia mater, and the adjacent astrocytic neuroglial processes. It is reabsorbed into the venous circulation at the arachnoid granulations (of PACCHIONI).

Obstruction of the flow of cerebrospinal fluid can occur at sites where the ventricles narrow: at the interventricular foramina, the cerebral aqueduct, and the median and lateral apertures. If flow is restricted, e.g., as a result of a developmental abnormality or of inflammation, an internal hydrocephalus can occur. If the subarachnoid space is dilated, e.g., as with brain atrophy, an external hydrocephalus can result.

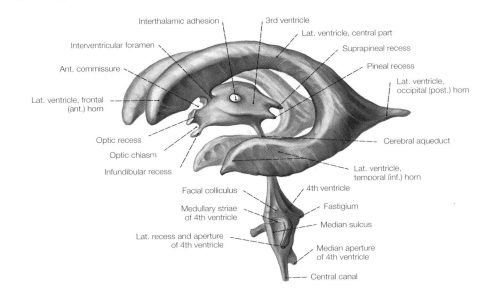

Fig. 518 The ventricles of the brain, viewed obliquely from the left side, in a cast specimen.

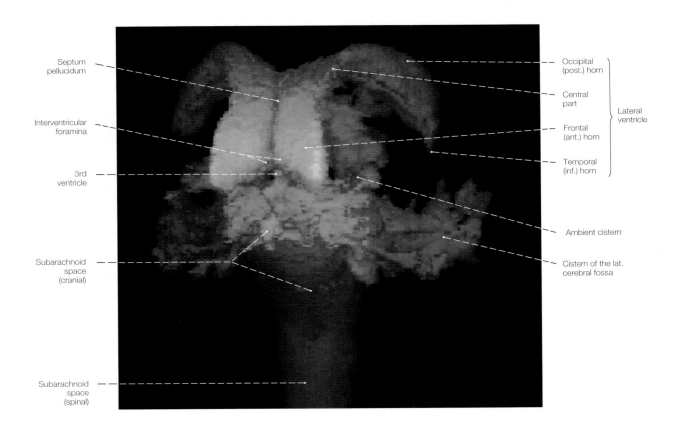

Fig. 519 The ventricles of the brain and the subarachnoid space. Three dimensional reconstruction from a magnetic resonance image (MRI), viewed from the left.

Of the subarachnoid spaces, only the cisterns at the base of the brain and the space around the spinal cord are visible.

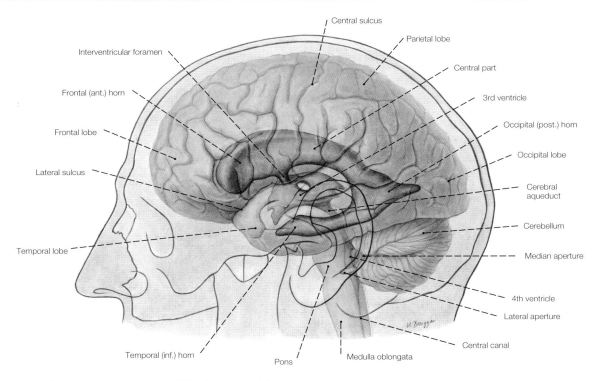

Fig. 520 The ventricles of the brain projected onto the surface of the brain, lateral aspect.

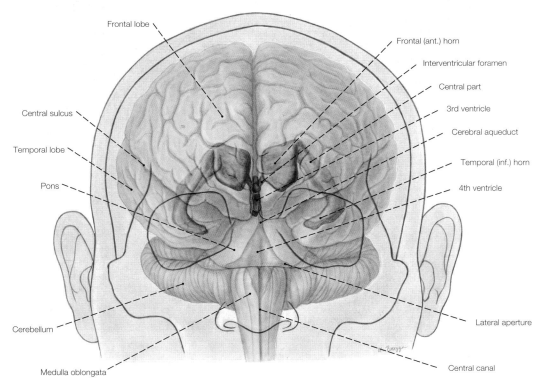

Fig. 521 The ventricles of the brain projected onto the surface of the brain, anterior aspect.

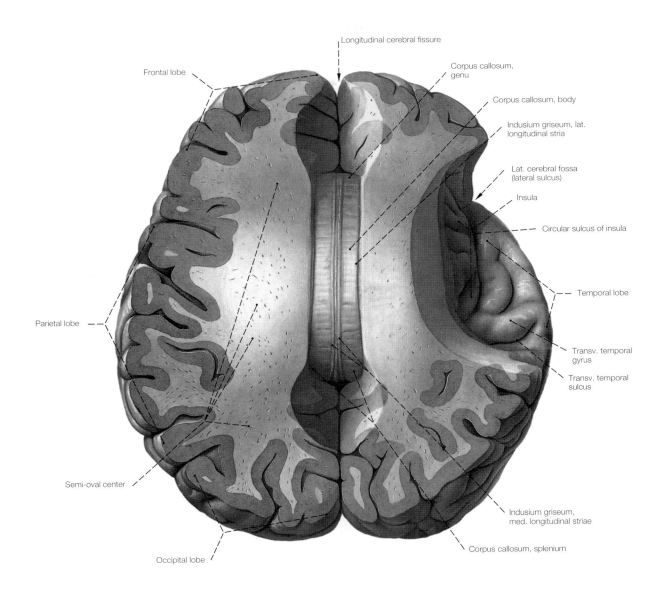

Longitudinal cerebral fissure

Frontal lobe

Corpus callosum,
genu

Corpus callosum, body

Indusium griseum, lat.
longitudinal stria

Lat. cerebral fossa
(lateral sulcus)

Insula

Circular sulcus of insula

Parietal lobe

Temporal lobe

Transv. temporal
gyrus

Transv. temporal
sulcus

Semi-oval center

Indusium griseum,
med. longitudinal striae

Corpus callosum, splenium

Occipital lobe

Fig. 522 The corpus callosum and insula, viewed
from above. The superior parts of the cerebral
hemispheres and a part of the right frontal and
parietal lobes have been removed.

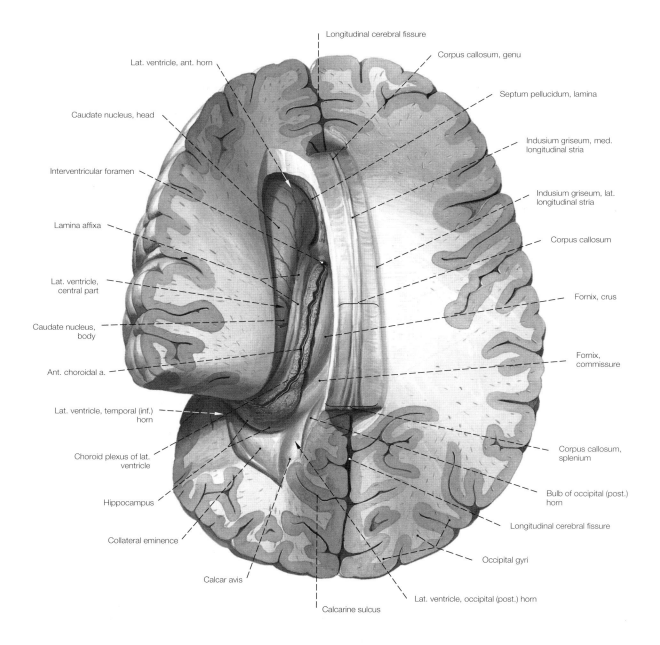

Longitudinal cerebral fissure

Corpus callosum, genu

Lat. ventricle, ant. horn

Septum pellucidum, lamina

Caudate nucleus, head

Indusium griseum, med. longitudinal stria

Interventricular foramen

Indusium griseum, lat. longitudinal stria

Lamina affixa

Corpus callosum

Lat. ventricle, central part

Fornix, crus

Caudate nucleus, body

Fornix, commissure

Ant. choroidal a.

Lat. ventricle, temporal (inf.) horn

Choroid plexus of lat. ventricle

Corpus callosum, splenium

Hippocampus

Bulb of occipital (post.) horn

Collateral eminence

Longitudinal cerebral fissure

Calcar avis

Occipital gyri

Calcarine sulcus

Lat. ventricle, occipital (post.) horn

Fig. 523 The lateral ventricle, viewed from above. A large part of the left cerebral hemisphere has been removed.

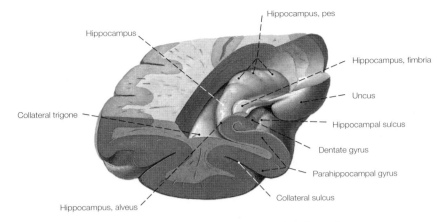

Hippocampus, pes

Hippocampus

Hippocampus, fimbria

Uncus

Collateral trigone

Hippocampal sulcus

Dentate gyrus

Parahippocampal gyrus

Collateral sulcus

Hippocampus, alveus

Fig. 524 Temporal (inferior) horn of the left lateral ventricle, viewed from posterior and above. Frontal section after removal of the roof of the ventricle.

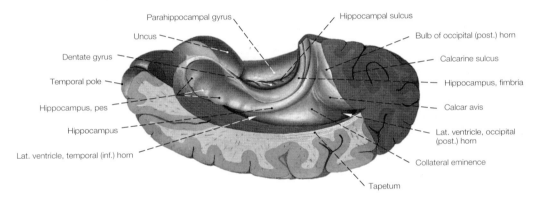

Parahippocampal gyrus

Hippocampal sulcus

Uncus

Bulb of occipital (post.) horn

Dentate gyrus

Calcarine sulcus

Temporal pole

Hippocampus, fimbria

Hippocampus, pes

Calcar avis

Hippocampus

Lat. ventricle, occipital (post.) horn

Lat. ventricle, temporal (inf.) horn

Collateral eminence

Tapetum

Fig. 525 Temporal (inferior) horn of the lateral ventricle, viewed from the left and above. Frontal section after opening the temporal wall.

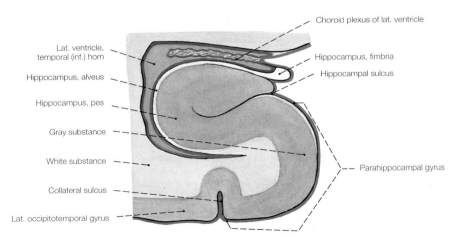

Choroid plexus of lat. ventricle

Lat. ventricle, temporal (inf.) horn

Hippocampus, fimbria

Hippocampus, alveus

Hippocampal sulcus

Hippocampus, pes

Gray substance

White substance

Parahippocampal gyrus

Collateral sulcus

Lat. occipitotemporal gyrus

Fig. 526 Temporal (inferior) horn of the lateral ventricle. Schematic frontal section.

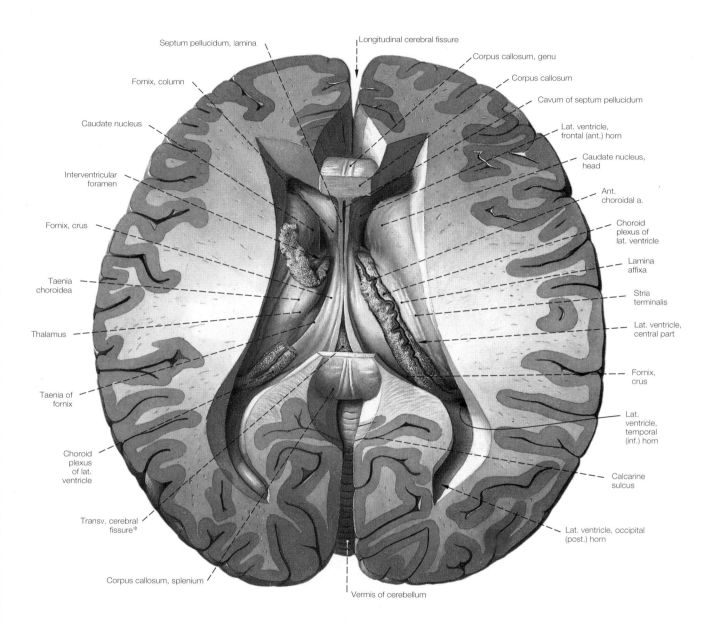

Septum pellucidum, lamina

Fornix, column

Caudate nucleus

Interventricular foramen

Fornix, crus

Taenia choroidea

Thalamus

Taenia of fornix

Choroid plexus of lat. ventricle

Transv. cerebral fissure*

Corpus callosum, splenium

Longitudinal cerebral fissure

Corpus callosum, genu

Corpus callosum

Cavum of septum pellucidum

Lat. ventricle, frontal (ant.) horn

Caudate nucleus, head

Ant. choroidal a.

Choroid plexus of lat. ventricle

Lamina affixa

Stria terminalis

Lat. ventricle, central part

Fornix, crus

Lat. ventricle, temporal (inf.) horn

Calcarine sulcus

Lat. ventricle, occipital (post.) horn

Vermis of cerebellum

Fig. 527 The lateral ventricles, viewed from above. The upper part of the cerebral hemispheres and the body of the corpus callosum have been removed.

* Also: Telodiencephalic fissure

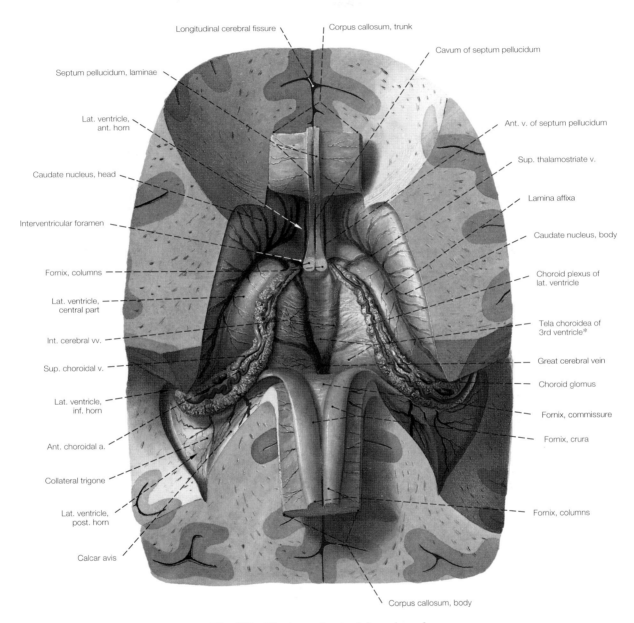

Longitudinal cerebral fissure

Corpus callosum, trunk

Cavum of septum pellucidum

Septum pellucidum, laminae

Ant. v. of septum pellucidum

Lat. ventricle, ant. horn

Sup. thalamostriate v.

Caudate nucleus, head

Lamina affixa

Interventricular foramen

Caudate nucleus, body

Fornix, columns

Choroid plexus of lat. ventricle

Lat. ventricle, central part

Tela choroidea of 3rd ventricle*

Int. cerebral vv.

Great cerebral vein

Sup. choroidal v.

Choroid glomus

Lat. ventricle, inf. horn

Fornix, commissure

Ant. choroidal a.

Fornix, crura

Collateral trigone

Lat. ventricle, post. horn

Fornix, columns

Calcar avis

Corpus callosum, body

Fig. 528 The lateral ventricles, viewed from above. The trunk of the corpus callosum and the columns of the fornix have been sectioned and reflected.

* Forms part of the roof of the third ventricle

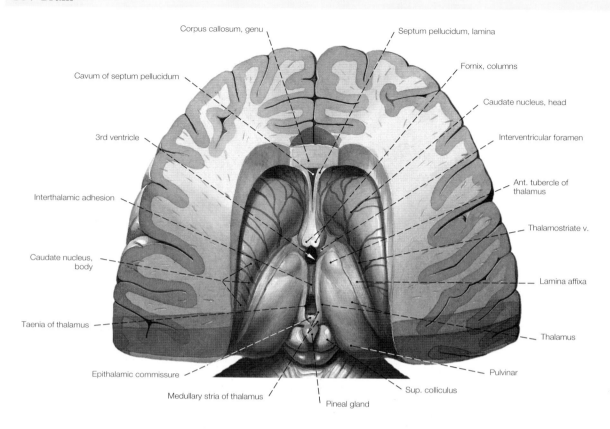

Corpus callosum, genu

Septum pellucidum, lamina

Cavum of septum pellucidum

Fornix, columns

Caudate nucleus, head

3rd ventricle

Interventricular foramen

Ant. tubercle of thalamus

Interthalamic adhesion

Thalamostriate v.

Caudate nucleus, body

Lamina affixa

Taenia of thalamus

Thalamus

Epithalamic commissure

Pulvinar

Medullary stria of thalamus

Sup. colliculus

Pineal gland

Fig. 529 The lateral ventricles and the third ventricle, viewed from above. Part of the cerebral hemispheres, the trunk of the corpus callosum, the fornix, as well as the choroid plexus and the tela choroidea of the third ventricle have been removed.

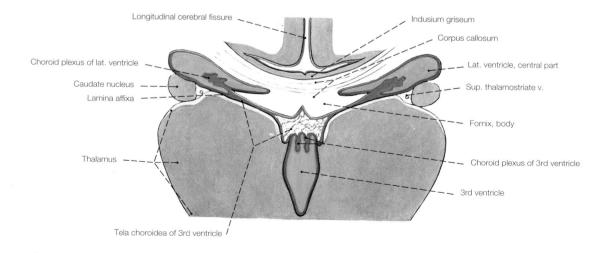

Longitudinal cerebral fissure

Indusium griseum

Corpus callosum

Choroid plexus of lat. ventricle

Lat. ventricle, central part

Caudate nucleus

Sup. thalamostriate v.

Lamina affixa

Fornix, body

Thalamus

Choroid plexus of 3rd ventricle

3rd ventricle

Tela choroidea of 3rd ventricle

Fig. 530 The central part of the lateral ventricle and the third ventricle, schematic frontal section.

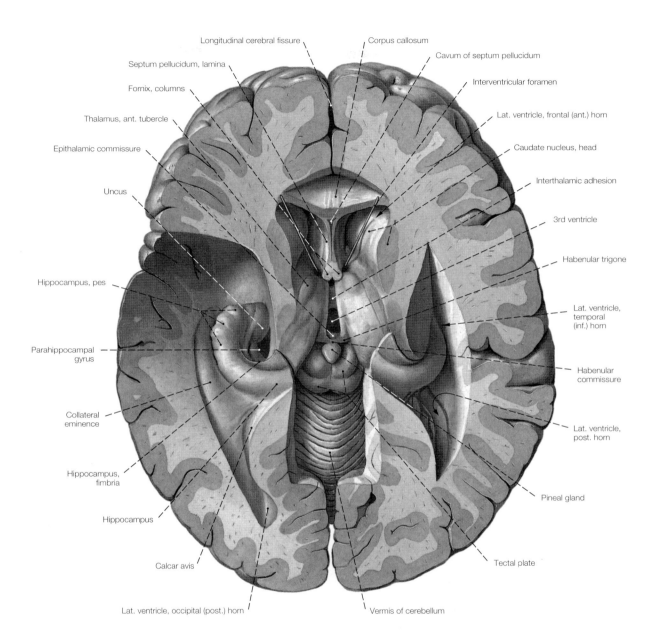

Longitudinal cerebral fissure

Corpus callosum

Septum pellucidum, lamina

Cavum of septum pellucidum

Fornix, columns

Interventricular foramen

Thalamus, ant. tubercle

Lat. ventricle, frontal (ant.) horn

Epithalamic commissure

Caudate nucleus, head

Interthalamic adhesion

Uncus

3rd ventricle

Habenular trigone

Hippocampus, pes

Lat. ventricle, temporal (inf.) horn

Parahippocampal gyrus

Habenular commissure

Collateral eminence

Lat. ventricle, post. horn

Hippocampus, fimbria

Hippocampus

Pineal gland

Calcar avis

Tectal plate

Lat. ventricle, occipital (post.) horn

Vermis of cerebellum

Fig. 531 The lateral ventricles and the third ventricle, viewed from above. Part of the cerebral hemispheres, the corpus callosum, the fornix as well as the choroid plexus, and the tela choroidea of the third ventricle have been removed.

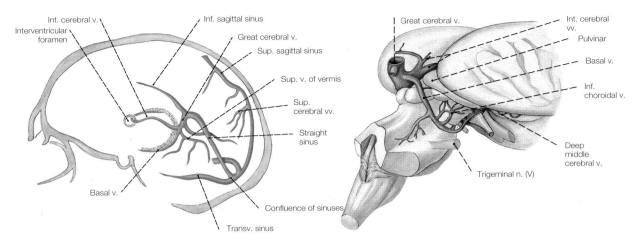

Fig. 532 labels:
Int. cerebral v.
Interventricular foramen
Inf. sagittal sinus
Great cerebral v.
Sup. sagittal sinus
Sup. v. of vermis
Sup. cerebral vv.
Straight sinus
Basal v.
Confluence of sinuses
Transv. sinus

Fig. 533 labels:
Great cerebral v.
Int. cerebral vv.
Pulvinar
Basal v.
Inf. choroidal v.
Deep middle cerebral v.
Trigeminal n. (V)

Fig. 532 The deep cerebral veins and sinuses of the dura mater, lateral aspect. Schematic from a phlebogram of the sinuses.

Fig. 533 The deep cerebral veins, viewed posterolaterally.

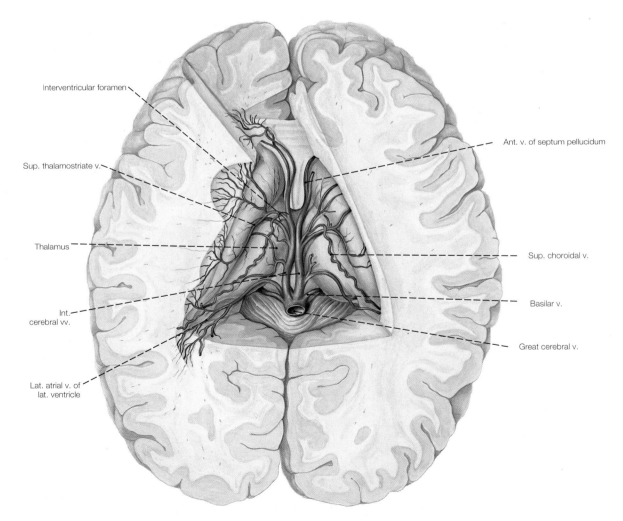

Fig. 534 labels:
Interventricular foramen
Ant. v. of septum pellucidum
Sup. thalamostriate v.
Thalamus
Sup. choroidal v.
Int. cerebral vv.
Basilar v.
Great cerebral v.
Lat. atrial v. of lat. ventricle

Fig. 534 The deep cerebral veins, viewed from above. The upper layer of the tela choroidea of the third ventricle has been removed.

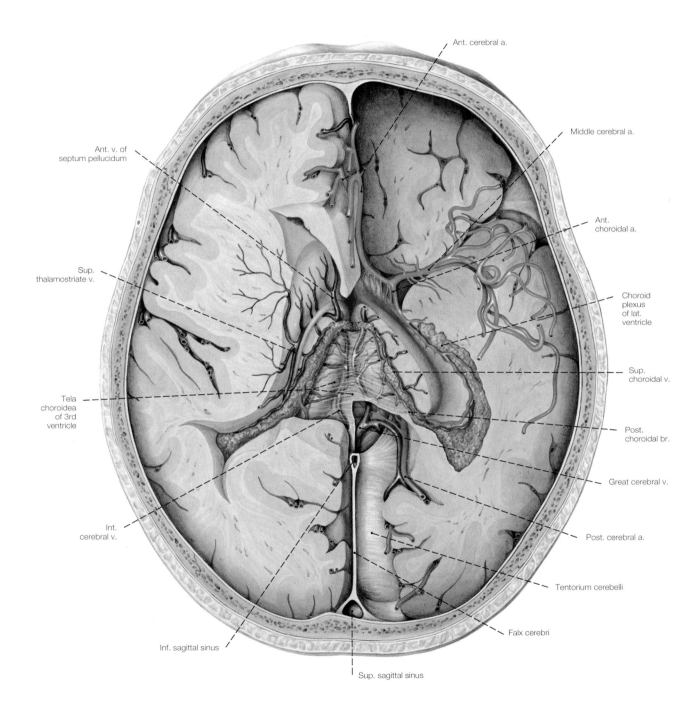

Ant. cerebral a.

Ant. v. of
septum pellucidum

Middle cerebral a.

Ant.
choroidal a.

Sup.
thalamostriate v.

Choroid
plexus
of lat.
ventricle

Sup.
choroidal v.

Tela
choroidea
of 3rd
ventricle

Post.
choroidal br.

Great cerebral v.

Int.
cerebral v.

Post. cerebral a.

Tentorium cerebelli

Inf. sagittal sinus

Falx cerebri

Sup. sagittal sinus

Fig. 535 Cerebral arteries and veins, viewed from
above. Parts of the cerebral hemispheres, the corpus
callosum and the fornix have been removed.

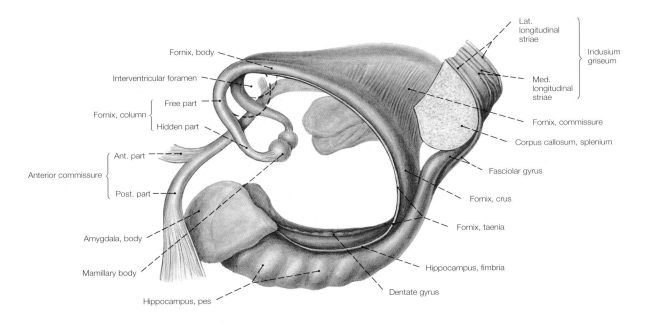

Lat. longitudinal striae

Indusium griseum

Fornix, body

Interventricular foramen

Med. longitudinal striae

Free part

Fornix, column

Fornix, commissure

Hidden part

Corpus callosum, splenium

Ant. part

Fasciolar gyrus

Anterior commissure

Fornix, crus

Post. part

Fornix, taenia

Amygdala, body

Hippocampus, fimbria

Mamillary body

Dentate gyrus

Hippocampus, pes

Fig. 536   The two fornices and the anterior commissure, viewed from the left posteriorly in a spatial schematic.

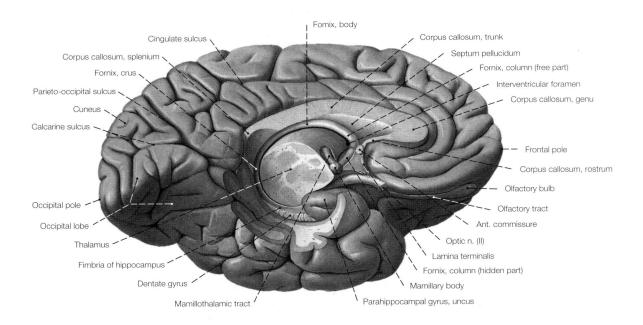

Fornix, body

Cingulate sulcus

Corpus callosum, trunk

Septum pellucidum

Corpus callosum, splenium

Fornix, column (free part)

Fornix, crus

Interventricular foramen

Parieto-occipital sulcus

Corpus callosum, genu

Cuneus

Calcarine sulcus

Frontal pole

Corpus callosum, rostrum

Olfactory bulb

Olfactory tract

Occipital pole

Ant. commissure

Occipital lobe

Optic n. (II)

Thalamus

Lamina terminalis

Fimbria of hippocampus

Fornix, column (hidden part)

Dentate gyrus

Mamillary body

Parahippocampal gyrus, uncus

Mamillothalamic tract

Fig. 537   The left fornix, viewed medially from below. The corpus callosum and the anterior commissure have been sectioned in the median plane after removal of the inferior part of the diencephalon and partial removal of the medial parts of the parahippocampal gyrus.

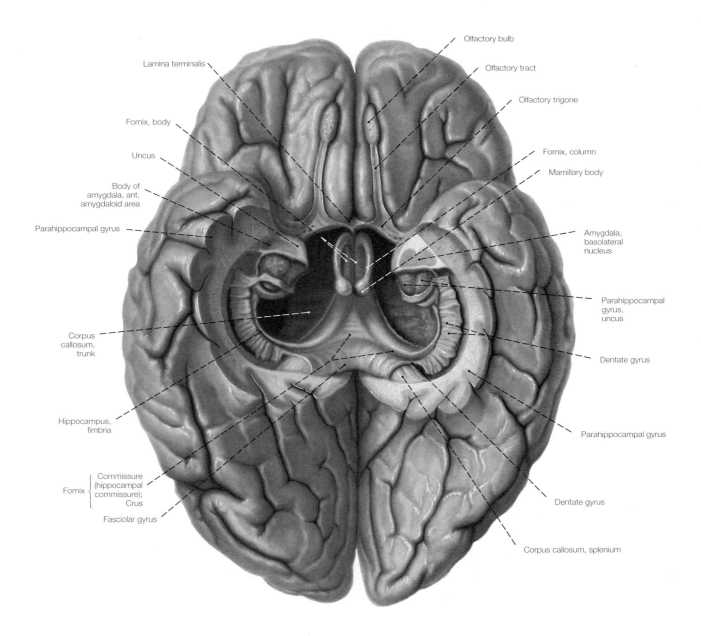

Olfactory bulb

Olfactory tract

Olfactory trigone

Lamina terminalis

Fornix, body

Uncus

Body of
amygdala, ant.
amygdaloid area

Fornix, column

Mamillary body

Parahippocampal gyrus

Amygdala,
basolateral
nucleus

Parahippocampal
gyrus,
uncus

Corpus
callosum,
trunk

Dentate gyrus

Hippocampus,
fimbria

Parahippocampal gyrus

Fornix {
Commissure
(hippocampal
commissure);
Crus

Fasciolar gyrus

Dentate gyrus

Corpus callosum, splenium

Fig. 538 The fornix, viewed from
below. Basal parts of the brain have
been removed.

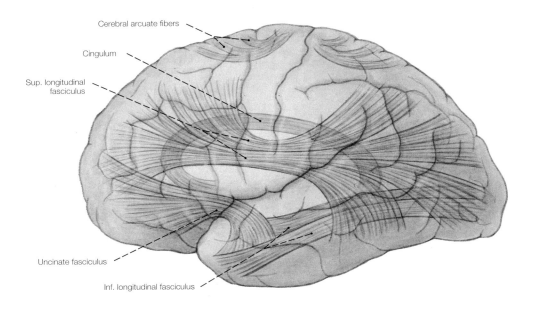

Cerebral arcuate fibers

Cingulum

Sup. longitudinal
fasciculus

Uncinate fasciculus

Inf. longitudinal fasciculus

Fig. 539 Association fibers projected onto the
cerebral hemisphere, viewed from the left.

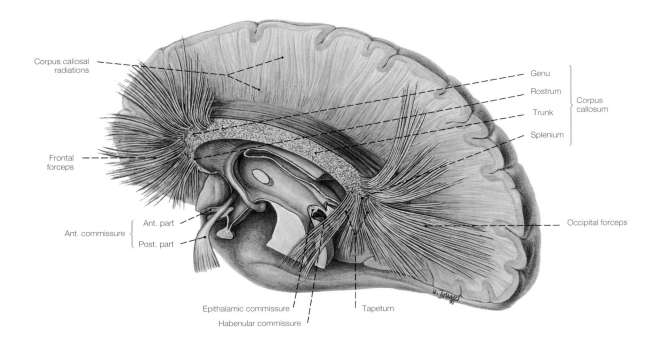

Corpus callosal
radiations

Frontal
forceps

Ant. commissure { Ant. part
Post. part

Epithalamic commissure
Habenular commissure

Tapetum

Genu
Rostrum
Trunk
Splenium

Corpus
callosum

Occipital forceps

Fig. 540 Commissural fibers of the cerebrum,
viewed from the left. Spatial overview after
extensive sectioning of the corpus callosum in the
paramedian plane. Individual corpus callosal fibers
are shown.

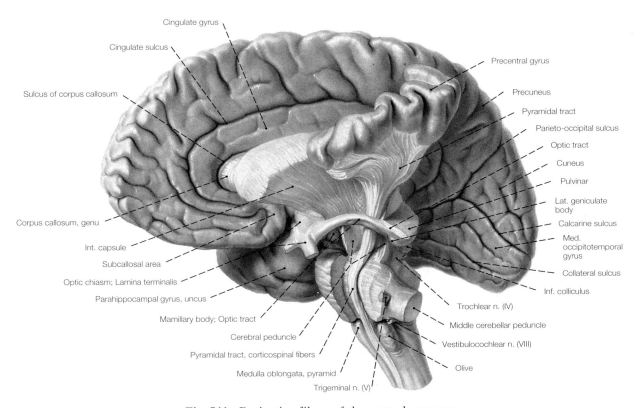

Cingulate gyrus

Cingulate sulcus

Sulcus of corpus callosum

Corpus callosum, genu

Int. capsule

Subcallosal area

Optic chiasm; Lamina terminalis

Parahippocampal gyrus, uncus

Mamillary body; Optic tract

Cerebral peduncle

Pyramidal tract, corticospinal fibers

Medulla oblongata, pyramid

Trigeminal n. (V)

Precentral gyrus

Precuneus

Pyramidal tract

Parieto-occipital sulcus

Optic tract

Cuneus

Pulvinar

Lat. geniculate body

Calcarine sulcus

Med. occipitotemporal gyrus

Collateral sulcus

Inf. colliculus

Trochlear n. (IV)

Middle cerebellar peduncle

Vestibulocochlear n. (VIII)

Olive

Fig. 541 Projection fibers of the central nervous system, viewed from the left. The internal capsule and the pyramidal tract have been exposed in this fiber preparation.

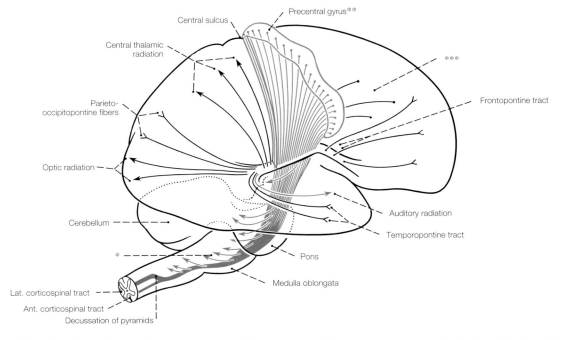

Central sulcus

Precentral gyrus**

Central thalamic radiation

***

Parieto-occipitopontine fibers

Frontopontine tract

Optic radiation

Cerebellum

*

Auditory radiation

Temporopontine tract

Pons

Lat. corticospinal tract

Ant. corticospinal tract

Decussation of pyramids

Medulla oblongata

Fig. 542 The internal capsule and the pyramidal tract. Functional overview, viewed from the right.

* Fibers to the superior and inferior colliculi and the nuclei of the hindbrain
** Perikarya of the pyramidal tract (corticospinal tract)
*** Perikarya of areas 6 and 8 (premotor cortex)

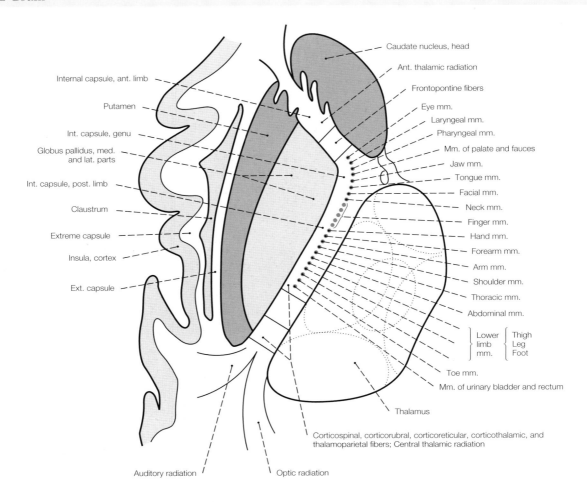

Internal capsule, ant. limb

Putamen

Int. capsule, genu

Globus pallidus, med.
and lat. parts

Int. capsule, post. limb

Claustrum

Extreme capsule

Insula, cortex

Ext. capsule

Caudate nucleus, head

Ant. thalamic radiation

Frontopontine fibers

Eye mm.

Laryngeal mm.

Pharyngeal mm.

Mm. of palate and fauces

Jaw mm.

Tongue mm.

Facial mm.

Neck mm.

Finger mm.

Hand mm.

Forearm mm.

Arm mm.

Shoulder mm.

Thoracic mm.

Abdominal mm.

Lower limb mm. { Thigh Leg Foot

Toe mm.

Mm. of urinary bladder and rectum

Thalamus

Corticospinal, corticorubral, corticoreticular, corticothalamic, and
thalamoparietal fibers; Central thalamic radiation

Auditory radiation

Optic radiation

Fig. 543 The internal capsule, functional organization.

Organization of the Internal Capsule and its Arterial Supply

Arterial Supply

Anterior limb
  Ant. thalamic radiation*
  Frontopontine fibers

Ant. cerebral a., precommunical part,
  long central a.

Genu
  Corticobulbar fibers
Posterior limb
  Thalamolenticular part
    Corticospinal fibers
    Corticorubral fibers
    Corticoreticular fibers
    Corticothalamic fibers
    Thalamoparietal fibers*
    Central thalamic radiation*
  Sublenticular part
    Optic radiation
    Auditory radiation
    Corticotectal fibers
    Temporopontine fibers
  Retrolenticular part
    Post. thalamic radiation*
    Parieto-occipitopontine tract

Middle cerebral a., sphenoid part, anterolat.
  central aa.;
Internal carotid a., cerebral part, ant. choroidal a.

* Together these fibers constitute the corona radiata.

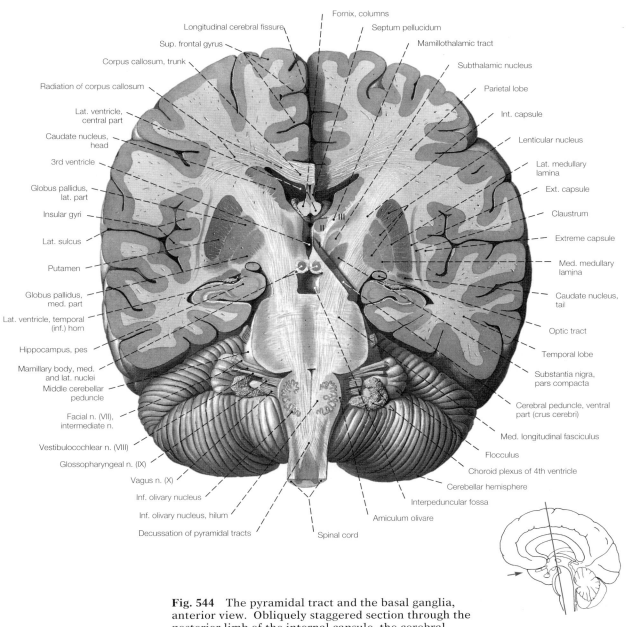

Fornix, columns
Longitudinal cerebral fissure
Septum pellucidum
Sup. frontal gyrus
Mamillothalamic tract
Corpus callosum, trunk
Subthalamic nucleus
Radiation of corpus callosum
Parietal lobe
Lat. ventricle, central part
Int. capsule
Caudate nucleus, head
Lenticular nucleus
3rd ventricle
Lat. medullary lamina
Globus pallidus, lat. part
Ext. capsule
Insular gyri
Claustrum
Lat. sulcus
Extreme capsule
Putamen
Med. medullary lamina
Globus pallidus, med. part
Caudate nucleus, tail
Lat. ventricle, temporal (inf.) horn
Optic tract
Hippocampus, pes
Temporal lobe
Mamillary body, med. and lat. nuclei
Substantia nigra, pars compacta
Middle cerebellar peduncle
Cerebral peduncle, ventral part (crus cerebri)
Facial n. (VII), intermediate n.
Med. longitudinal fasciculus
Vestibulocochlear n. (VIII)
Flocculus
Glossopharyngeal n. (IX)
Choroid plexus of 4th ventricle
Vagus n. (X)
Cerebellar hemisphere
Inf. olivary nucleus
Interpeduncular fossa
Inf. olivary nucleus, hilum
Amiculum olivare
Decussation of pyramidal tracts
Spinal cord

Fig. 544 The pyramidal tract and the basal ganglia, anterior view. Obliquely staggered section through the posterior limb of the internal capsule, the cerebral peduncles, and the spinal cord.

I–III	=	Thalamic nuclear groups:
I	=	Medial nuclei
II	=	Anterior nuclei
III	=	Ventral nuclei

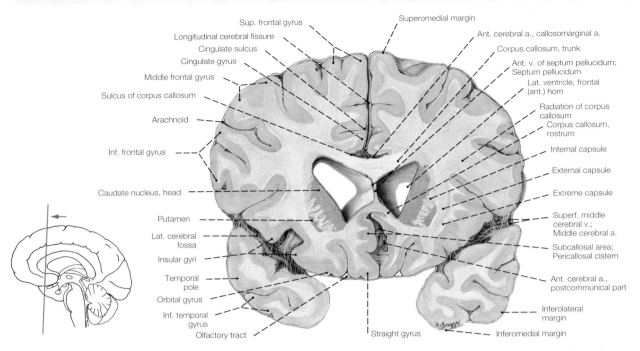

Fig. 545 The brain. Frontal section at the level of the anterior part of the frontal horn of the lateral ventricle, posterior aspect.

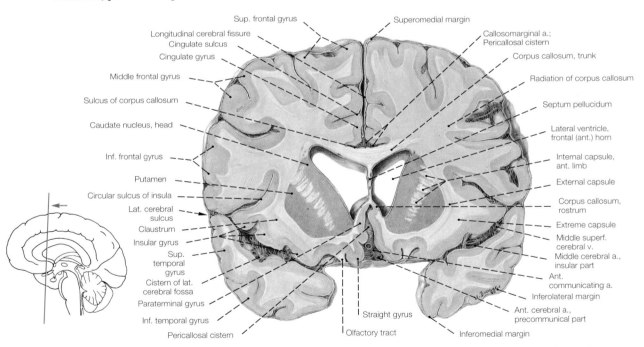

Fig. 546 The brain. Frontal section at the level of the posterior part of the anterior horn of the lateral ventricle, posterior aspect.

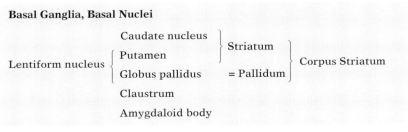

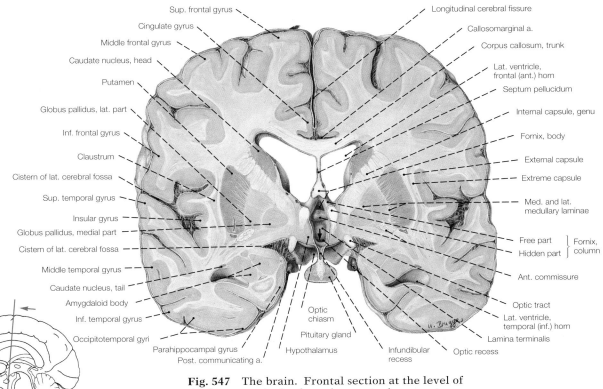

Sup. frontal gyrus
Cingulate gyrus
Middle frontal gyrus
Caudate nucleus, head
Putamen
Globus pallidus, lat. part
Inf. frontal gyrus
Claustrum
Cistern of lat. cerebral fossa
Sup. temporal gyrus
Insular gyrus
Globus pallidus, medial part
Cistern of lat. cerebral fossa
Middle temporal gyrus
Caudate nucleus, tail
Amygdaloid body
Inf. temporal gyrus
Occipitotemporal gyri
Parahippocampal gyrus
Post. communicating a.

Longitudinal cerebral fissure
Callosomarginal a.
Corpus callosum, trunk
Lat. ventricle, frontal (ant.) horn
Septum pellucidum
Internal capsule, genu
Fornix, body
External capsule
Extreme capsule
Med. and lat. medullary laminae
Free part ⎫ Fornix,
Hidden part ⎭ column
Ant. commissure
Optic tract
Lat. ventricle, temporal (inf.) horn
Lamina terminalis

Optic chiasm
Pituitary gland
Hypothalamus
Infundibular recess
Optic recess

Fig. 547 The brain. Frontal section at the level of the interventricular foramina, posterior aspect.

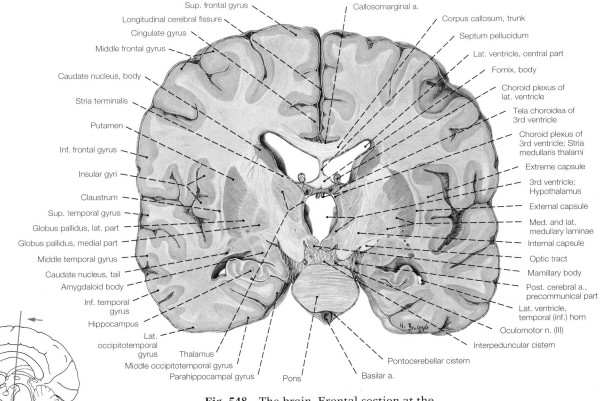

Sup. frontal gyrus
Longitudinal cerebral fissure
Cingulate gyrus
Middle frontal gyrus
Caudate nucleus, body
Stria terminalis
Putamen
Inf. frontal gyrus
Insular gyri
Claustrum
Sup. temporal gyrus
Globus pallidus, lat. part
Globus pallidus, medial part
Middle temporal gyrus
Caudate nucleus, tail
Amygdaloid body
Inf. temporal gyrus
Hippocampus
Lat. occipitotemporal gyrus
Middle occipitotemporal gyrus
Parahippocampal gyrus

Callosomarginal a.
Corpus callosum, trunk
Septum pellucidum
Lat. ventricle, central part
Fornix, body
Choroid plexus of lat. ventricle
Tela choroidea of 3rd ventricle
Choroid plexus of 3rd ventricle; Stria medullaris thalami
Extreme capsule
3rd ventricle; Hypothalamus
External capsule
Med. and lat. medullary laminae
Internal capsule
Optic tract
Mamillary body
Post. cerebral a., precommunical part
Lat. ventricle, temporal (inf.) horn
Oculomotor n. (III)
Interpeduncular cistern

Thalamus
Pons
Basilar a.
Pontocerebellar cistern

Fig. 548 The brain. Frontal section at the level of the mamillary bodies, posterior aspect.

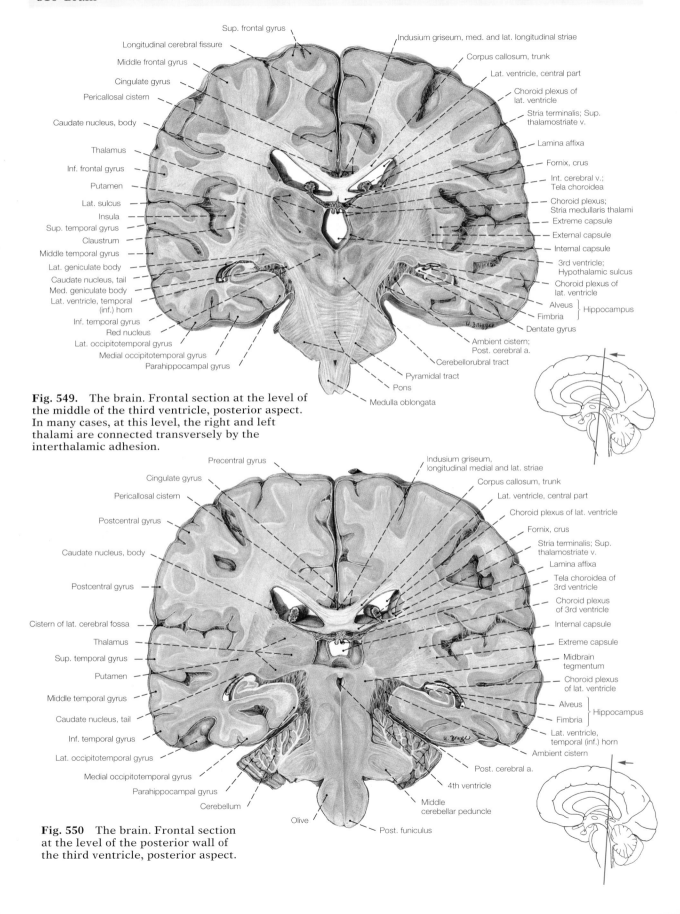

Fig. 549. The brain. Frontal section at the level of the middle of the third ventricle, posterior aspect. In many cases, at this level, the right and left thalami are connected transversely by the interthalamic adhesion.

Sup. frontal gyrus
Longitudinal cerebral fissure
Middle frontal gyrus
Cingulate gyrus
Pericallosal cistern
Caudate nucleus, body
Thalamus
Inf. frontal gyrus
Putamen
Lat. sulcus
Insula
Sup. temporal gyrus
Claustrum
Middle temporal gyrus
Lat. geniculate body
Caudate nucleus, tail
Med. geniculate body
Lat. ventricle, temporal (inf.) horn
Inf. temporal gyrus
Red nucleus
Lat. occipitotemporal gyrus
Medial occipitotemporal gyrus
Parahippocampal gyrus

Indusium griseum, med. and lat. longitudinal striae
Corpus callosum, trunk
Lat. ventricle, central part
Choroid plexus of lat. ventricle
Stria terminalis; Sup. thalamostriate v.
Lamina affixa
Fornix, crus
Int. cerebral v.; Tela choroidea
Choroid plexus; Stria medullaris thalami
Extreme capsule
External capsule
Internal capsule
3rd ventricle; Hypothalamic sulcus
Choroid plexus of lat. ventricle
Alveus } Hippocampus
Fimbria }
Dentate gyrus
Ambient cistern; Post. cerebral a.
Cerebellorubral tract
Pyramidal tract
Pons
Medulla oblongata

Fig. 550 The brain. Frontal section at the level of the posterior wall of the third ventricle, posterior aspect.

Precentral gyrus
Cingulate gyrus
Pericallosal cistern
Postcentral gyrus
Caudate nucleus, body
Postcentral gyrus
Cistern of lat. cerebral fossa
Thalamus
Sup. temporal gyrus
Putamen
Middle temporal gyrus
Caudate nucleus, tail
Inf. temporal gyrus
Lat. occipitotemporal gyrus
Medial occipitotemporal gyrus
Parahippocampal gyrus
Cerebellum
Olive

Indusium griseum, longitudinal medial and lat. striae
Corpus callosum, trunk
Lat. ventricle, central part
Choroid plexus of lat. ventricle
Fornix, crus
Stria terminalis; Sup. thalamostriate v.
Lamina affixa
Tela choroidea of 3rd ventricle
Choroid plexus of 3rd ventricle
Internal capsule
Extreme capsule
Midbrain tegmentum
Choroid plexus of lat. ventricle
Alveus } Hippocampus
Fimbria }
Lat. ventricle, temporal (inf.) horn
Ambient cistern
Post. cerebral a.
4th ventricle
Middle cerebellar peduncle
Post. funiculus

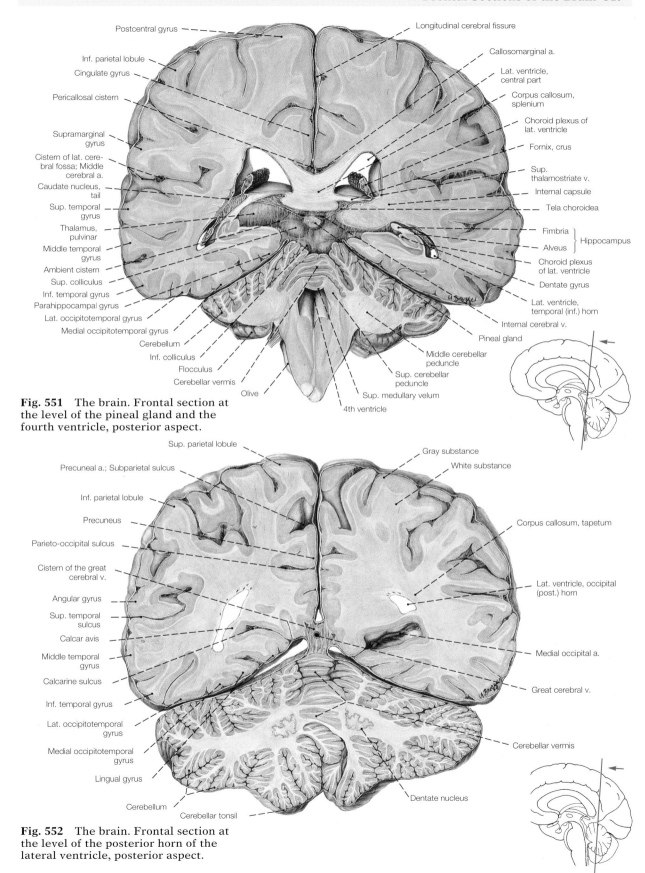

Postcentral gyrus

Longitudinal cerebral fissure

Callosomarginal a.

Inf. parietal lobule

Cingulate gyrus

Lat. ventricle, central part

Pericallosal cistern

Corpus callosum, splenium

Choroid plexus of lat. ventricle

Supramarginal gyrus

Fornix, crus

Cistern of lat. cerebral fossa; Middle cerebral a.

Sup. thalamostriate v.

Caudate nucleus, tail

Internal capsule

Sup. temporal gyrus

Tela choroidea

Thalamus, pulvinar

Fimbria

Middle temporal gyrus

Alveus

Hippocampus

Ambient cistern

Choroid plexus of lat. ventricle

Sup. colliculus

Dentate gyrus

Inf. temporal gyrus

Parahippocampal gyrus

Lat. ventricle, temporal (inf.) horn

Lat. occipitotemporal gyrus

Internal cerebral v.

Medial occipitotemporal gyrus

Pineal gland

Cerebellum

Middle cerebellar peduncle

Inf. colliculus

Flocculus

Sup. cerebellar peduncle

Cerebellar vermis

Olive

Sup. medullary velum

4th ventricle

Fig. 551 The brain. Frontal section at the level of the pineal gland and the fourth ventricle, posterior aspect.

Sup. parietal lobule

Gray substance

Precuneal a.; Subparietal sulcus

White substance

Inf. parietal lobule

Precuneus

Corpus callosum, tapetum

Parieto-occipital sulcus

Cistern of the great cerebral v.

Lat. ventricle, occipital (post.) horn

Angular gyrus

Sup. temporal sulcus

Calcar avis

Middle temporal gyrus

Medial occipital a.

Calcarine sulcus

Inf. temporal gyrus

Great cerebral v.

Lat. occipitotemporal gyrus

Medial occipitotemporal gyrus

Lingual gyrus

Cerebellar vermis

Cerebellum

Cerebellar tonsil

Dentate nucleus

Fig. 552 The brain. Frontal section at the level of the posterior horn of the lateral ventricle, posterior aspect.

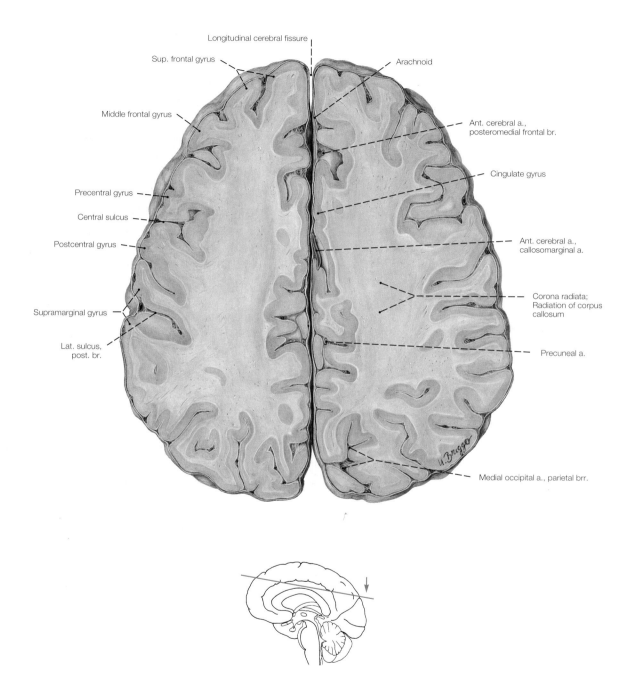

Longitudinal cerebral fissure

Sup. frontal gyrus

Middle frontal gyrus

Precentral gyrus

Central sulcus

Postcentral gyrus

Supramarginal gyrus

Lat. sulcus,
post. br.

Arachnoid

Ant. cerebral a.,
posteromedial frontal br.

Cingulate gyrus

Ant. cerebral a.,
callosomarginal a.

Corona radiata;
Radiation of corpus
callosum

Precuneal a.

Medial occipital a., parietal brr.

Fig. 553 The brain. Horizontal section immediately above the corpus callosum, viewed from above. In Figs. 545–561, the subarachnoid space appears somewhat enlarged, particularly in the region of the sulci of the hemispheres, due to the fact that these specimens were taken from elderly persons.

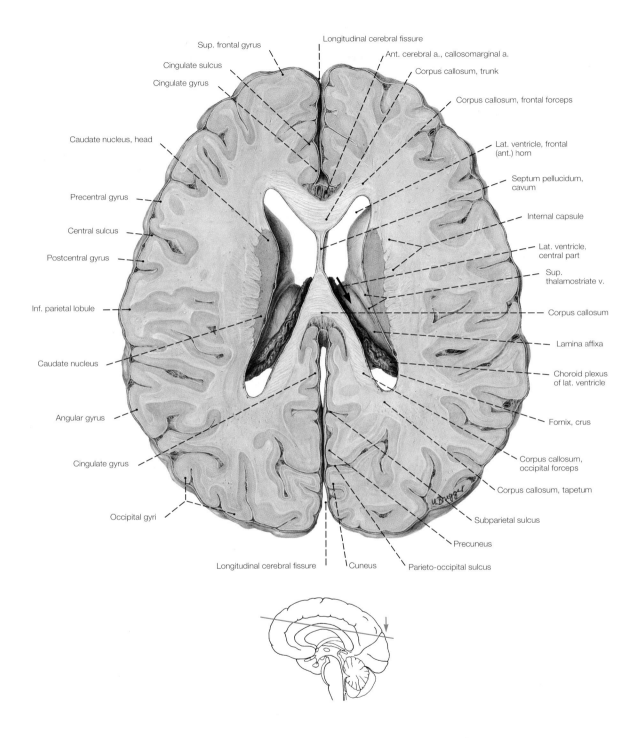

Sup. frontal gyrus

Cingulate sulcus

Cingulate gyrus

Caudate nucleus, head

Precentral gyrus

Central sulcus

Postcentral gyrus

Inf. parietal lobule

Caudate nucleus

Angular gyrus

Cingulate gyrus

Occipital gyri

Longitudinal cerebral fissure

Longitudinal cerebral fissure

Ant. cerebral a., callosomarginal a.

Corpus callosum, trunk

Corpus callosum, frontal forceps

Lat. ventricle, frontal (ant.) horn

Septum pellucidum, cavum

Internal capsule

Lat. ventricle, central part

Sup. thalamostriate v.

Corpus callosum

Lamina affixa

Choroid plexus of lat. ventricle

Fornix, crus

Corpus callosum, occipital forceps

Corpus callosum, tapetum

Subparietal sulcus

Precuneus

Cuneus

Parieto-occipital sulcus

Fig. 554 The brain. Horizontal section at the level of the middle part of the lateral ventricle, viewed from above.

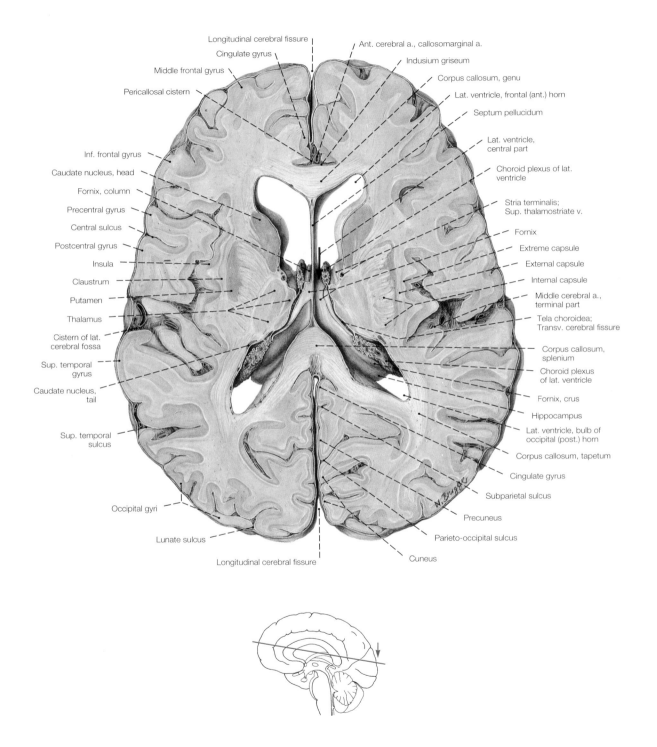

Longitudinal cerebral fissure
Cingulate gyrus
Middle frontal gyrus
Pericallosal cistern
Inf. frontal gyrus
Caudate nucleus, head
Fornix, column
Precentral gyrus
Central sulcus
Postcentral gyrus
Insula
Claustrum
Putamen
Thalamus
Cistern of lat. cerebral fossa
Sup. temporal gyrus
Caudate nucleus, tail
Sup. temporal sulcus
Occipital gyri
Lunate sulcus
Longitudinal cerebral fissure

Ant. cerebral a., callosomarginal a.
Indusium griseum
Corpus callosum, genu
Lat. ventricle, frontal (ant.) horn
Septum pellucidum
Lat. ventricle, central part
Choroid plexus of lat. ventricle
Stria terminalis; Sup. thalamostriate v.
Fornix
Extreme capsule
External capsule
Internal capsule
Middle cerebral a., terminal part
Tela choroidea; Transv. cerebral fissure
Corpus callosum, splenium
Choroid plexus of lat. ventricle
Fornix, crus
Hippocampus
Lat. ventricle, bulb of occipital (post.) horn
Corpus callosum, tapetum
Cingulate gyrus
Subparietal sulcus
Precuneus
Parieto-occipital sulcus
Cuneus

Fig. 555 The brain. Horizontal section at the level of the floor of the central part of the lateral ventricle, viewed from above.

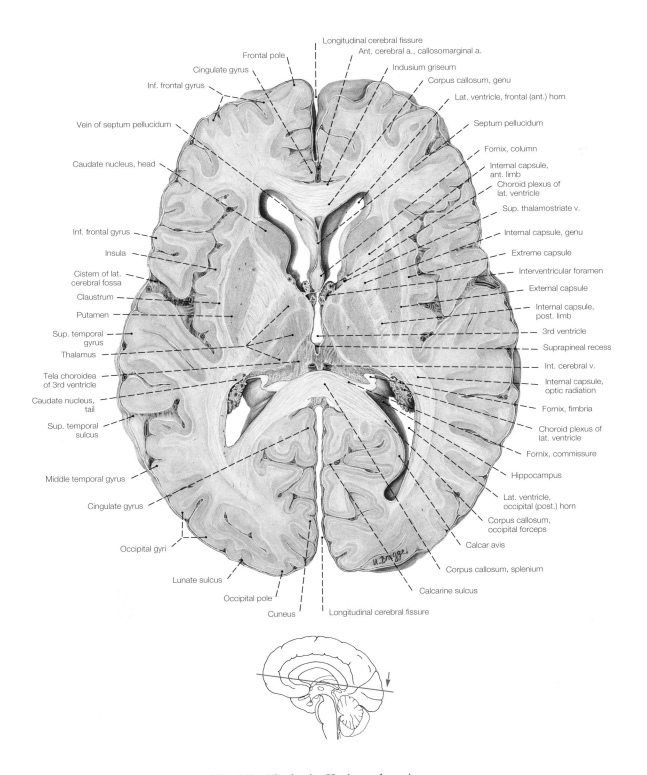

Longitudinal cerebral fissure

Frontal pole

Ant. cerebral a., callosomarginal a.

Cingulate gyrus

Indusium griseum

Inf. frontal gyrus

Corpus callosum, genu

Lat. ventricle, frontal (ant.) horn

Vein of septum pellucidum

Septum pellucidum

Fornix, column

Caudate nucleus, head

Internal capsule, ant. limb

Choroid plexus of lat. ventricle

Sup. thalamostriate v.

Inf. frontal gyrus

Internal capsule, genu

Insula

Extreme capsule

Cistern of lat. cerebral fossa

Interventricular foramen

Claustrum

External capsule

Putamen

Internal capsule, post. limb

Sup. temporal gyrus

3rd ventricle

Thalamus

Suprapineal recess

Tela choroidea of 3rd ventricle

Int. cerebral v.

Caudate nucleus, tail

Internal capsule, optic radiation

Sup. temporal sulcus

Fornix, fimbria

Choroid plexus of lat. ventricle

Middle temporal gyrus

Fornix, commissure

Cingulate gyrus

Hippocampus

Lat. ventricle, occipital (post.) horn

Occipital gyri

Corpus callosum, occipital forceps

Lunate sulcus

Calcar avis

Occipital pole

Corpus callosum, splenium

Cuneus

Calcarine sulcus

Longitudinal cerebral fissure

Fig. 556 The brain. Horizontal section at the level of the upper part of the third ventricle, viewed from above.

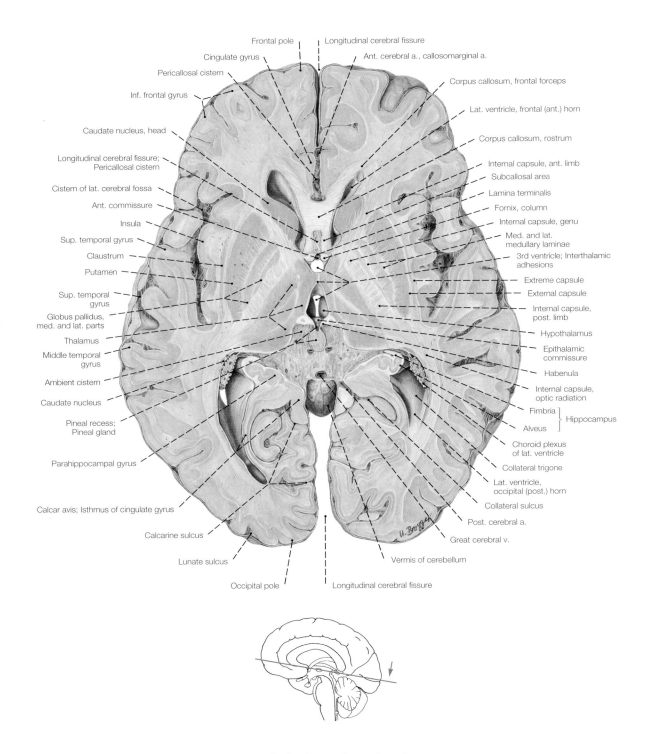

Frontal pole

Longitudinal cerebral fissure

Cingulate gyrus

Ant. cerebral a., callosomarginal a.

Pericallosal cistern

Corpus callosum, frontal forceps

Inf. frontal gyrus

Lat. ventricle, frontal (ant.) horn

Caudate nucleus, head

Corpus callosum, rostrum

Longitudinal cerebral fissure; Pericallosal cistern

Internal capsule, ant. limb

Cistern of lat. cerebral fossa

Subcallosal area

Ant. commissure

Lamina terminalis

Insula

Fornix, column

Sup. temporal gyrus

Internal capsule, genu

Claustrum

Med. and lat. medullary laminae

Putamen

3rd ventricle; Interthalamic adhesions

Sup. temporal gyrus

Extreme capsule

External capsule

Globus pallidus, med. and lat. parts

Internal capsule, post. limb

Thalamus

Hypothalamus

Middle temporal gyrus

Epithalamic commissure

Ambient cistern

Habenula

Caudate nucleus

Internal capsule, optic radiation

Pineal recess; Pineal gland

Fimbria

Alveus

Hippocampus

Parahippocampal gyrus

Choroid plexus of lat. ventricle

Collateral trigone

Lat. ventricle, occipital (post.) horn

Calcar avis; Isthmus of cingulate gyrus

Collateral sulcus

Calcarine sulcus

Post. cerebral a.

Lunate sulcus

Great cerebral v.

Vermis of cerebellum

Occipital pole

Longitudinal cerebral fissure

U. Brugger

Fig. 557 The brain. Horizontal section through the middle of the third ventricle at the level of the interthalamic adhesion, viewed from above.

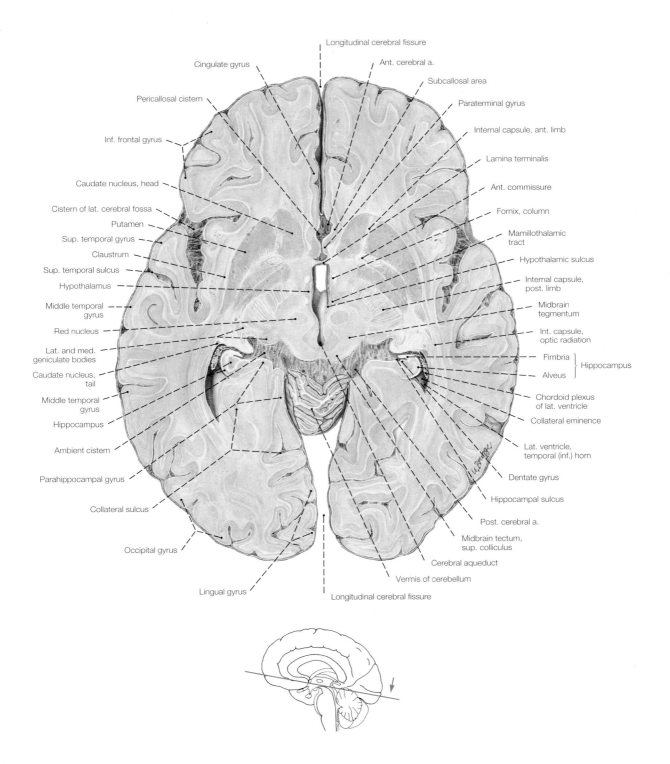

Longitudinal cerebral fissure

Cingulate gyrus

Ant. cerebral a.

Subcallosal area

Pericallosal cistern

Paraterminal gyrus

Internal capsule, ant. limb

Inf. frontal gyrus

Lamina terminalis

Caudate nucleus, head

Ant. commissure

Cistern of lat. cerebral fossa

Fornix, column

Putamen

Mamillothalamic tract

Sup. temporal gyrus

Hypothalamic sulcus

Claustrum

Internal capsule, post. limb

Sup. temporal sulcus

Hypothalamus

Midbrain tegmentum

Middle temporal gyrus

Int. capsule, optic radiation

Red nucleus

Fimbria

Lat. and med. geniculate bodies

Hippocampus

Alveus

Caudate nucleus, tail

Chordoid plexus of lat. ventricle

Middle temporal gyrus

Collateral eminence

Hippocampus

Lat. ventricle, temporal (inf.) horn

Ambient cistern

Dentate gyrus

Parahippocampal gyrus

Hippocampal sulcus

Collateral sulcus

Post. cerebral a.

Occipital gyrus

Midbrain tectum, sup. colliculus

Cerebral aqueduct

Lingual gyrus

Vermis of cerebellum

Longitudinal cerebral fissure

Fig. 558 The brain. Horizontal section through the third ventricle at the level of its communication with the cerebral aqueduct, viewed from above.

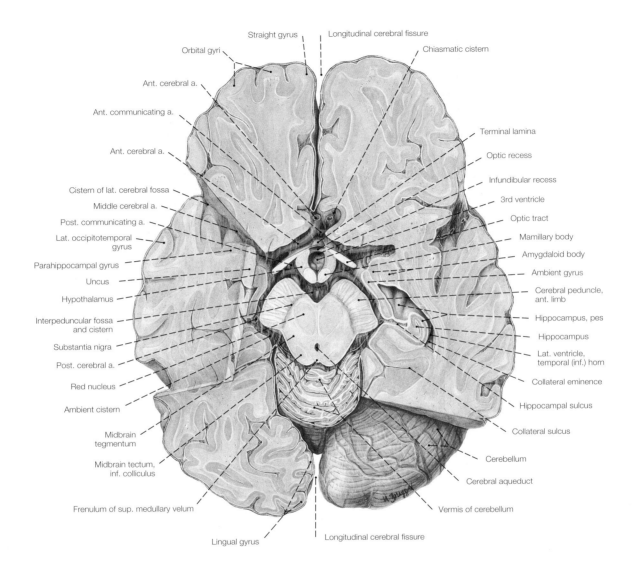

Straight gyrus

Longitudinal cerebral fissure

Orbital gyri

Chiasmatic cistern

Ant. cerebral a.

Terminal lamina

Ant. communicating a.

Optic recess

Ant. cerebral a.

Infundibular recess

Cistern of lat. cerebral fossa

3rd ventricle

Middle cerebral a.

Optic tract

Post. communicating a.

Mamillary body

Lat. occipitotemporal gyrus

Amygdaloid body

Parahippocampal gyrus

Ambient gyrus

Uncus

Cerebral peduncle, ant. limb

Hypothalamus

Hippocampus, pes

Interpeduncular fossa and cistern

Hippocampus

Substantia nigra

Lat. ventricle, temporal (inf.) horn

Post. cerebral a.

Collateral eminence

Red nucleus

Hippocampal sulcus

Ambient cistern

Collateral sulcus

Midbrain tegmentum

Cerebellum

Midbrain tectum, inf. colliculus

Cerebral aqueduct

Frenulum of sup. medullary velum

Vermis of cerebellum

Lingual gyrus

Longitudinal cerebral fissure

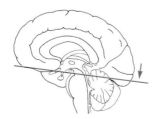

Fig. 559 The brain. Staggered horizontal section through the floor of the third ventricle at the level of the mamillary bodies, viewed from above.

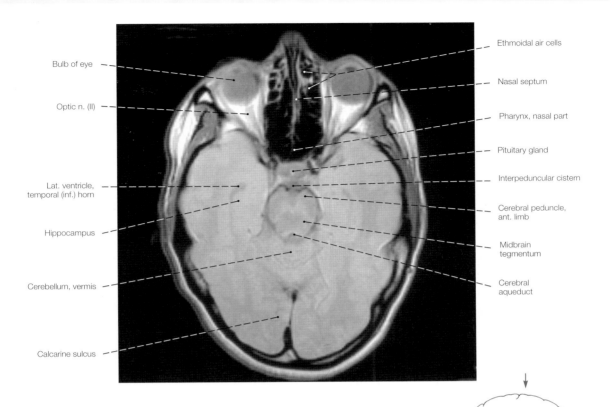

Bulb of eye

Optic n. (II)

Lat. ventricle, temporal (inf.) horn

Hippocampus

Cerebellum, vermis

Calcarine sulcus

Ethmoidal air cells

Nasal septum

Pharynx, nasal part

Pituitary gland

Interpeduncular cistern

Cerebral peduncle, ant. limb

Midbrain tegmentum

Cerebral aqueduct

Fig. 560 The brain. Magnetic resonance image (MRI) of a horizontal section at the level of the midbrain and the inferior horn of the lateral ventricle, viewed from above.

561
562
560

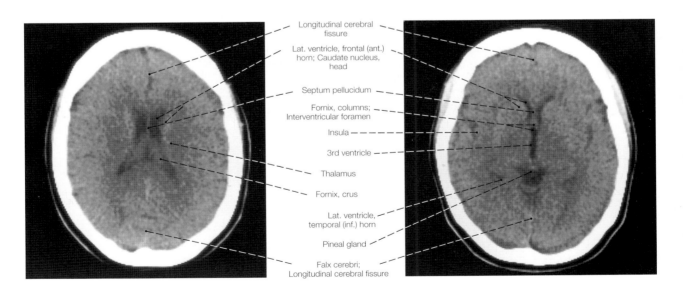

Longitudinal cerebral fissure

Lat. ventricle, frontal (ant.) horn; Caudate nucleus, head

Septum pellucidum

Fornix, columns; Interventricular foramen

Insula

3rd ventricle

Thalamus

Fornix, crus

Lat. ventricle, temporal (inf.) horn

Pineal gland

Falx cerebri; Longitudinal cerebral fissure

Fig. 561 The brain. Computed tomography (CT) scan of a horizontal section at the level of the floor of the middle part of the lateral ventricle, viewed from above.

Fig. 562 The brain. Computed tomography (CT) scan of a horizontal section at the level of the third ventricle and the exit of the inferior horn of the lateral ventricle, viewed from above.

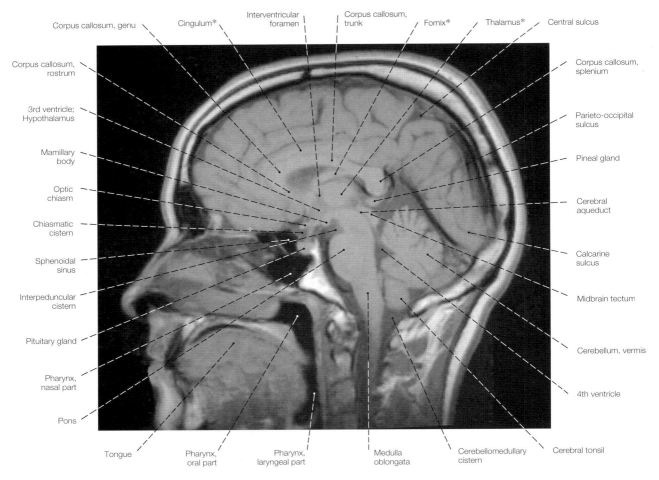

Corpus callosum, genu — Cingulum* — Interventricular foramen — Corpus callosum, trunk — Fornix* — Thalamus* — Central sulcus

Corpus callosum, rostrum

3rd ventricle; Hypothalamus

Mamillary body

Optic chiasm

Chiasmatic cistern

Sphenoidal sinus

Interpeduncular cistern

Pituitary gland

Pharynx, nasal part

Pons

Corpus callosum, splenium

Parieto-occipital sulcus

Pineal gland

Cerebral aqueduct

Calcarine sulcus

Midbrain tectum

Cerebellum, vermis

4th ventricle

Tongue — Pharynx, oral part — Pharynx, laryngeal part — Medulla oblongata — Cerebellomedullary cistern — Cerebral tonsil

Fig. 563 The brain. Magnetic resonance image (MRI) of a median section. Due to the "partial volume effect," the contour of structures marked with an asterisk (*) has been somewhat distorted.

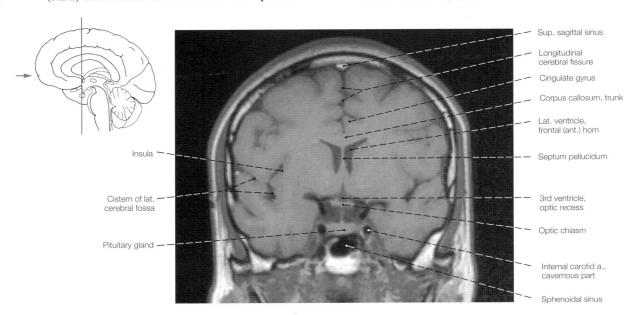

Sup. sagittal sinus

Longitudinal cerebral fissure

Cingulate gyrus

Corpus callosum, trunk

Lat. ventricle, frontal (ant.) horn

Septum pellucidum

3rd ventricle, optic recess

Optic chiasm

Internal carotid a., cavernous part

Sphenoidal sinus

Insula

Cistern of lat. cerebral fossa

Pituitary gland

Fig. 564 The brain. Magnetic resonance image (MRI) of a frontal section at the level of the anterior part of the third ventricle.

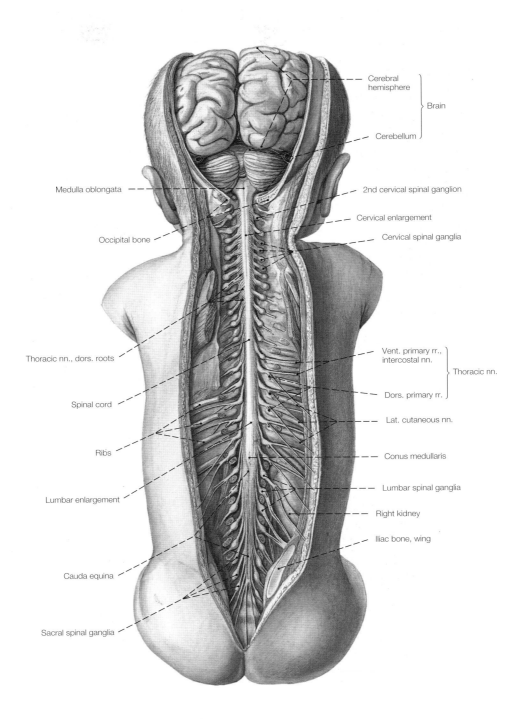

Cerebral
hemisphere

Brain

Cerebellum

Medulla oblongata

2nd cervical spinal ganglion

Cervical enlargement

Occipital bone

Cervical spinal ganglia

Thoracic nn., dors. roots

Vent. primary rr.,
intercostal nn.

Thoracic nn.

Spinal cord

Dors. primary rr.

Lat. cutaneous nn.

Ribs

Conus medullaris

Lumbar enlargement

Lumbar spinal ganglia

Right kidney

Iliac bone, wing

Cauda equina

Sacral spinal ganglia

Fig. 565   Brain, spinal cord, and spinal nerves in
situ in a newborn, dorsal aspect. The dorsal wall of
the vertebral canal has been excised, the
intervertebral foramina have been opened and the
spinal dura mater removed.

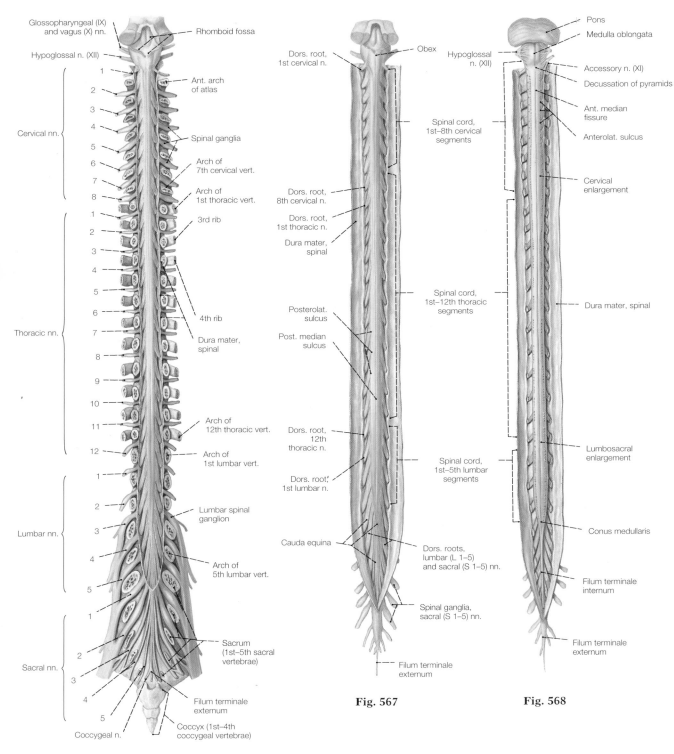

Glossopharyngeal (IX) and vagus (X) nn.
Rhomboid fossa
Hypoglossal n. (XII)
Cervical nn.
1
2
3
4
5
6
7
8
Ant. arch of atlas
Spinal ganglia
Arch of 7th cervical vert.
Arch of 1st thoracic vert.
3rd rib
Thoracic nn.
1
2
3
4
5
6
7
8
9
10
11
12
4th rib
Dura mater, spinal
Arch of 12th thoracic vert.
Arch of 1st lumbar vert.
Lumbar nn.
1
2
3
4
5
Lumbar spinal ganglion
Arch of 5th lumbar vert.
Sacral nn.
1
2
3
4
5
Sacrum (1st–5th sacral vertebrae)
Filum terminale externum
Coccygeal n.
Coccyx (1st–4th coccygeal vertebrae)

Fig. 566 Spinal cord and spinal nerves, dorsal aspect. The spinal cord in situ after opening of the vertebral canal, the intervertebral foramina and the dura mater.

Dors. root, 1st cervical n.
Obex
Hypoglossal n. (XII)
Pons
Medulla oblongata
Accessory n. (XI)
Decussation of pyramids
Ant. median fissure
Anterolat. sulcus
Spinal cord, 1st–8th cervical segments
Dors. root, 8th cervical n.
Dors. root, 1st thoracic n.
Dura mater, spinal
Cervical enlargement
Posterolat. sulcus
Post. median sulcus
Spinal cord, 1st–12th thoracic segments
Dura mater, spinal
Dors. root, 12th thoracic n.
Dors. root, 1st lumbar n.
Spinal cord, 1st–5th lumbar segments
Lumbosacral enlargement
Cauda equina
Dors. roots, lumbar (L 1–5) and sacral (S 1–5) nn.
Conus medullaris
Spinal ganglia, sacral (S 1–5) nn.
Filum terminale internum
Filum terminale externum
Filum terminale externum

Fig. 567

Fig. 568

Fig. 567 Spinal cord and spinal nerves, dorsal view. The vertebral canal and the dura mater have been opened.

Fig. 568 Spinal cord and spinal nerves, ventral view. The vertebral canal and the dura mater have been opened.

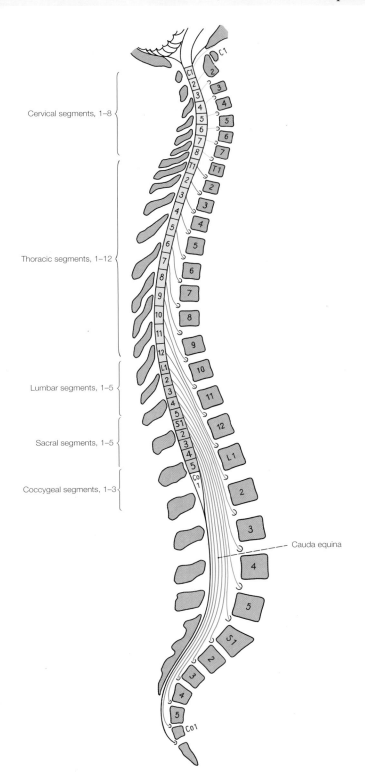

Fig. 569 Spinal cord segments, in a schematic median section viewed from the left. Regional groups of segments are indicated by different colors. In the newborn, the spinal cord extends two vertebral segments further caudally

(see Fig. 565). Note that the cervical region contains 8 8 segments. Because spinal cord segments are numbered according to the spinal nerves and the uppermost spinal nerve is counted as the first cervical nerve, there are 8 cervical segments.

Cervical segments, 1–8

Thoracic segments, 1–12

Lumbar segments, 1–5

Sacral segments, 1–5

Coccygeal segments, 1–3

Cauda equina

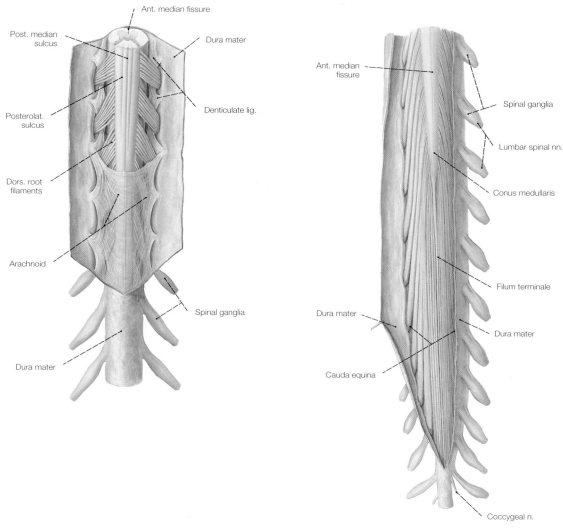

Fig. 570 The spinal cord and its meninges, dorsal view. The subarachnoid space has been opened.

Fig. 571 The spinal cord, showing its caudal portion with the cauda equina, ventral view. The subarachnoid space has been opened.

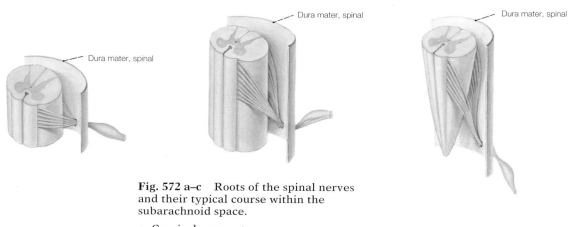

Fig. 572 a–c Roots of the spinal nerves and their typical course within the subarachnoid space.

a Cervical segment
b Thoracic segment
c Lumbar segment

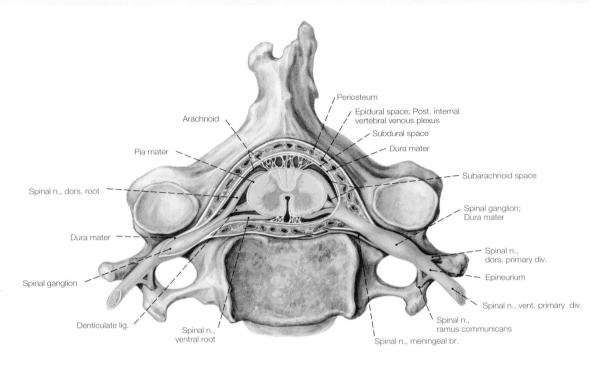

Fig. 573 Contents of the vertebral canal. A cross section at the level of the fifth cervical vertebra, viewed from above.

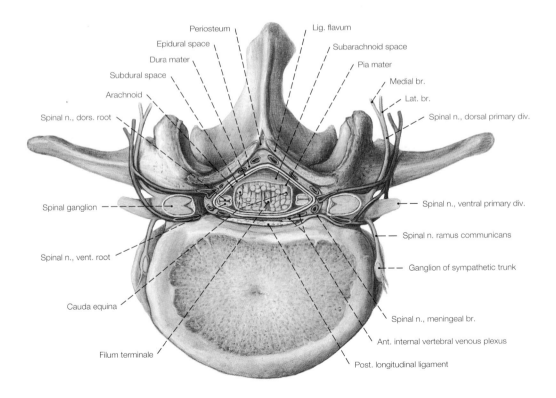

Fig. 574 Contents of the vertebral canal. A cross section at the level of the third lumbar vertebra, viewed from above.

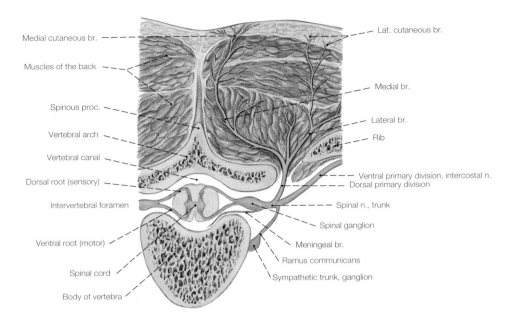

Medial cutaneous br.

Muscles of the back

Spinous proc.

Vertebral arch

Vertebral canal

Dorsal root (sensory)

Intervertebral foramen

Ventral root (motor)

Spinal cord

Body of vertebra

Lat. cutaneous br.

Medial br.

Lateral br.

Rib

Ventral primary division, intercostal n.

Dorsal primary division

Spinal n., trunk

Spinal ganglion

Meningeal br.

Ramus communicans

Sympathetic trunk, ganglion

Fig. 575 A spinal nerve in the thoracic region; schematic.

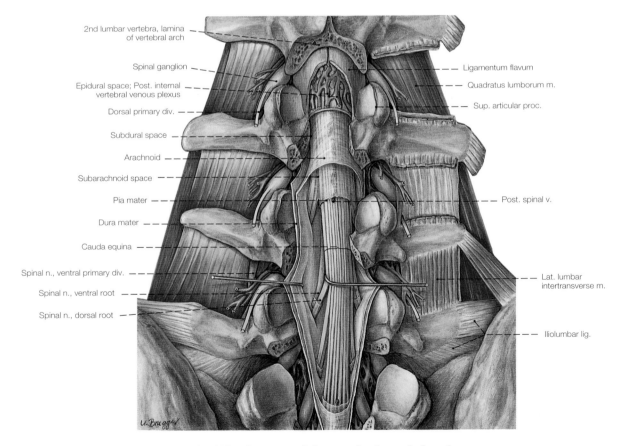

2nd lumbar vertebra, lamina of vertebral arch

Spinal ganglion

Epidural space; Post. internal vertebral venous plexus

Dorsal primary div.

Subdural space

Arachnoid

Subarachnoid space

Pia mater

Dura mater

Cauda equina

Spinal n., ventral primary div.

Spinal n., ventral root

Spinal n., dorsal root

Ligamentum flavum

Quadratus lumborum m.

Sup. articular proc.

Post. spinal v.

Lat. lumbar intertransverse m.

Iliolumbar lig.

U. Brugger

Fig. 576 Contents of the vertebral canal, dorsal view. The lumbar and lumbosacral regions after removal of the vertebral arches.

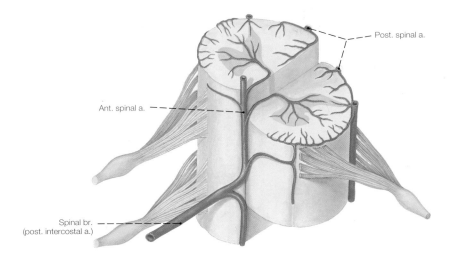

Fig. 577 Arteries of the spinal cord, schematic.

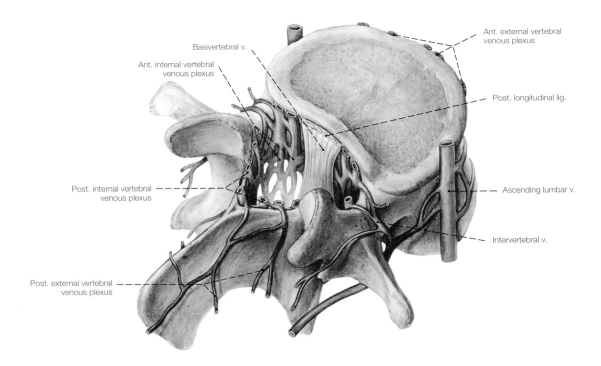

Fig. 578 Veins of the vertebral canal, showing the venous plexuses.

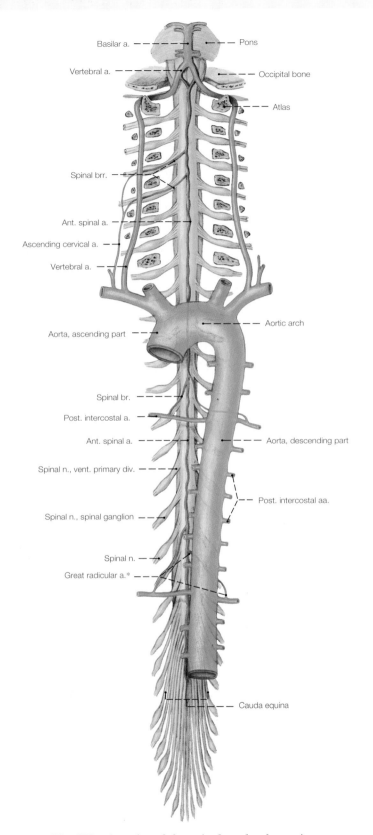

Basilar a.

Pons

Vertebral a.

Occipital bone

Atlas

Spinal brr.

Ant. spinal a.

Ascending cervical a.

Vertebral a.

Aortic arch

Aorta, ascending part

Spinal br.

Post. intercostal a.

Ant. spinal a.

Aorta, descending part

Spinal n., vent. primary div.

Post. intercostal aa.

Spinal n., spinal ganglion

Spinal n.

Great radicular a.*

Cauda equina

Fig. 579   Arteries of the spinal cord, schematic.

* Clinical: Artery of ADAMKIEWICZ

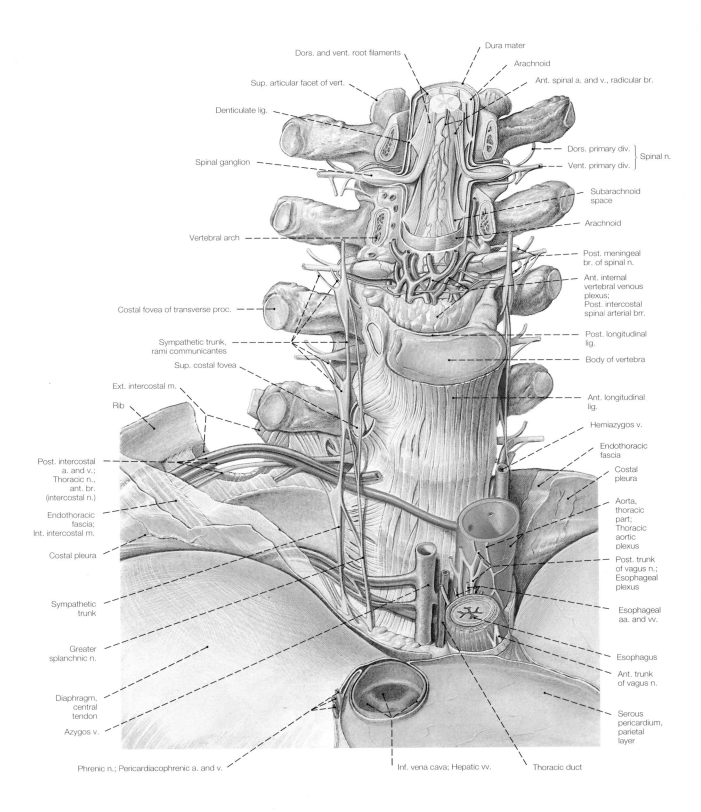

Fig. 580 Contents of the vertebral canal, ventral aspect. Stepwise exposure of the thoracic region.

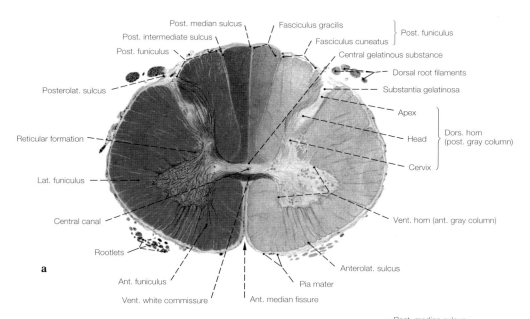

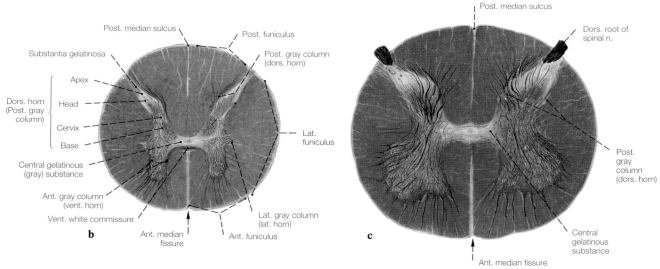

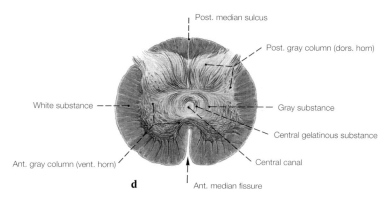

Fig. 581 a–d Spinal cord. Cross sections with myelin stain.

a Cervical part
b Thoracic part
c Lumbar part
d Sacral part

Substantia gelatinosa

Posteromarginal nucleus

Proper sensory nucleus

Post. gray column
(dors. horn)

Dorsal (thoracic) nucleus
(of Clarke)

Lat. column (lat. horn)

Intermediolat. nucleus
(autonomic)

Ant. gray column
(vent. horn)

Nuclei

Central canal

Intermediate central gray substance

I
II
III
IV
V
VII
VIII
IX
X

Fig. 582 Spinal cord, showing the laminar organization of the gray substance in this typical example at the tenth thoracic segment (T10), as determined cytoarchitectonically (laminae I–X, REXED, 1952). The formation and number of layers vary at individual spinal cord segments.

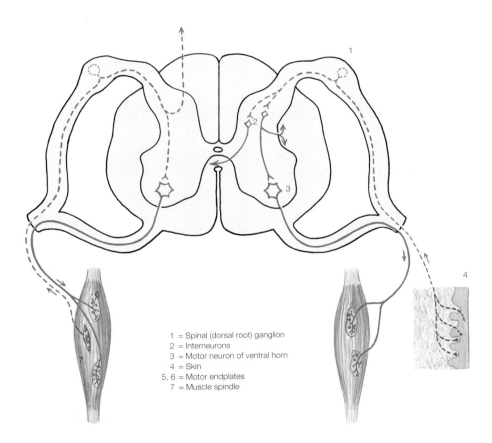

1 = Spinal (dorsal root) ganglion
2 = Interneurons
3 = Motor neuron of ventral horn
4 = Skin
5, 6 = Motor endplates
7 = Muscle spindle

Fig. 583 Reflexes of the spinal cord. Left: the segmental myotatic or stretch reflex (bineuronal, monosynaptic, proprioceptive, e.g., patellar tendon reflex, Achilles tendon reflex, etc.). Right: the multisegmental reflex (multineuronal, multisynaptic, e.g., abdominal reflex, cremasteric reflex, plantar reflex, etc.).

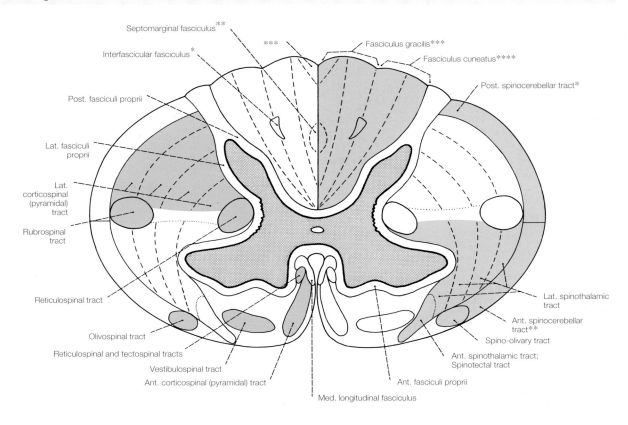

Fig. 584 Spinal cord. Diagram of the organization of the white substance in this typical example at a lower cervical segment. Sensory (ascending) afferent tracts are blue, motor (descending) efferent tracts are red.

*   Clinical: FLECHSIG's fasciculus
**   Clinical: GOWER's column
***   Clinical: GOLL's column
**** Clinical: BURDACH's fasciculus

The regions indicated by +, ++ and +++, designate descending collateral tracts of the posterior fasciculi.

\+   SCHULTZE's comma tract (cervical part)
\++   FLECHSIG's oval area (thoracic part)
\+++ PHILLIPE-GOMBAULT's triangle (lumbar part, sacral part)

Cellular Structure of the Spinal Cord

Root Neurons

Efferent (motor) root neurons (cell bodies in the gray substance, axons in the ventral root)
– multipolar, motor root cells (motoneurons)
– multipolar, visceral root cells (C8–L3: connections to the sympathetic trunk; S2–S5: connections to the pelvic parasympathetic ganglia)

Afferent (sensory) root neurons (cell bodies in the spinal ganglia, central processes in the dorsal root)
– pseudounipolar, sensory root cells (form the funiculus posterior, connections with the anterior, lateral and posterior columns)

Interneuronal and column cells

Interneurons (multipolar cells in the gray substance)
– Internuncial cells in the strict sense (homolateral connections)
– Commissural cells (contralateral connections)
– Association cells (short segmental connections in the fasciculi proprii)

Column cells (multipolar cells; cell bodies in the gray substance, long ascending or descending axons, form the tracts of the funiculi).

Long Tracts of the Spinal Cord

Ascending Tracts

Pathways for epicritic sensibility (tactile pathway) (Precise differentiation of pressure and touch, vibration, position sense)

Neuron I (uncrossed)
    From receptors (exteroceptors) in the skin and mucosa, the periosteum, the joints as well as muscle spindles, etc. to the nucleus cuneatus and nucleus gracilis in the medulla oblongata: Fasciculus cuneatus and fasciculus gracilis (neurons, cell bodies in the spinal ganglia); ascending collaterals (see Fig. 584).

Neuron II (crossed)
    From the medulla oblongata to the thalamus (medial lemniscus, perikarya in the nucleus cuneatus and in the nucleus gracilis), branches to the cerebellum (cuneocerebellar tract).

Neuron III (uncrossed)
    From the thalamus to the cerebral cortex, especially to the postcentral gyrus (thalamocortical fibers, cell bodies in the thalamus).

Pathways for protopathic sensibility (pain pathway) (Pain, temperature, general pressure sensation)

Neuron I (uncrossed)
    From receptors (exteroceptors) in the skin, mucosa, etc. to the central nucleus of the posterior funiculi, laminae I, IV, VII and VIII (neurons, perikarya in the spinal ganglia).

Neuron II (crossed, some fibers possibly uncrossed)
    From the posterior horn to the thalamus, in the reticular formation and to the midbrain tectum (anterior and lateral spinothalamic tracts, spinoreticular tract, spinotectal tract; cell bodies in the posterior funiculi).

Neuron III (uncrossed)
    From thalamus to cerebral cortex, especially to the postcentral gyrus (thalamocortical fibers, cell bodies in the thalamus), and also to parts of the medial geniculate body.

Pathways for unconscious deep sensibility (Unconscious, but precise spatial differentiation as a prerequisite for movement coordination by the cerebellum)

Via the anterior cerebellar tract
Neuron I (uncrossed)
    From receptors (proprioceptors) in muscles, tendons, and connective tissue to the dorsal (thoracic) nucleus of Clarke of the posterior columns (neurons, cell bodies in the spinal ganglia)

Neuron II (mostly crossed)
    From the posterior horn to the cerebellum, especially to the anterior part of the cerebellar vermis through the superior cerebellar peduncle (anterior spinocerebellar tract, cell bodies in the dorsal (thoracic) nucleus of Clarke)

Via the posterior cerebellar tract
Neuron I (uncrossed)
    From end organs (proprioceptors) in muscles, tendons, and connective tissue to the nuclei of the posterior and anterior columns (neurons, cell bodies in the spinal ganglia).

Neuron II (probably uncrossed)
    From the posterior horn to the cerebellum through the inferior cerebellar peduncle (posterior spinocerebellar tract, cell bodies in the posterior horn).

Descending Tracts

The motor system encompasses a large number of nuclear regions and tracts. The "final common path" is the lower motor neuron. For didactic reasons, we maintain here the traditional organization because of the acknowledged complexity of the system.

Corticospinal ("Pyramidal tract") systems
Central neuron I (crossed and uncrossed)
    From the cerebral cortex through the internal capsule and the cerebral peduncles to interneurons in the anterior and posterior columns (lateral corticospinal tract, anterior corticospinal tract, cell bodies in precentral gyrus). Branches to the cranial nerve nuclei (corticonuclear tract and corticobulbar tract).

Peripheral neuron II (lower motor neuron)
    From the anterior horn to the motor endplates of the skeletal musculature (motor neurons, cell bodies in the anterior horn).

"Extrapyramidal" motor system
Central neuron I (crossed and uncrossed)
    From the cerebral cortex, especially the precentral gyrus and those cortical areas anterior to it, with synapses in the telencephalic nuclei, thalamus, subthalamic nucleus, nucleus ruber, substantia nigra, cerebellum, etc. and collaterals directed to the interneurons of the anterior columns (rubrospinal tract, medial and lateral vestibulospinal tracts, reticulospinal tract, tectospinal tract).

Peripheral neuron II (lower motor neuron)
    From the anterior horn to the motor endplates of the skeletal musculature (motor neurons, cell bodies in the anterior horn).

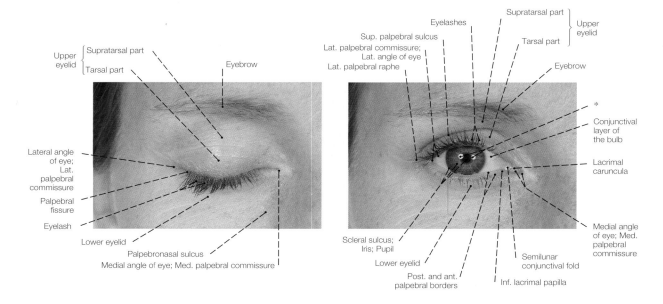

Fig. 585 The right eyelids (palpebrae) in the closed position, anterior view.

Fig. 586 The right eye and eyelids (palpebrae), in the open position, anterior view.

* Light conditioned pupillary reflex

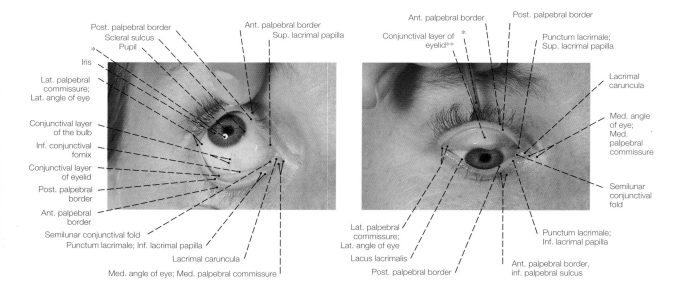

Fig. 587 The right eye and eyelids (palpebrae), anterior view. The palpebral fissure is enlarged as the eyelids are pulled apart. The gaze is oriented superiorly and laterally.

* Light conditioned pupillary reflex

Fig. 588 The right eye and eyelids (palpebrae), anterior view. The upper lid is everted. The gaze is oriented downward.

Eversion of the upper lid is occasionally hindered by the stiffness of the tarsus (**). Eversion is required, for example, to remove foreign bodies from the eye and can be facilitated with the aid of a small hook with a curved end (*).

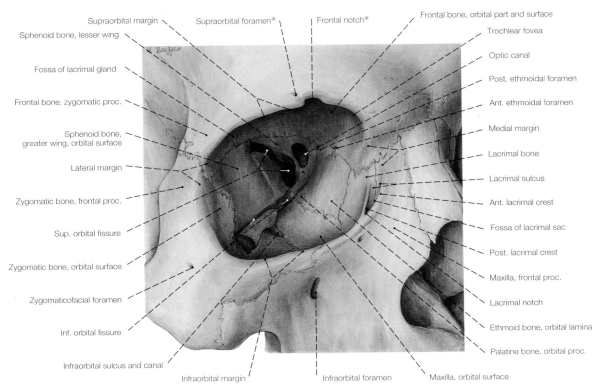

Supraorbital margin

Sphenoid bone, lesser wing

Fossa of lacrimal gland

Frontal bone, zygomatic proc.

Sphenoid bone, greater wing, orbital surface

Lateral margin

Zygomatic bone, frontal proc.

Sup. orbital fissure

Zygomatic bone, orbital surface

Zygomaticofacial foramen

Inf. orbital fissure

Infraorbital sulcus and canal

Supraorbital foramen*

Frontal notch*

Infraorbital margin

Infraorbital foramen

Maxilla, orbital surface

Frontal bone, orbital part and surface

Trochlear fovea

Optic canal

Post. ethmoidal foramen

Ant. ethmoidal foramen

Medial margin

Lacrimal bone

Lacrimal sulcus

Ant. lacrimal crest

Fossa of lacrimal sac

Post. lacrimal crest

Maxilla, frontal proc.

Lacrimal notch

Ethmoid bone, orbital lamina

Palatine bone, orbital proc.

Fig. 589 The right orbit, anterolateral view.

* These structures can be present as foramina or as notches.

The walls of the orbit are designated as: superior, lateral, inferior, and medial.

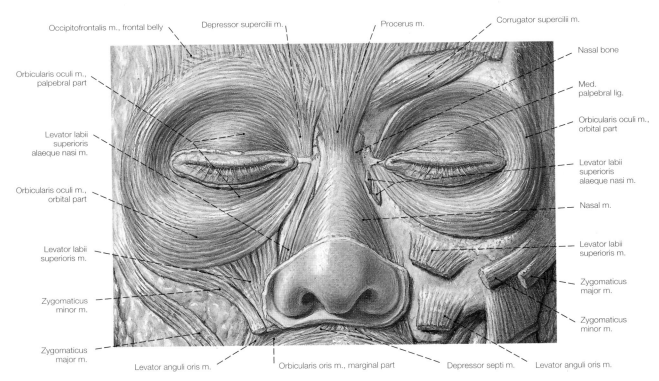

Occipitofrontalis m., frontal belly

Depressor supercilii m.

Procerus m.

Corrugator supercilii m.

Orbicularis oculi m., palpebral part

Levator labii superioris alaeque nasi m.

Orbicularis oculi m., orbital part

Levator labii superioris m.

Zygomaticus minor m.

Zygomaticus major m.

Levator anguli oris m.

Orbicularis oris m., marginal part

Depressor septi m.

Nasal bone

Med. palpebral lig.

Orbicularis oculi m., orbital part

Levator labii superioris alaeque nasi m.

Nasal m.

Levator labii superioris m.

Zygomaticus major m.

Zygomaticus minor m.

Levator anguli oris m.

Fig. 590 The facial muscles in the region of the eye, anterior view.

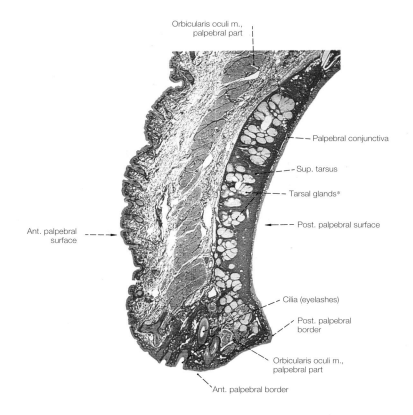

Orbicularis oculi m.,
palpebral part

Palpebral conjunctiva

Sup. tarsus

Tarsal glands*

Post. palpebral surface

Ant. palpebral
surface

Cilia (eyelashes)

Post. palpebral
border

Orbicularis oculi m.,
palpebral part

Ant. palpebral border

Fig. 591   The upper eyelid. Photograph of a
microscopic specimen; azan stain, sagittal section,
magnified.

* Clinical: MEIBOMian gland

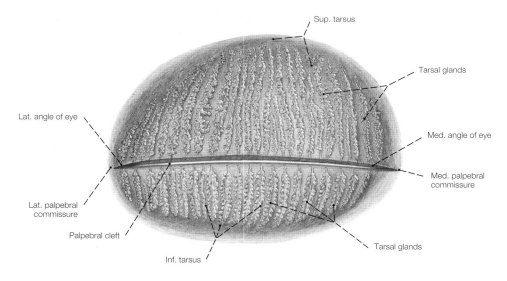

Sup. tarsus

Tarsal glands

Med. angle of eye

Med. palpebral
commissure

Lat. angle of eye

Lat. palpebral
commissure

Palpebral cleft

Tarsal glands

Inf. tarsus

Fig. 592   The left eyelids (palpebrae), posterior
view. A translucent specimen showing the
excretory ductules of the tarsal glands on the
inner surface of the eyelids.

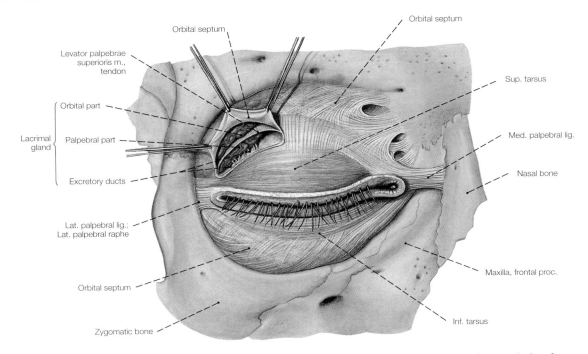

Orbital septum

Levator palpebrae superioris m., tendon

Orbital part

Lacrimal gland

Palpebral part

Excretory ducts

Lat. palpebral lig.; Lat. palpebral raphe

Orbital septum

Zygomatic bone

Orbital septum

Sup. tarsus

Med. palpebral lig.

Nasal bone

Maxilla, frontal proc.

Inf. tarsus

Fig. 593 The entrance to the right orbit, with eyelids and lacrimal gland, anterior view. The orbicularis oculi muscle has been removed and the orbital septum exposed. The aponeurosis of the levator palpebrae superioris muscle has been sectioned to expose the palpebral part of the lacrimal gland.

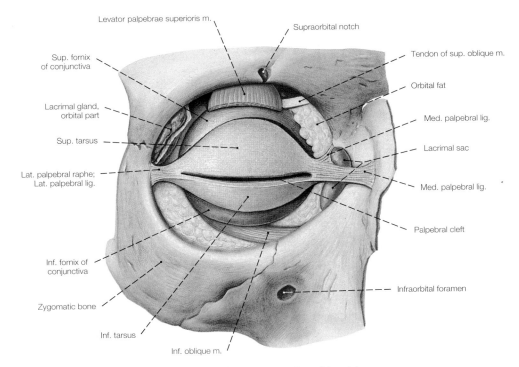

Levator palpebrae superioris m.

Supraorbital notch

Sup. fornix of conjunctiva

Lacrimal gland, orbital part

Sup. tarsus

Lat. palpebral raphe; Lat. palpebral lig.

Inf. fornix of conjunctiva

Zygomatic bone

Inf. tarsus

Inf. oblique m.

Tendon of sup. oblique m.

Orbital fat

Med. palpebral lig.

Lacrimal sac

Med. palpebral lig.

Palpebral cleft

Infraorbital foramen

Fig. 594 The entrance to the right orbit with eyelids, anterior view. The orbital septum has been removed and the levator palpebrae superioris muscle sectioned.

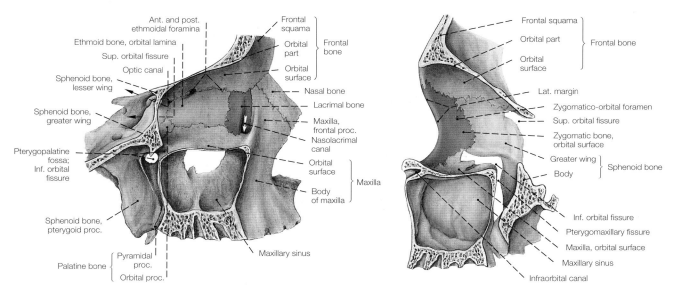

Fig. 595 Medial wall of the right orbit, lateral view. Exposure by a vertical section in the plane of the axis of the orbit.

Fig. 596 Lateral wall of the right orbit, medial view. Exposure by a vertical section in the plane of the axis of the orbit.

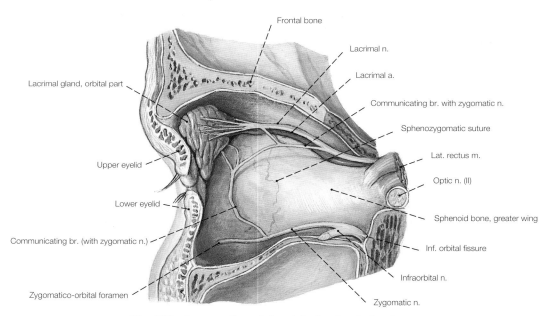

Fig. 597 Innervation of the right lacrimal gland, medial view. The lateral wall of the orbit has been exposed by a vertical section.

Lacrimal Apparatus

The lacrimal fluid is conveyed from the lacrimal gland by the excretory ductules beneath the conjunctiva. When the lids blink, fluid is distributed over the cornea and gathers in the lacus lacrimalis along the posterior border of the lower lid. The lacrimal ducts take up the fluid at their orifices, the puncta lacrimalia, which are immersed in the lacus lacrimalis, in part by capillary action, and transport the fluid to the lacrimal sac.

The nasolacrimal canal, which is about 20 mm long and 5 mm wide, contains the nasolacrimal duct. The duct begins in the fossa of the lacrimal sac and extends to the inferior nasal meatus under the inferior nasal concha where it ends in an orifice protected by a fold of mucous membrane, the lacrimal fold. In the newborn the nasal orifice of the nasolacrimal duct may be closed by a membrane.

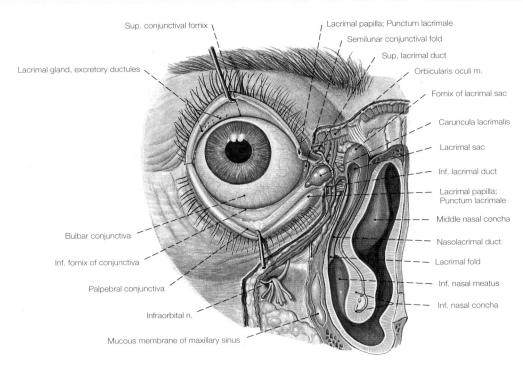

Sup. conjunctival fornix

Lacrimal gland, excretory ductules

Bulbar conjunctiva

Inf. fornix of conjunctiva

Palpebral conjunctiva

Infraorbital n.

Mucous membrane of maxillary sinus

Lacrimal papilla; Punctum lacrimale

Semilunar conjunctival fold

Sup. lacrimal duct

Orbicularis oculi m.

Fornix of lacrimal sac

Caruncula lacrimalis

Lacrimal sac

Inf. lacrimal duct

Lacrimal papilla; Punctum lacrimale

Middle nasal concha

Nasolacrimal duct

Lacrimal fold

Inf. nasal meatus

Inf. nasal concha

Fig. 598 The right lacrimal apparatus, anterior view. The palpebrae have been pulled away from the eyeball. The nasolacrimal duct has been opened down to its orifice in the inferior nasal meatus.

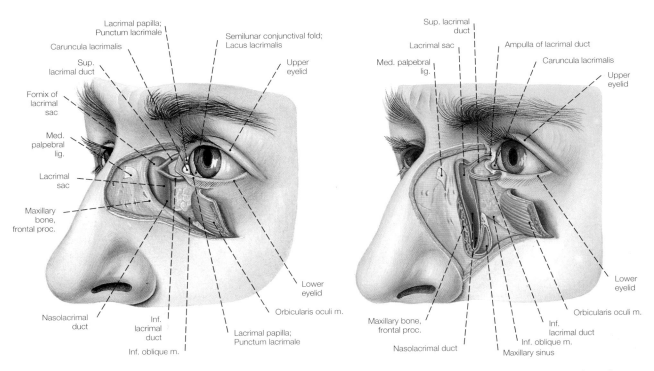

Lacrimal papilla; Punctum lacrimale

Caruncula lacrimalis

Sup. lacrimal duct

Fornix of lacrimal sac

Med. palpebral lig.

Lacrimal sac

Maxillary bone, frontal proc.

Semilunar conjunctival fold; Lacus lacrimalis

Upper eyelid

Lower eyelid

Orbicularis oculi m.

Lacrimal papilla; Punctum lacrimale

Nasolacrimal duct

Inf. lacrimal duct

Inf. oblique m.

Fig. 599 The left lacrimal apparatus, viewed from the anterolateral aspect. The orbicularis oculi muscle has been detached from the maxilla and the medial palpebral ligament has been sectioned.

Sup. lacrimal duct

Lacrimal sac

Med. palpebral lig.

Ampulla of lacrimal duct

Caruncula lacrimalis

Upper eyelid

Lower eyelid

Orbicularis oculi m.

Inf. lacrimal duct

Inf. oblique m.

Maxillary sinus

Maxillary bone, frontal proc.

Nasolacrimal duct

Fig. 600 The left lacrimal apparatus, viewed from the anterolateral aspect. The nasolacrimal duct and the nasolacrimal canal have been opened.

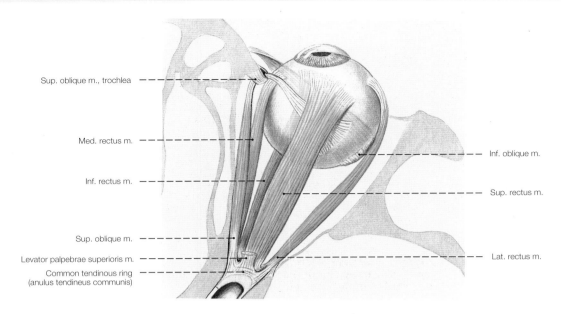

Sup. oblique m., trochlea

Med. rectus m.

Inf. rectus m.

Sup. oblique m.

Levator palpebrae superioris m.

Common tendinous ring
(anulus tendineus communis)

Inf. oblique m.

Sup. rectus m.

Lat. rectus m.

Fig. 601 The ocular muscles in a schematic of the right eye, viewed from above. The axis of the eyeball is directed sagittally, while the muscles orient themselves along the axis of the orbital cavity.

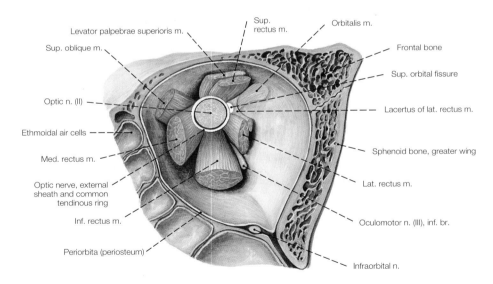

Levator palpebrae superioris m.

Sup. oblique m.

Optic n. (II)

Ethmoidal air cells

Med. rectus m.

Optic nerve, external sheath and common tendinous ring

Inf. rectus m.

Periorbita (periosteum)

Sup. rectus m.

Orbitalis m.

Frontal bone

Sup. orbital fissure

Lacertus of lat. rectus m.

Sphenoid bone, greater wing

Lat. rectus m.

Oculomotor n. (III), inf. br.

Infraorbital n.

Fig. 602 The ocular muscles, anterior view. A frontal section through the left orbit, showing their origins from the common tendinous ring (anulus tendineus communis). The optic nerve (II) has been sectioned.

Innervation of the Ocular Muscles

Oculomotor nerve (III)
  Levator palpebrae superioris m.
  Superior rectus m.
  Medial rectus m.
  Inferior rectus m.
  Inferior oblique m.

Trochlear nerve (IV)
  Superior oblique m.

Abducens nerve (VI)
  Lateral rectus m.

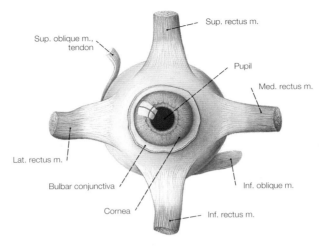

Fig. 603 The right ocular muscles, anterior aspect. The insertions of the muscles have been deflected from the eyeball.

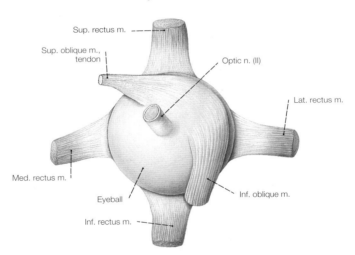

Fig. 604 The right ocular muscles, posterior aspect. The insertions of the muscles have been deflected from the eyeball.

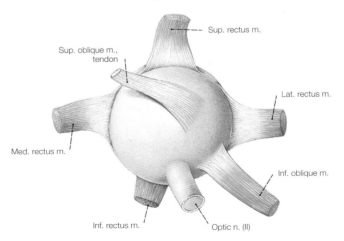

Fig. 605 The right ocular muscles, viewed posteriorly from above. The insertions of the muscles have been deflected from the eyeball.

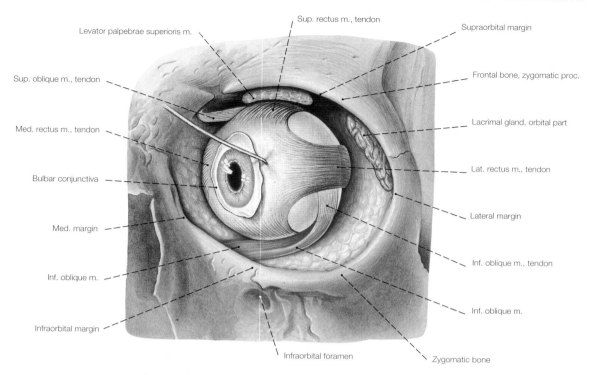

Levator palpebrae superioris m.

Sup. oblique m., tendon

Med. rectus m., tendon

Bulbar conjunctiva

Med. margin

Inf. oblique m.

Infraorbital margin

Sup. rectus m., tendon

Supraorbital margin

Frontal bone, zygomatic proc.

Lacrimal gland, orbital part

Lat. rectus m., tendon

Lateral margin

Inf. oblique m., tendon

Inf. oblique m.

Infraorbital foramen

Zygomatic bone

Fig. 606 The left ocular muscles, anterior aspect. The palpebrae, the orbicularis oculi muscle, and the orbital septum have been removed, and the eyeball is abducted medially.

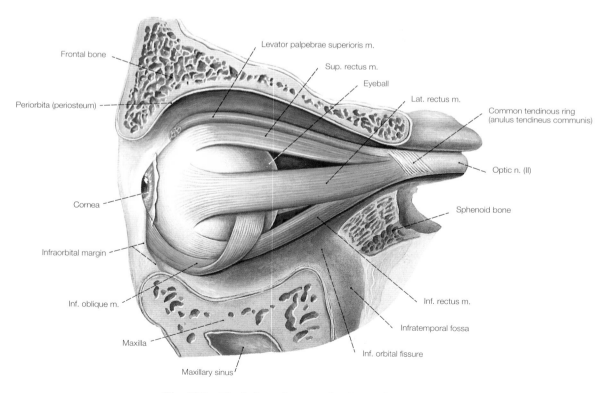

Frontal bone

Periorbita (periosteum)

Cornea

Infraorbital margin

Inf. oblique m.

Maxilla

Maxillary sinus

Levator palpebrae superioris m.

Sup. rectus m.

Eyeball

Lat. rectus m.

Common tendinous ring (anulus tendineus communis)

Optic n. (II)

Sphenoid bone

Inf. rectus m.

Infratemporal fossa

Inf. orbital fissure

Fig. 607 The left ocular muscles, lateral aspect. The lateral wall of the orbit has been removed.

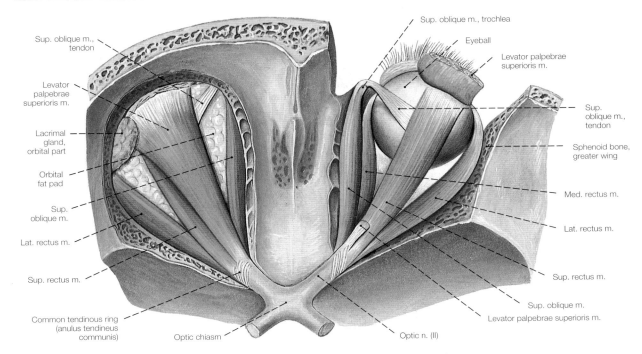

Sup. oblique m., tendon

Levator palpebrae superioris m.

Lacrimal gland, orbital part

Orbital fat pad

Sup. oblique m.

Lat. rectus m.

Sup. rectus m.

Common tendinous ring (anulus tendineus communis)

Optic chiasm

Sup. oblique m., trochlea

Eyeball

Levator palpebrae superioris m.

Sup. oblique m., tendon

Sphenoid bone, greater wing

Med. rectus m.

Lat. rectus m.

Sup. rectus m.

Sup. oblique m.

Levator palpebrae superioris m.

Optic n. (II)

Fig. 608 The ocular muscles. The roofs of both orbits have been removed, the optic canals have been opened and the right levator palpebrae superioris muscle has been partially removed.

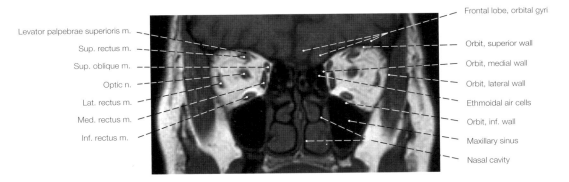

Levator palpebrae superioris m.

Sup. rectus m.

Sup. oblique m.

Optic n.

Lat. rectus m.

Med. rectus m.

Inf. rectus m.

Frontal lobe, orbital gyri

Orbit, superior wall

Orbit, medial wall

Orbit, lateral wall

Ethmoidal air cells

Orbit, inf. wall

Maxillary sinus

Nasal cavity

Fig. 609 The ocular muscles, anterior aspect. Computed tomography (CT) scan of a frontal section at the level of the middle of the orbits.

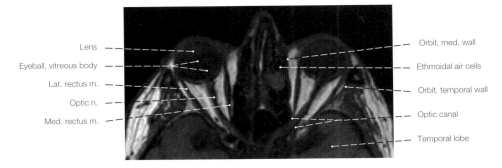

Lens

Eyeball, vitreous body

Lat. rectus m.

Optic n.

Med. rectus m.

Orbit, med. wall

Ethmoidal air cells

Orbit, temporal wall

Optic canal

Temporal lobe

Fig. 610 The eyeball and the ocular muscles, viewed from above. Computed tomography (CT) scan of a cross section at the level of the optic nerve (II).

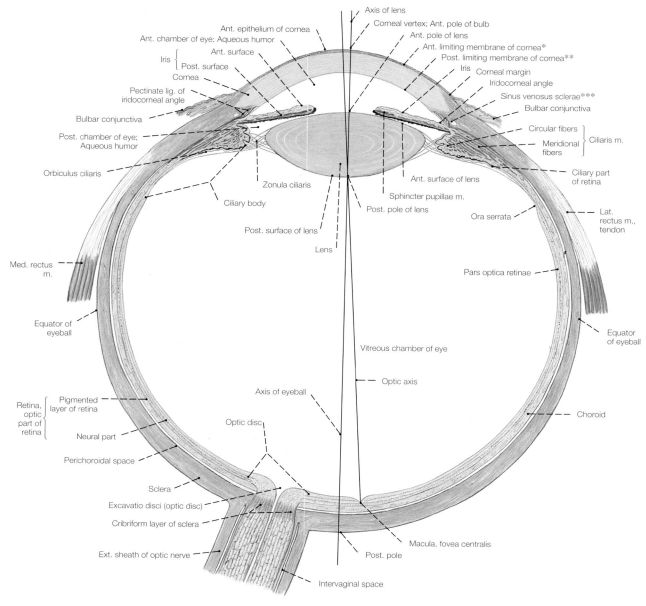

Fig. 611 The eyeball. Schematic horizontal section at the level of the exit of the optic nerve (II).

*   Clinical: BOWMAN's membrane
**   Clinical: membrane of DESCEMET
*** Clinical: canal of SCHLEMM

Measurements of the Eyeball
(Average values from the anatomical and ophthalmological literature)

External bulbar axis	24.0 mm	Radius of curvature of sclera	13.0 mm
Internal bulbar axis	22.5 mm	Radius of curvature of cornea	7.8 mm
Thickness of cornea	0.5 mm	Power of entire eye (distance vision)	59 diopters
Depth of anterior chamber	3.6 mm	Power of cornea	43 diopters
Thickness of lens	3.6 mm	Power of lens (distance vision)	19 diopters
Distance between lens and retina	15.6 mm	Interpupillary distance	61–69 mm
Thickness of retina	0.3 mm		

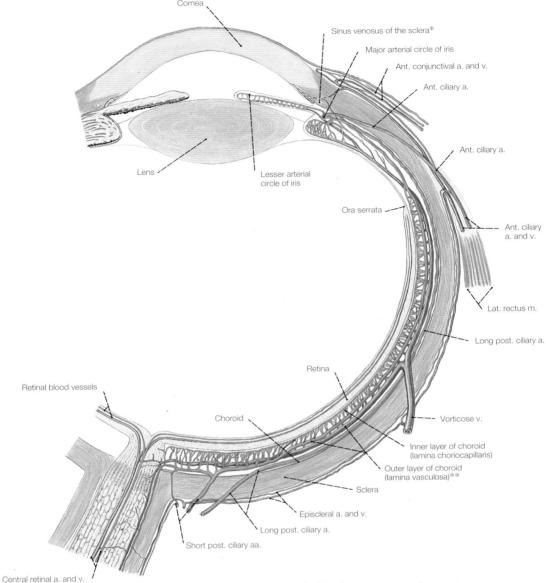

Cornea

Sinus venosus of the sclera*

Major arterial circle of iris

Ant. conjunctival a. and v.

Ant. ciliary a.

Ant. ciliary a.

Lens

Lesser arterial circle of iris

Ora serrata

Ant. ciliary a. and v.

Lat. rectus m.

Long post. ciliary a.

Retina

Retinal blood vessels

Choroid

Vorticose v.

Inner layer of choroid (lamina choriocapillaris)

Outer layer of choroid (lamina vasculosa)**

Sclera

Episcleral a. and v.

Long post. ciliary a.

Short post. ciliary aa.

Central retinal a. and v.

Fig. 612 The blood vessels of the eyeball, schematic overview.

* Clinical: Canal of SCHLEMM
** Clinical: Uvea

Tunics of the Eye

External, fibrous tunic
- Cornea (pronounced curvature, translucent)
- Sclera (lesser curvature, opaque, bluish-white in infancy, yellowish-white in senescence)

Intermediate, vascular tunic
- Iris, with central circular opening, the pupil
- Ciliary body with ciliary muscle, ciliary processes, ciliary zonule with suspensory ligament, and the zonular space
- Choroid

Internal tunic (retina)
- Anterior non-neural part (from the pupillary-iridial border to the ora serrata)
  Iridial part of retina (single layered, heavily pigmented epithelium)
  Ciliary part of retina (single layered, unpigmented epithelium)
- Posterior neural part, optic part of retina (stratified)
  Neuron I: Vision cells (Rods—brightness; cones—color)
  Neuron II: Bipolar ganglion cells within the retina (ganglion of the retina)
  Neuron III: Multipolar ganglion cells (optic ganglion), whose long axons form the optic nerve (II) and connect to the visual centers of the brain via the optic tract

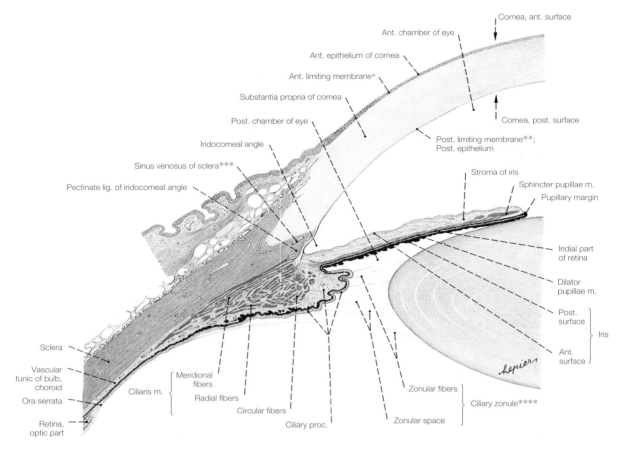

Fig. 613 The eyeball. A schematic horizontal section at the level of the middle of the pupil.

* Clinical: membrane of BOWMAN
** Clinical: membrane of DESCEMET
*** Clinical: canal of SCHLEMM
**** Clinical: zonule of ZINN

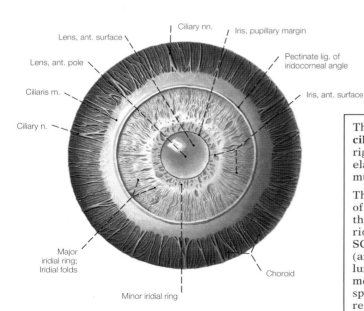

Fig. 614 The iris and the pupil, anterior aspect (400%). The cornea and sclera have been removed.

The ring-shaped suspensory ligament of the lens, **ciliary zonule (zonule of Zinn),** consists of delicate, rigid fibers, which are kept under tension by the elasticity of the lens itself and also by the ciliary muscle.

The **aqueous humor** is produced by the epithelium of the ciliary processes in the posterior chamber of the eye, and flows through the pupil into the anterior chamber, where it drains into the canal of SCHLEMM in the region of the iridocorneal angle (angle of the anterior chamber). Here the reticulum trabeculare (also known as the pectinate ligament) forms a dense network with interstitial spaces. Constriction of the iridocorneal angle can restrict the drainage of aqueous humor, resulting in an elevation of the interocular pressure (glaucoma).

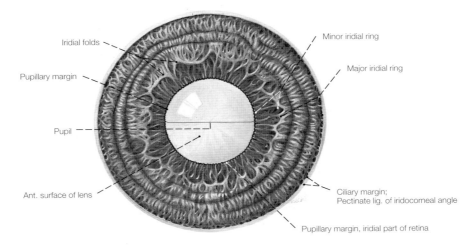

Iridial folds

Pupillary margin

Pupil

Ant. surface of lens

Minor iridial ring

Major iridial ring

Ciliary margin;
Pectinate lig. of iridocorneal angle

Pupillary margin, iridial part of retina

Fig. 615 The iris, anterior view (500%). The cornea has been removed.

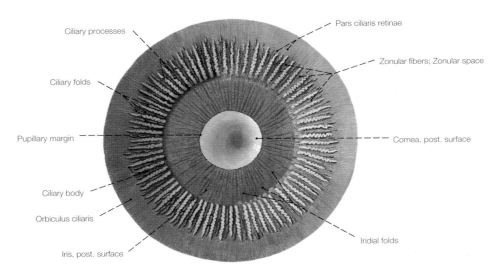

Ciliary processes

Ciliary folds

Pupillary margin

Ciliary body

Orbiculus ciliaris

Iris, post. surface

Pars ciliaris retinae

Zonular fibers; Zonular space

Cornea, post. surface

Iridial folds

Fig. 616 The iris, posterior view (300%). The iris has been detached at the ciliary margin.

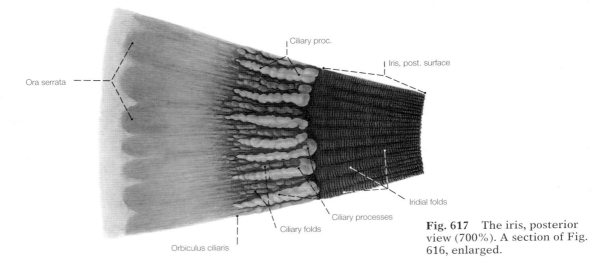

Ora serrata

Ciliary proc.

Iris, post. surface

Iridial folds

Orbiculus ciliaris

Ciliary folds

Ciliary processes

Fig. 617 The iris, posterior view (700%). A section of Fig. 616, enlarged.

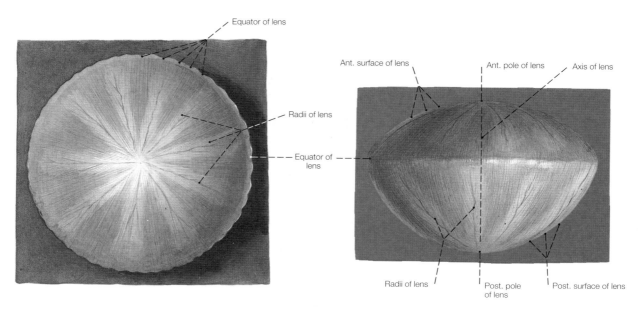

Fig. 618 The lens of the eye, anterior view (600%). Under specific optical conditions, the adult specimen can show a "lens star with multiple radiations" while the lens from a newborn shows a "lens star with three radiations."

Fig. 619 The lens of the eye, viewed from the equator (600%).

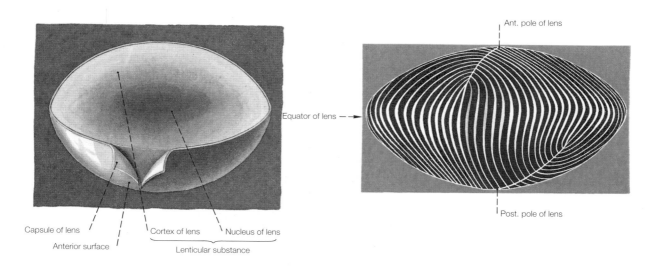

Fig. 620 The lens of the eye, viewed from the equator (600%). The lens has been halved meridionally and its capsule partially removed.

Fig. 621 The lens of the eye of a newborn, viewed from the equator (800%). Schematic representation of the lens fibers. The anterior and posterior lens stars are displaced 60° from each other.

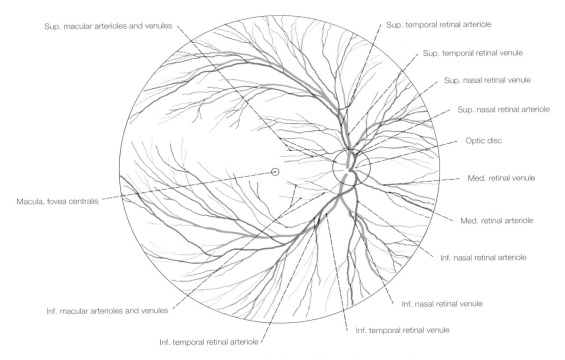

Sup. macular arterioles and venules

Sup. temporal retinal arteriole

Sup. temporal retinal venule

Sup. nasal retinal venule

Sup. nasal retinal arteriole

Optic disc

Med. retinal venule

Macula, fovea centralis

Med. retinal arteriole

Inf. nasal retinal arteriole

Inf. macular arterioles and venules

Inf. nasal retinal venule

Inf. temporal retinal venule

Inf. temporal retinal arteriole

Fig. 622 Blood vessels of the right retina, anterior view of the fundus of the eye (400%).

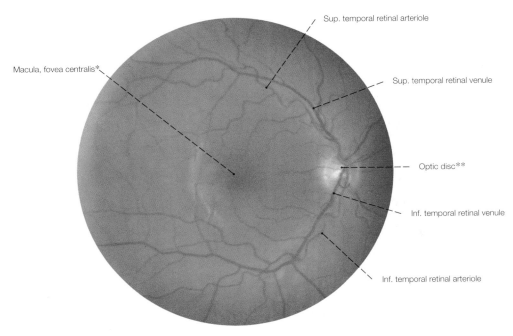

Sup. temporal retinal arteriole

Macula, fovea centralis*

Sup. temporal retinal venule

Optic disc**

Inf. temporal retinal venule

Inf. temporal retinal arteriole

Fig. 623 The fundus of the right eye, anterior view (600%). Ophthalmoscopic view of the central region.

* Clinical: Yellow spot
** Clinical: Papilla or blind spot

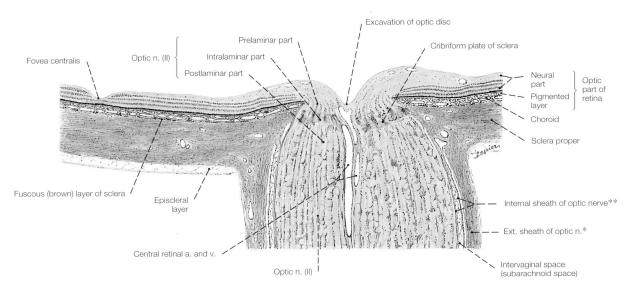

Fig. 624 The optic nerve (II). Horizontal section through its site of exit from the eyeball (1000%).

The optic nerve is covered by the cranial dura mater* and also by the arachnoid and pia mater**.

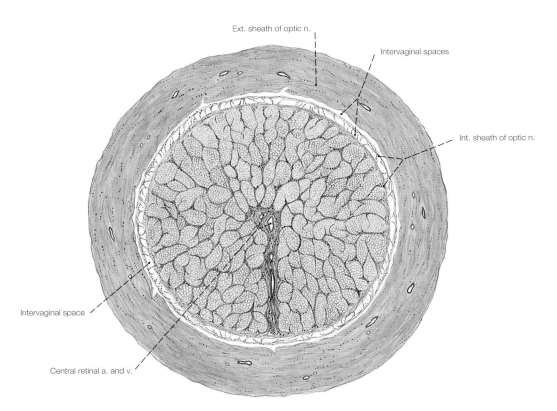

Fig. 625 The optic nerve (II). Cross section close to the eyeball (1500%).

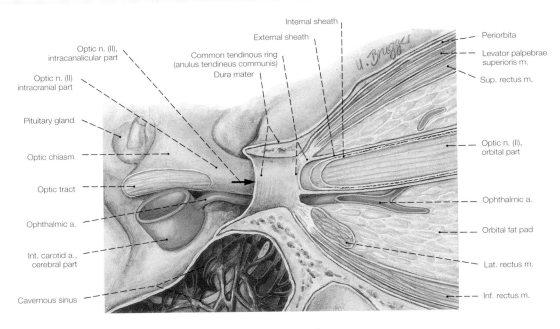

Internal sheath
External sheath
Common tendinous ring
(anulus tendineus communis)
Dura mater
u. Brüggs
Periorbita
Levator palpebrae
superioris m.
Sup. rectus m.

Optic n. (II),
intracanalicular part
Optic n. (II)
intracranial part
Pituitary gland
Optic chiasm
Optic tract
Ophthalmic a.
Int. carotid a.,
cerebral part
Cavernous sinus

Optic n. (II),
orbital part
Ophthalmic a.
Orbital fat pad
Lat. rectus m.
Inf. rectus m.

Fig. 626 The right optic nerve
(II), lateral aspect (200%). The
optic canal has been opened.

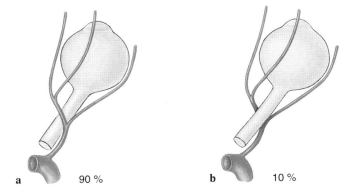

a   90 %   b   10 %

Fig. 627 a, b Variations of the right
ophthalmic artery, viewed from above.

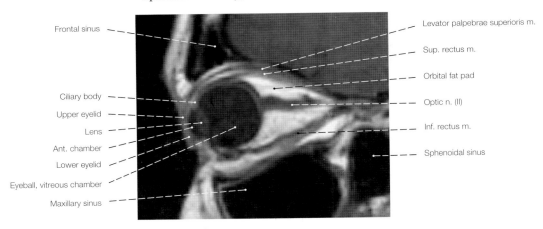

Frontal sinus

Ciliary body
Upper eyelid
Lens
Ant. chamber
Lower eyelid
Eyeball, vitreous chamber
Maxillary sinus

Levator palpebrae superioris m.
Sup. rectus m.
Orbital fat pad
Optic n. (II)
Inf. rectus m.
Sphenoidal sinus

Fig. 628 The right orbit, lateral aspect. Magnetic
resonance image (MRI) of a vertical section along the
optic nerve (II).

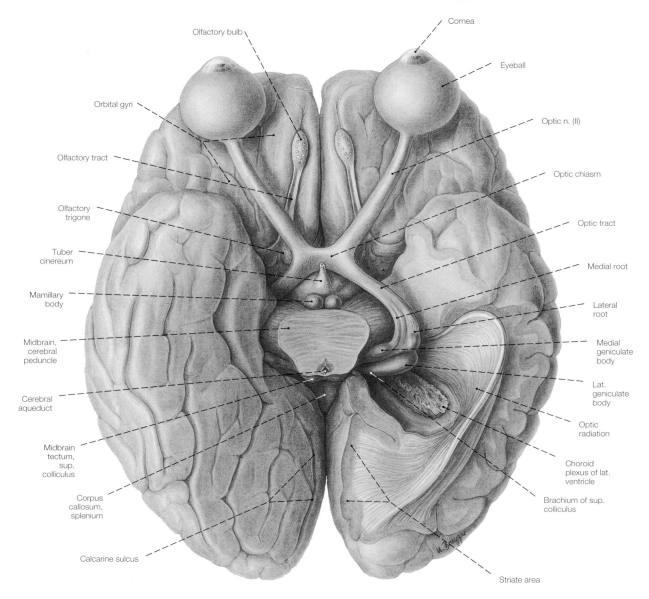

Olfactory bulb

Cornea

Eyeball

Orbital gyri

Optic n. (II)

Olfactory tract

Optic chiasm

Olfactory trigone

Optic tract

Tuber cinereum

Medial root

Mamillary body

Lateral root

Midbrain, cerebral peduncle

Medial geniculate body

Cerebral aqueduct

Lat. geniculate body

Optic radiation

Midbrain tectum, sup. colliculus

Choroid plexus of lat. ventricle

Corpus callosum, splenium

Brachium of sup. colliculus

Calcarine sulcus

Striate area

Fig. 629 The brain and the visual pathway, viewed from below. The midbrain and the pons have been sectioned obliquely and the left temporal and occipital lobes have been partially removed.

Visual Pathway

Neuron I: Rods and cones of the retina

Neuron II: Bipolar ganglion cells of the retina (cell bodies in the retinal ganglion)

Neuron III: Multipolar ganglion cells of the retina (cell bodies in the optic ganglion). The axons of the optic ganglion cells extend primarily to the lateral geniculate body (lateral root), although several fibers also extend to the medial geniculate body (medial root), to the hypothalamus, and to the cerebral cortex. They course in the optic nerve to the optic chiasm, where the fibers from the nasal part of the ocular fundus cross to the opposite side. Each optic tract contains fibers which transmit information from the contralateral half of the visual field.

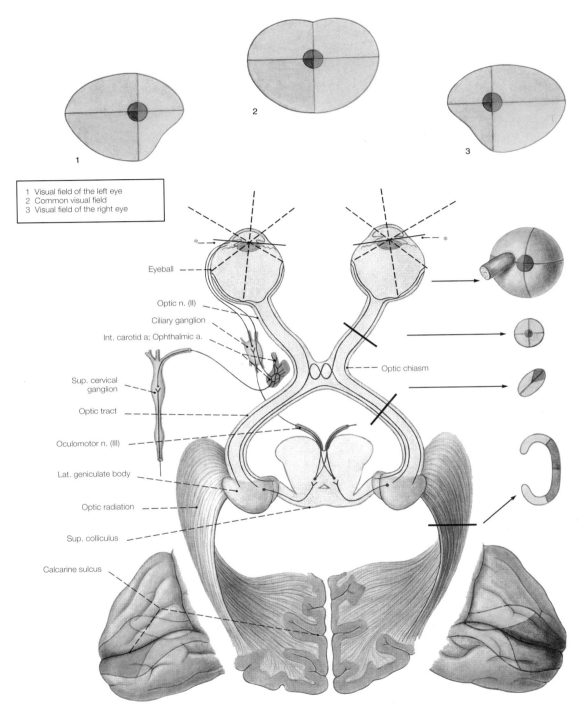

1 Visual field of the left eye
2 Common visual field
3 Visual field of the right eye

Eyeball

Optic n. (II)

Ciliary ganglion

Int. carotid a; Ophthalmic a.

Sup. cervical ganglion

Optic tract

Oculomotor n. (III)

Lat. geniculate body

Optic radiation

Sup. colliculus

Calcarine sulcus

Optic chiasm

Fig. 630 The visual pathway, viewed from above in a schematic overview. The medial surfaces of the occipital lobes are shown. The central part of the visual field has a disproportionately large projection area. Colors refer to the visual field quadrants.

∗ Plane of refraction of light

Visual Pathway—continued

Neuron IV: Its axons travel primarily from the lateral geniculate body to areas 17 and 18 of the cerebral cortex in the region surrounding the calcarine sulcus (striate area).

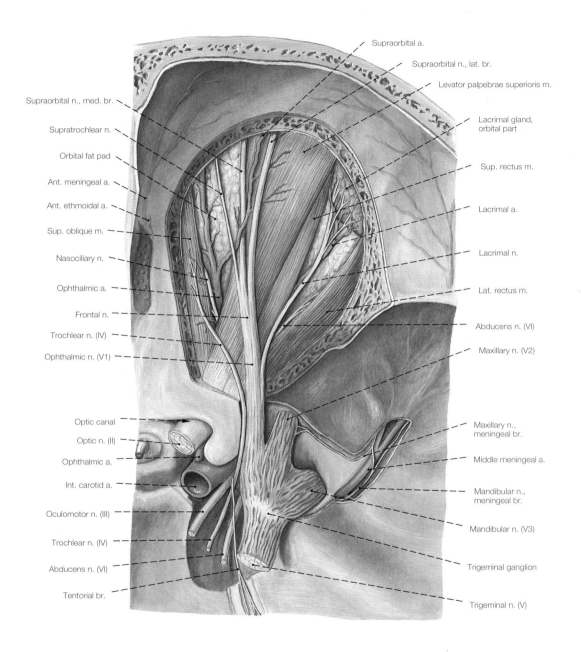

Supraorbital a.

Supraorbital n., lat. br.

Levator palpebrae superioris m.

Lacrimal gland, orbital part

Sup. rectus m.

Lacrimal a.

Lacrimal n.

Lat. rectus m.

Abducens n. (VI)

Maxillary n. (V2)

Maxillary n., meningeal br.

Middle meningeal a.

Mandibular n., meningeal br.

Mandibular n. (V3)

Trigeminal ganglion

Trigeminal n. (V)

Supraorbital n., med. br.

Supratrochlear n.

Orbital fat pad

Ant. meningeal a.

Ant. ethmoidal a.

Sup. oblique m.

Nasociliary n.

Ophthalmic a.

Frontal n.

Trochlear n. (IV)

Ophthalmic n. (V1)

Optic canal

Optic n. (II)

Ophthalmic a.

Int. carotid a.

Oculomotor n. (III)

Trochlear n. (IV)

Abducens n. (VI)

Tentorial br.

Fig. 631 Arteries and nerves of the right orbit, viewed from above. The roof of the orbit has been removed and the superior orbital fissure opened.

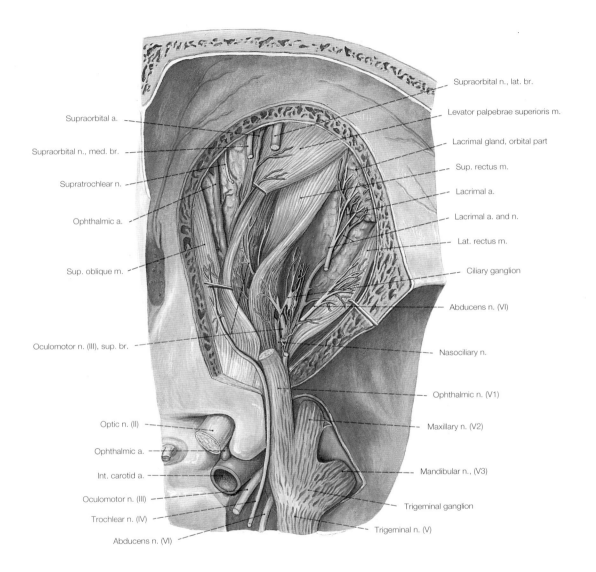

Supraorbital n., lat. br.

Levator palpebrae superioris m.

Lacrimal gland, orbital part

Sup. rectus m.

Lacrimal a.

Lacrimal a. and n.

Lat. rectus m.

Ciliary ganglion

Abducens n. (VI)

Nasociliary n.

Ophthalmic n. (V1)

Maxillary n. (V2)

Mandibular n., (V3)

Trigeminal ganglion

Trigeminal n. (V)

Supraorbital a.

Supraorbital n., med. br.

Supratrochlear n.

Ophthalmic a.

Sup. oblique m.

Oculomotor n. (III), sup. br.

Optic n. (II)

Ophthalmic a.

Int. carotid a.

Oculomotor n. (III)

Trochlear n. (IV)

Abducens n. (VI)

Fig. 632 Arteries and nerves of the right orbit, viewed from above. The roof of the orbit has been excised, the superior orbital fissure has been opened, and the frontal nerve partially removed. The ciliary ganglion has been exposed by retracting the levator palpebrae superioris and the superior rectus muscles.

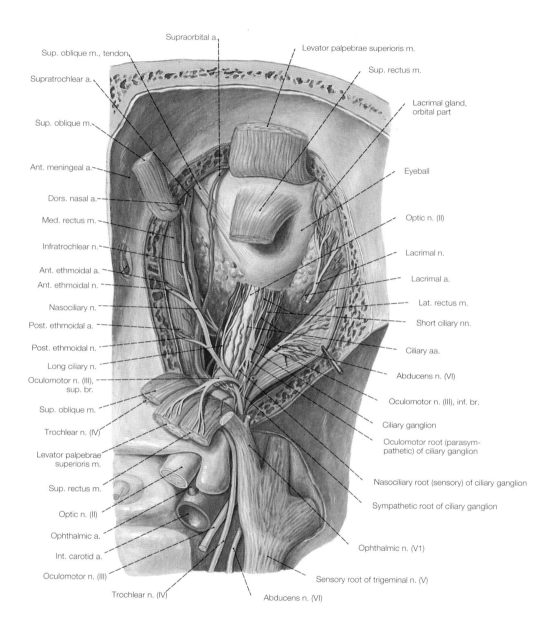

Supraorbital a.

Sup. oblique m., tendon

Supratrochlear a.

Sup. oblique m.

Ant. meningeal a.

Dors. nasal a.

Med. rectus m.

Infratrochlear n.

Ant. ethmoidal a.

Ant. ethmoidal n.

Nasociliary n.

Post. ethmoidal a.

Post. ethmoidal n.

Long ciliary n.

Oculomotor n. (III), sup. br.

Sup. oblique m.

Trochlear n. (IV)

Levator palpebrae superioris m.

Sup. rectus m.

Optic n. (II)

Ophthalmic a.

Int. carotid a.

Oculomotor n. (III)

Trochlear n. (IV)

Abducens n. (VI)

Levator palpebrae superioris m.

Sup. rectus m.

Lacrimal gland, orbital part

Eyeball

Optic n. (II)

Lacrimal n.

Lacrimal a.

Lat. rectus m.

Short ciliary nn.

Ciliary aa.

Abducens n. (VI)

Oculomotor n. (III), inf. br.

Ciliary ganglion

Oculomotor root (parasympathetic) of ciliary ganglion

Nasociliary root (sensory) of ciliary ganglion

Sympathetic root of ciliary ganglion

Ophthalmic n. (V1)

Sensory root of trigeminal n. (V)

Fig. 633 Arteries and nerves of the right orbit, viewed from above. The roof of the orbit has been excised, the superior orbital fissure has been opened, and the levator palpebrae superioris, superior rectus, and superior oblique muscles have been partially removed. The lateral rectus muscle has been retracted laterally.

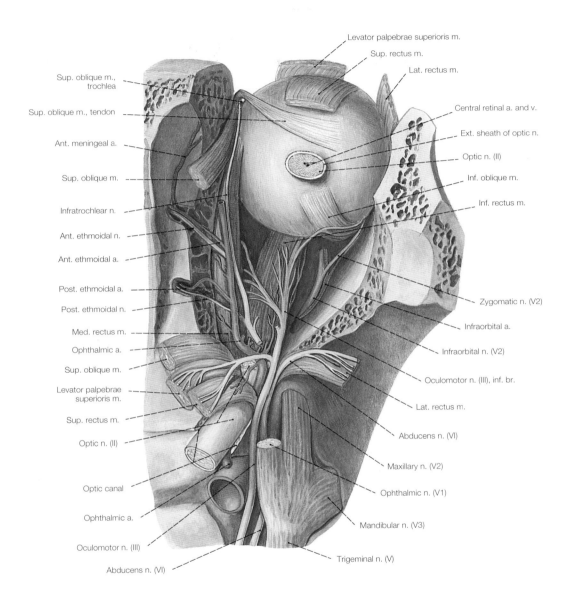

Levator palpebrae superioris m.

Sup. rectus m.

Lat. rectus m.

Sup. oblique m., trochlea

Sup. oblique m., tendon

Ant. meningeal a.

Sup. oblique m.

Infratrochlear n.

Ant. ethmoidal n.

Ant. ethmoidal a.

Post. ethmoidal a.

Post. ethmoidal n.

Med. rectus m.

Ophthalmic a.

Sup. oblique m.

Levator palpebrae superioris m.

Sup. rectus m.

Optic n. (II)

Optic canal

Ophthalmic a.

Oculomotor n. (III)

Abducens n. (VI)

Central retinal a. and v.

Ext. sheath of optic n.

Optic n. (II)

Inf. oblique m.

Inf. rectus m.

Zygomatic n. (V2)

Infraorbital a.

Infraorbital n. (V2)

Oculomotor n. (III), inf. br.

Lat. rectus m.

Abducens n. (VI)

Maxillary n. (V2)

Ophthalmic n. (V1)

Mandibular n. (V3)

Trigeminal n. (V)

Fig. 634 Arteries and nerves of the right orbit, viewed from above. The roof of the orbit has been excised, the superior orbital fissure and the optic canal have been opened, and the ophthalmic nerve and the ocular muscles, except for the inferior oblique muscle, have been removed.

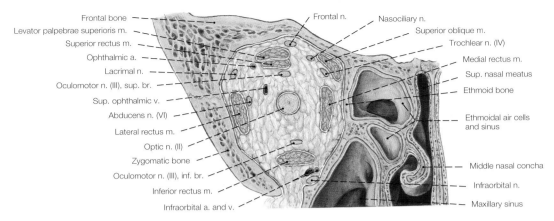

Frontal bone
Levator palpebrae superioris m.
Superior rectus m.
Ophthalmic a.
Lacrimal n.
Oculomotor n. (III), sup. br.
Sup. ophthalmic v.
Abducens n. (VI)
Lateral rectus m.
Optic n. (II)
Zygomatic bone
Oculomotor n. (III), inf. br.
Inferior rectus m.
Infraorbital a. and v.

Frontal n.
Nasociliary n.
Superior oblique m.
Trochlear n. (IV)
Medial rectus m.
Sup. nasal meatus
Ethmoid bone
Ethmoidal air cells and sinus
Middle nasal concha
Infraorbital n.
Maxillary sinus

Fig. 635 The right orbit, anterior view. Frontal section at the level of the middle of the extracranial course of the optic nerve (II).

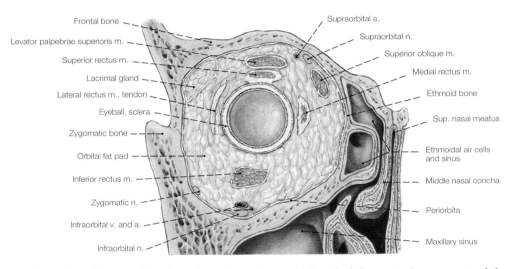

Frontal bone
Levator palpebrae superioris m.
Superior rectus m.
Lacrimal gland
Lateral rectus m., tendon
Eyeball, sclera
Zygomatic bone
Orbital fat pad
Inferior rectus m.
Zygomatic n.
Infraorbital v. and a.
Infraorbital n.

Supraorbital a.
Supraorbital n.
Superior oblique m.
Medial rectus m.
Ethmoid bone
Sup. nasal meatus
Ethmoidal air cells and sinus
Middle nasal concha
Periorbita
Maxillary sinus

Fig. 636 The right orbit, anterior view. Frontal section at the level of the posterior segment of the orbit behind the tendinous insertion of the inferior oblique muscle.

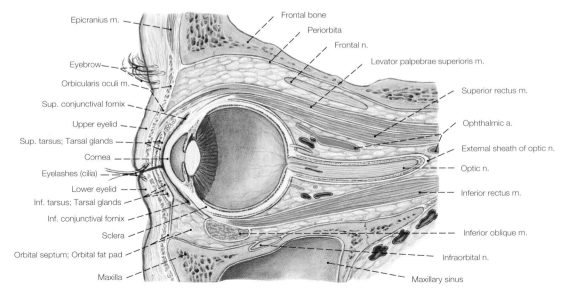

Epicranius m.
Eyebrow
Orbicularis oculi m.
Sup. conjunctival fornix
Upper eyelid
Sup. tarsus; Tarsal glands
Cornea
Eyelashes (cilia)
Lower eyelid
Inf. tarsus; Tarsal glands
Inf. conjunctival fornix
Sclera
Orbital septum; Orbital fat pad
Maxilla

Frontal bone
Periorbita
Frontal n.
Levator palpebrae superioris m.
Superior rectus m.
Ophthalmic a.
External sheath of optic n.
Optic n.
Inferior rectus m.
Inferior oblique m.
Infraorbital n.
Maxillary sinus

Fig. 637 The left orbit, lateral view. Vertical section through the orbit and the optic nerve (II).

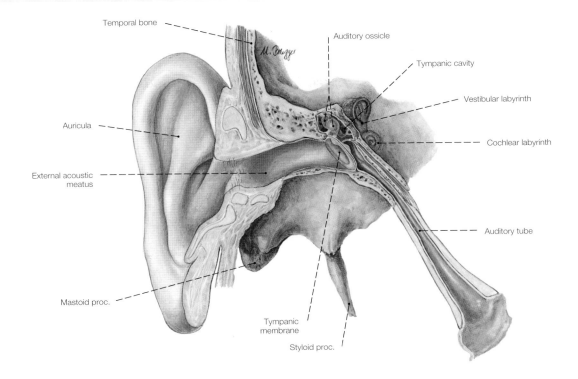

Temporal bone

Auditory ossicle

Tympanic cavity

Vestibular labyrinth

Auricula

Cochlear labyrinth

External acoustic
meatus

Auditory tube

Mastoid proc.

Tympanic
membrane

Styloid proc.

Fig. 638   The right ear, organ of hearing and
equilibration, anterior view (110%). Semischematic
overview with the tympanic cavity, the auditory tube
and part of the petrous portion of the temporal bone
opened.

The Parts of the Ear, Summary

External ear
Auricula or pinna
External acoustic meatus

Middle ear or tympanum
Tympanic cavity
Tympanic membrane
Auditory ossicles
Auditory tube

Internal ear or labyrinth
Membranous labyrinth
Vestibular labyrinth
Cochlear labyrinth
Osseous labyrinth
Vestibule
Bony semicircular canals
Cochlea
Internal acoustic meatus

The Parts of the Membranous Labyrinth, Summary (see p. 379)

Vestibular labyrinth
Perilymphatic space
Utricle
Semicircular ducts
Ant. semicircular duct
Post. semicircular duct
Lat. semicircular duct
Utriculosaccular duct
Endolymphatic duct
Saccus
Saccule
Ductus reuniens

Cochlear labyrinth
Perilymphatic space
Scala tympani
Scala vestibuli
Vestibular aqueduct
Cochlear aqueduct
Cochlear duct

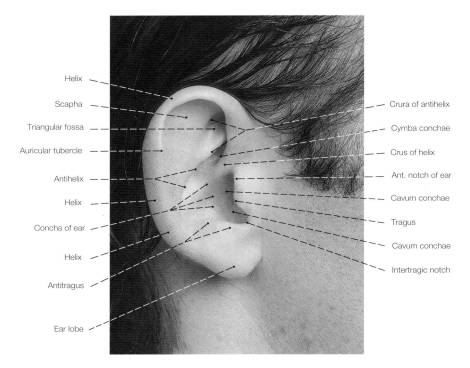

Helix

Scapha

Triangular fossa

Auricular tubercle

Antihelix

Helix

Concha of ear

Helix

Antitragus

Ear lobe

Crura of antihelix

Cymba conchae

Crus of helix

Ant. notch of ear

Cavum conchae

Tragus

Cavum conchae

Intertragic notch

Fig. 639   The right auricula,
lateral aspect.

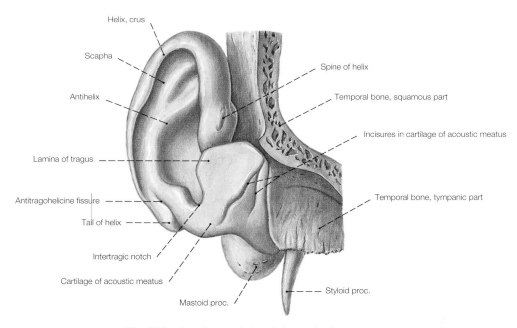

Helix, crus

Scapha

Antihelix

Lamina of tragus

Antitragohelicine fissure

Tail of helix

Intertragic notch

Cartilage of acoustic meatus

Mastoid proc.

Spine of helix

Temporal bone, squamous part

Incisures in cartilage of acoustic meatus

Temporal bone, tympanic part

Styloid proc.

Fig. 640   Cartilage of the right auricula,
viewed obliquely from anterior. Parts of
the temporal bone are shown after
removal of all soft tissue.

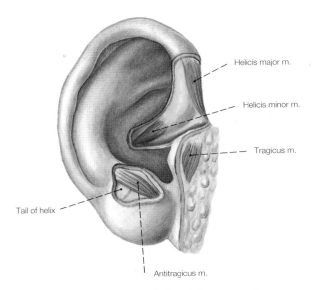

Fig. 641 Muscles of the right external ear, anterior view.

Helicis major m.

Helicis minor m.

Tragicus m.

Tail of helix

Antitragicus m.

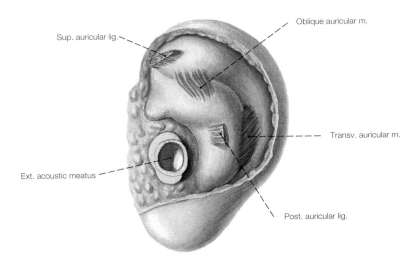

Fig. 642 Muscles of the right external ear, posterior view.

Sup. auricular lig.

Oblique auricular m.

Transv. auricular m.

Ext. acoustic meatus

Post. auricular lig.

Innervation of the External Ear

Vagus n., auricular br.:
Fundus of the external acoustic meatus and the posterior sickle-shaped part of the outer surface of the tympanic membrane

Great auricular n., posterior br. (C2/C3):
Posterior surface of the auricula

Great auricular n., anterior br. (C2/C3):
Anterior surface of the auricula

Mandibular n. (V3), auriculotemporal n., external acoustic meatus n., and tympanic membrane brr.:
Anterior root of the auricula, floor, anterior wall and roof of the external acoustic meatus as well as a large part of the tympanic membrane

Facial n. (VII), posterior auricular n., auricular br:
All muscles of the auricula

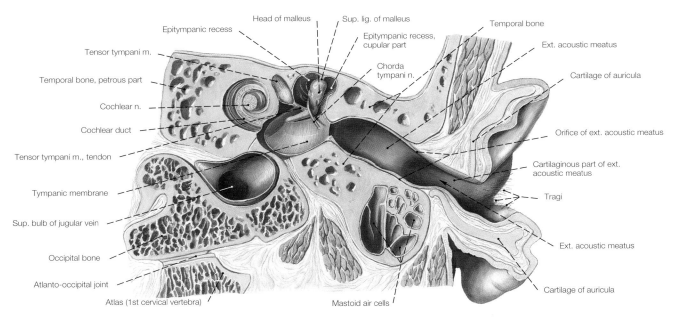

Fig. 643 The right external acoustic meatus, middle ear, and cochlea. Frontal section, posterior view.

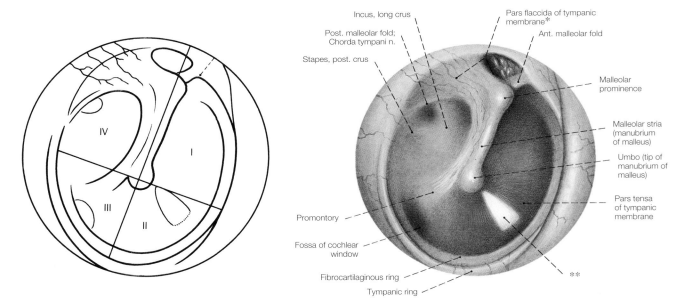

Fig. 644 The right tympanic membrane, lateral view. Diagram of the quadrants (cf. Fig. 645).

Fig. 645 The right tympanic membrane, lateral view (600%). Otoscopic image.

* Clinical: SHRAPNELL's membrane
** Typically occurring reflection of light

In order to obtain a complete overview of the cutaneous surface of the tympanic membrane with the otoscope, the external acoustic meatus must be stretched. This can be achieved by pulling the auricula posteriorly.

To facilitate orientation, the tympanic membrane is usually divided into four quadrants (I–IV).

The major axis of the tympanic membrane in an adult is 10–11 mm, the minor axis is approximately 9 mm.

The light source characteristically produces a triangular reflection of light in front of the umbo in the region of quadrant II.

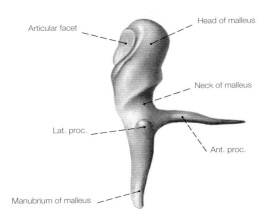

Articular facet

Head of malleus

Neck of malleus

Lat. proc.

Ant. proc.

Manubrium of malleus

Fig. 646 The right malleus,
lateral view (700%).

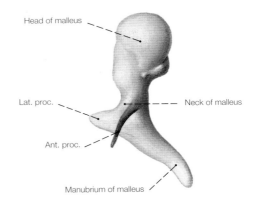

Head of malleus

Lat. proc.

Ant. proc.

Neck of malleus

Manubrium of malleus

Fig. 647 The right malleus,
anterior view (700%).

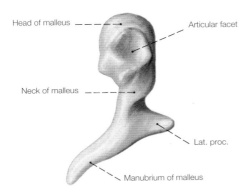

Head of malleus

Articular facet

Neck of malleus

Lat. proc.

Manubrium of malleus

Fig. 648 The right malleus,
posterior view (700%).

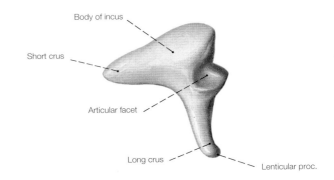

Body of incus

Short crus

Articular facet

Long crus

Lenticular proc.

Fig. 649 The right incus,
lateral view (700%).

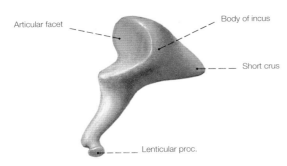

Articular facet

Body of incus

Short crus

Lenticular proc.

Fig. 650 The right incus,
medial view (700%).

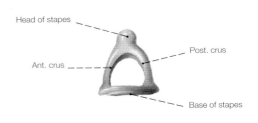

Head of stapes

Ant. crus

Post. crus

Base of stapes

Fig. 651 The right stapes,
viewed from above (700%).

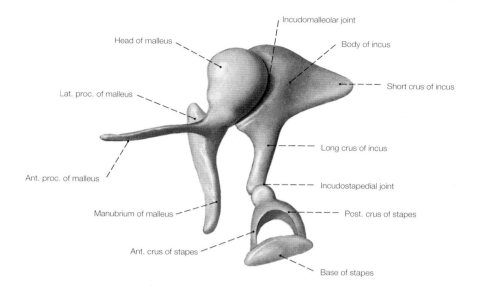

Incudomalleolar joint

Head of malleus

Body of incus

Short crus of incus

Lat. proc. of malleus

Long crus of incus

Ant. proc. of malleus

Incudostapedial joint

Manubrium of malleus

Post. crus of stapes

Ant. crus of stapes

Base of stapes

Fig. 652   The right auditory ossicles in their normal positions, viewed medially from above (700%).

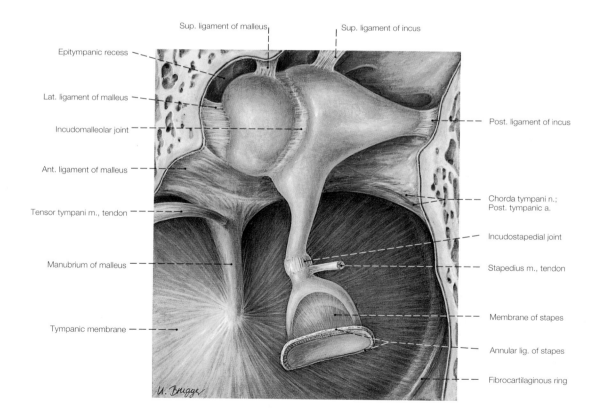

Sup. ligament of malleus

Sup. ligament of incus

Epitympanic recess

Lat. ligament of malleus

Post. ligament of incus

Incudomalleolar joint

Ant. ligament of malleus

Chorda tympani n.; Post. tympanic a.

Tensor tympani m., tendon

Incudostapedial joint

Manubrium of malleus

Stapedius m., tendon

Tympanic membrane

Membrane of stapes

Annular lig. of stapes

Fibrocartilaginous ring

U. Brügger

Fig. 653   Joints and ligaments of the right auditory ossicles, viewed medially from above. Covered by mucous membrane in situ.

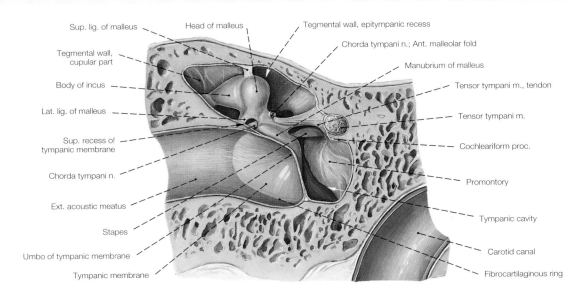

Fig. 654 The right tympanic cavity, anterior view. Frontal section.

Boundaries of the Tympanic Cavity and Their Clinical Significance

Name	Components	Adjacent Organs	Distinguishing Features	Clinical Complications
Tegmental wall (Roof)	Epitympanic recess, tegmen tympani of temporal bone, petrosquamous suture	Middle cranial fossa, meninges, temporal lobe	Vascular channels in the roof and suture: route for infections	Meningitis, abscess of temporal lobe
Jugular wall (Floor)	Styloid prominence	Jugular fossa, superior bulb of jugular vein	Variable form and size of air cells; bony lamina may be partially absent	Septic thrombosis of internal jugular vein (pyemia)
Labyrinthine wall (Medial wall)	Promontory, fenestrae cochleae and vestibuli, prominence of the facial canal	Membranous labyrinth, facial nerve (VII) [nervus intermediofacialis]		Infections of the labyrinth (deafness), facial paresis
Membranous wall (Lateral wall)	Tympanic membrane, manubrium mallei (chorda tympani)	External acoustic meatus, temporomandibular joint		Perforation of tympanic membrane (e.g., by careless cleaning)
Mastoid wall (Posterior wall)	Mastoid antrum, mastoid air cells, prominence of lat. semicircular canal, prominence of facial canal	Facial nerve (VII) [nervus intermediofacialis], sigmoid sinus, post. cranial fossa, cerebellum	Variable pneumatization of the mastoid process	Mastoiditis, sinus thrombosis, meningitis, cerebellar abscess, facial paresis
Carotid wall (Anterior wall)	Tympanic opening of auditory tube, musculotubular canal	Carotid canal, cavernous sinus, abducens nerve (VI), trigeminal ganglion	Apical pneumatization of the pyramid	Auditory tube as route for infection of apical air cells, abducens paresis, otitis of middle ear

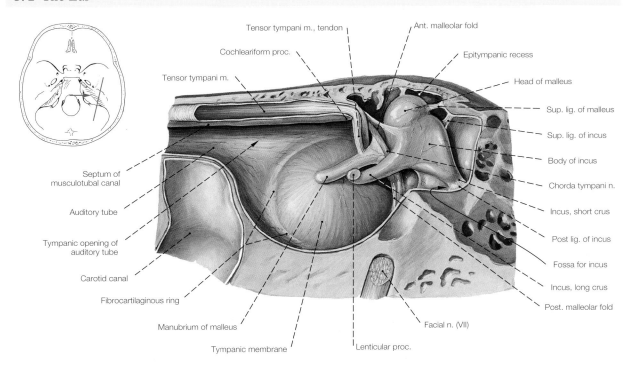

Tensor tympani m., tendon

Cochleariform proc.

Tensor tympani m.

Ant. malleolar fold

Epitympanic recess

Head of malleus

Sup. lig. of malleus

Sup. lig. of incus

Body of incus

Chorda tympani n.

Incus, short crus

Post lig. of incus

Fossa for incus

Incus, long crus

Post. malleolar fold

Septum of musculotubal canal

Auditory tube

Tympanic opening of auditory tube

Carotid canal

Fibrocartilaginous ring

Manubrium of malleus

Tympanic membrane

Lenticular proc.

Facial n. (VII)

Fig. 655 The lateral wall of the right tympanic cavity, medial view. Sagittal section after extensive removal of the auditory tube and the fascia of the tensor tympani muscle.

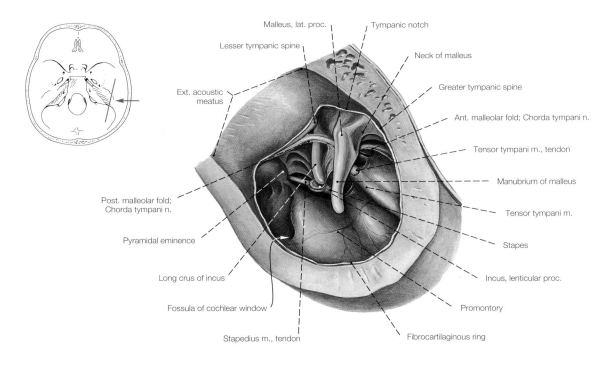

Malleus, lat. proc.

Tympanic notch

Lesser tympanic spine

Neck of malleus

Greater tympanic spine

Ext. acoustic meatus

Ant. malleolar fold; Chorda tympani n.

Tensor tympani m., tendon

Manubrium of malleus

Tensor tympani m.

Post. malleolar fold; Chorda tympani n.

Stapes

Pyramidal eminence

Incus, lenticular proc.

Long crus of incus

Promontory

Fossula of cochlear window

Fibrocartilaginous ring

Stapedius m., tendon

Fig. 656 The right tympanic cavity after removal of the tympanic membrane, lateral view.

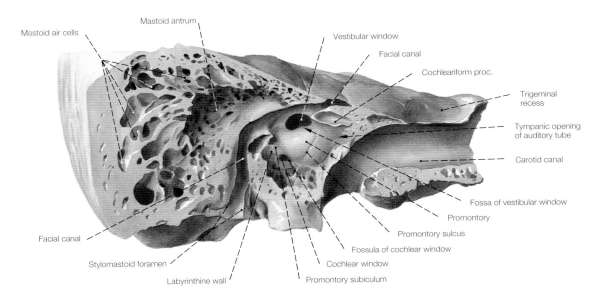

Mastoid air cells

Mastoid antrum

Vestibular window

Facial canal

Cochleariform proc.

Trigeminal recess

Tympanic opening of auditory tube

Carotid canal

Fossa of vestibular window

Promontory

Promontory sulcus

Fossula of cochlear window

Cochlear window

Promontory subiculum

Labyrinthine wall

Stylomastoid foramen

Facial canal

Fig. 657 The medial wall of the right tympanic cavity, anterolateral view (170%). The lateral wall has been removed as well as adjacent parts of the anterior and posterior walls. The facial canal and the carotid canal have been opened.

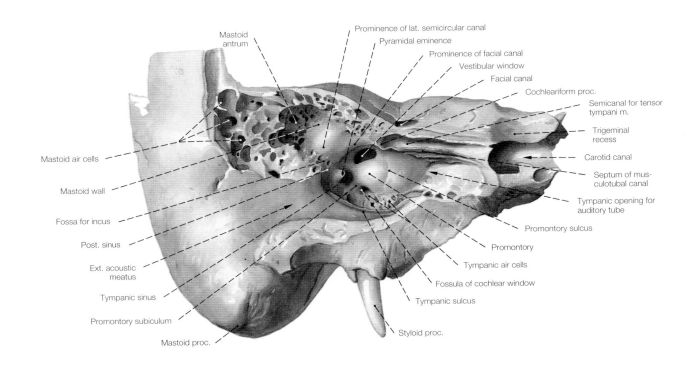

Mastoid antrum

Prominence of lat. semicircular canal

Pyramidal eminence

Prominence of facial canal

Vestibular window

Facial canal

Cochleariform proc.

Semicanal for tensor tympani m.

Trigeminal recess

Carotid canal

Septum of musculotubal canal

Tympanic opening for auditory tube

Promontory sulcus

Promontory

Tympanic air cells

Fossula of cochlear window

Tympanic sulcus

Styloid proc.

Mastoid air cells

Mastoid wall

Fossa for incus

Post. sinus

Ext. acoustic meatus

Tympanic sinus

Promontory subiculum

Mastoid proc.

Fig. 658 The medial wall of the right tympanic cavity, anterolateral view (170%). Vertical section in the long axis of the petrous part of the temporal bone.

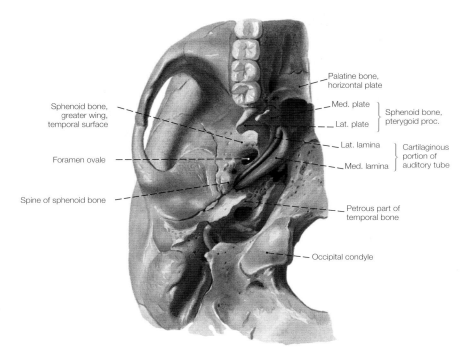

Fig. 659 Cartilage of the right auditory tube, viewed from below. Specimen shows the base of the skull.

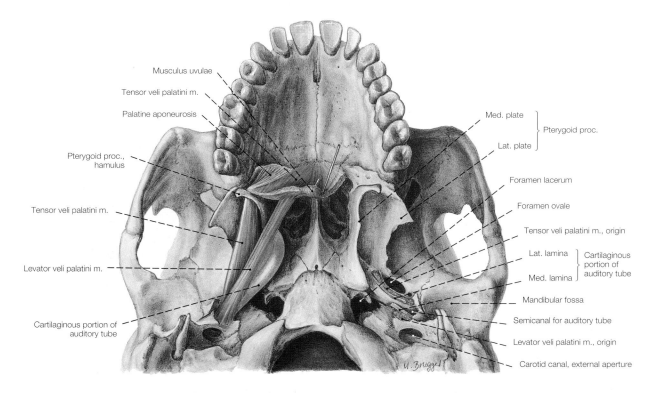

Fig. 660 The levator and tensor veli palatini muscles and the cartilage of the right auditory tube, viewed from below. Muscle origins are shown on the left side of the specimen. The soft palate has been retracted anteriorly.

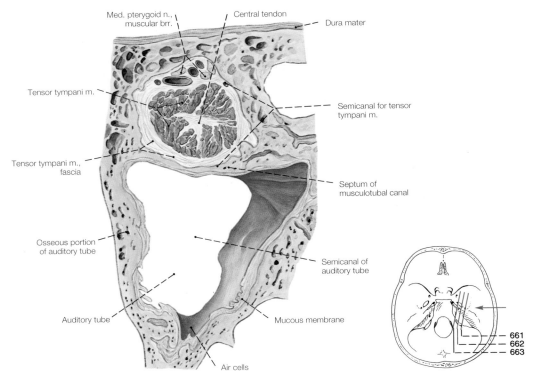

Med. pterygoid n., muscular brr.

Central tendon

Dura mater

Tensor tympani m.

Semicanal for tensor tympani m.

Tensor tympani m., fascia

Septum of musculotubal canal

Osseous portion of auditory tube

Semicanal of auditory tube

Auditory tube

Mucous membrane

Air cells

661
662
663

Fig. 661 The right auditory tube, lateral view (1500%). Cross section at the level of the osseous portion.

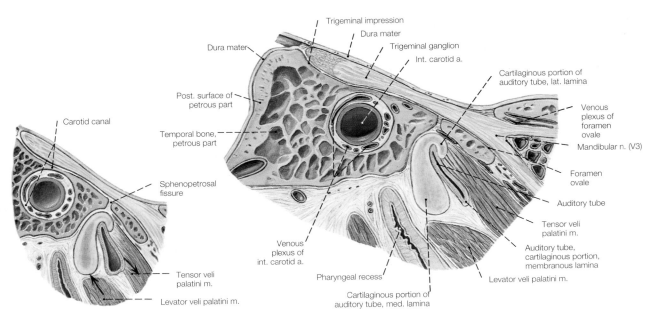

Trigeminal impression

Dura mater

Trigeminal ganglion

Int. carotid a.

Dura mater

Cartilaginous portion of auditory tube, lat. lamina

Post. surface of petrous part

Venous plexus of foramen ovale

Carotid canal

Mandibular n. (V3)

Temporal bone, petrous part

Foramen ovale

Sphenopetrosal fissure

Auditory tube

Tensor veli palatini m.

Venous plexus of int. carotid a.

Auditory tube, cartilaginous portion, membranous lamina

Tensor veli palatini m.

Pharyngeal recess

Levator veli palatini m.

Levator veli palatini m.

Cartilaginous portion of auditory tube, med. lamina

Fig. 662 The right auditory tube, lateral view (400%). Cross section at the level of the lateral part of the cartilaginous portion.

Fig. 663 The right auditory tube, lateral view (400%). Cross section at the level of the medial part of the cartilaginous portion.

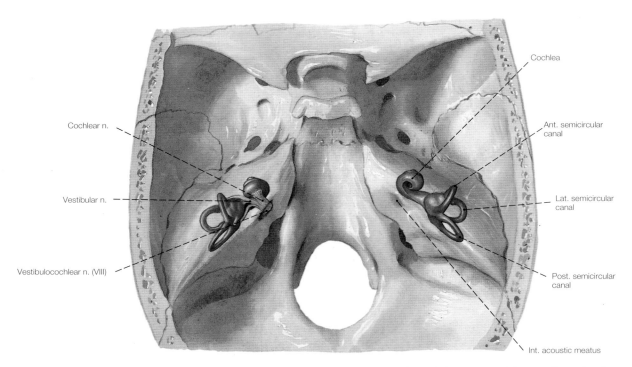

Cochlear n.

Vestibular n.

Vestibulocochlear n. (VIII)

Cochlea

Ant. semicircular canal

Lat. semicircular canal

Post. semicircular canal

Int. acoustic meatus

Fig. 664   The internal ear and the vestibulocochlear nerve (VIII), viewed from above. Casts of the osseous labyrinths in their natural position projected onto the petrous portion of the temporal bone. The axis of the cochlea is oriented from posteromedially above to anterolaterally below.

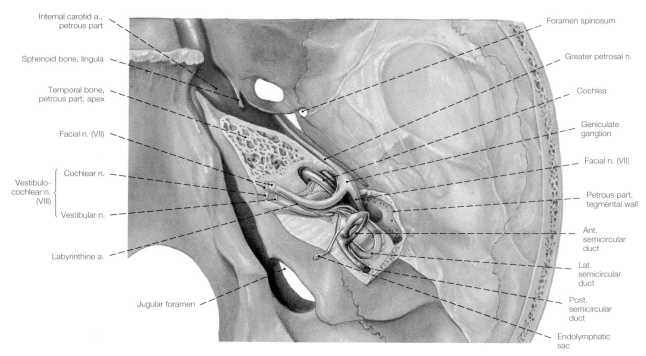

Internal carotid a., petrous part

Sphenoid bone, lingula

Temporal bone, petrous part, apex

Facial n. (VII)

Vestibulo-cochlear n. (VIII) { Cochlear n.

Vestibular n.

Labyrinthine a.

Jugular foramen

Foramen spinosum

Greater petrosal n.

Cochlea

Geniculate ganglion

Facial n. (VII)

Petrous part, tegmental wall

Ant. semicircular duct

Lat. semicircular duct

Post. semicircular duct

Endolymphatic sac

Fig. 665   The right internal ear with the facial (VII) and the vestibulocochlear (VIII) nerves, viewed from above. Parts of the petrous portion of the temporal bone have been stripped away. (See also p. 379)

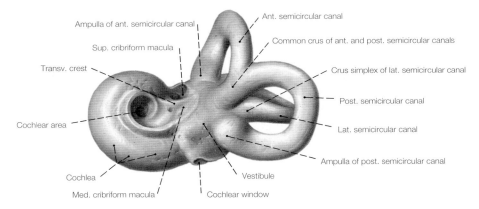

Ampulla of ant. semicircular canal

Sup. cribriform macula

Transv. crest

Cochlear area

Cochlea

Med. cribriform macula

Ant. semicircular canal

Common crus of ant. and post. semicircular canals

Crus simplex of lat. semicircular canal

Post. semicircular canal

Lat. semicircular canal

Ampulla of post. semicircular canal

Vestibule

Cochlear window

Fig. 666   The right osseous labyrinth, viewed posteriorly from above (300%). The bony covering of the membranous labyrinth has been hollowed out of the petrous part of the temporal bone.

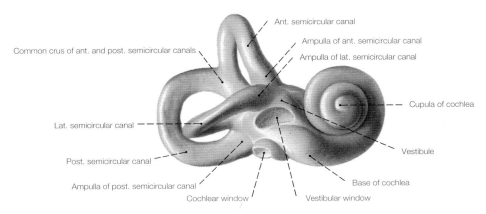

Common crus of ant. and post. semicircular canals

Ant. semicircular canal

Ampulla of ant. semicircular canal

Ampulla of lat. semicircular canal

Cupula of cochlea

Lat. semicircular canal

Post. semicircular canal

Ampulla of post. semicircular canal

Vestibule

Cochlear window

Vestibular window

Base of cochlea

Fig. 667   The right osseous labyrinth, lateral view (300%). The bony covering of the membranous labyrinth has been hollowed out of the petrous part of the temporal bone.

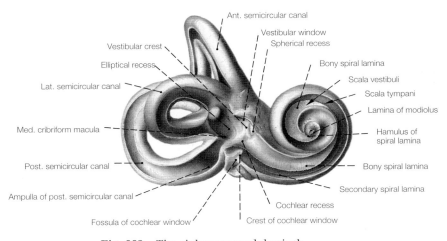

Vestibular crest

Elliptical recess

Lat. semicircular canal

Med. cribriform macula

Post. semicircular canal

Ampulla of post. semicircular canal

Fossula of cochlear window

Ant. semicircular canal

Vestibular window

Spherical recess

Bony spiral lamina

Scala vestibuli

Scala tympani

Lamina of modiolus

Hamulus of spiral lamina

Bony spiral lamina

Secondary spiral lamina

Cochlear recess

Crest of cochlear window

Fig. 668   The right osseous labyrinth, anterolateral view (300%). The semicircular canals and the cochlea have been opened.

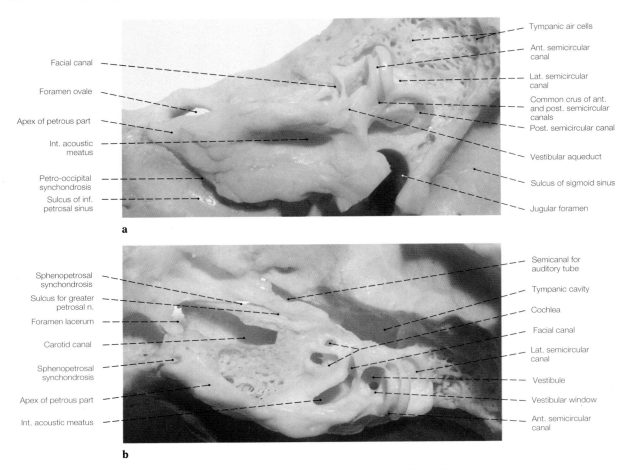

Tympanic air cells

Ant. semicircular canal

Lat. semicircular canal

Common crus of ant. and post. semicircular canals

Post. semicircular canal

Vestibular aqueduct

Sulcus of sigmoid sinus

Jugular foramen

Facial canal

Foramen ovale

Apex of petrous part

Int. acoustic meatus

Petro-occipital synchondrosis

Sulcus of inf. petrosal sinus

a

Sphenopetrosal synchondrosis

Sulcus for greater petrosal n.

Foramen lacerum

Carotid canal

Sphenopetrosal synchondrosis

Apex of petrous part

Int. acoustic meatus

Semicanal for auditory tube

Tympanic cavity

Cochlea

Facial canal

Lat. semicircular canal

Vestibule

Vestibular window

Ant. semicircular canal

b

Fig. 669 a, b The right osseous labyrinth, hollowed out of the petrous part of the temporal bone.

a viewed posteriorly from above (300%).
b viewed from above (300%).

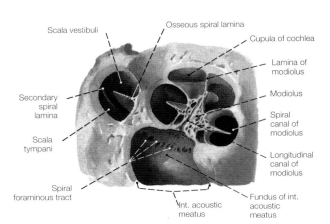

Scala vestibuli

Osseous spiral lamina

Cupula of cochlea

Lamina of modiolus

Modiolus

Spiral canal of modiolus

Longitudinal canal of modiolus

Fundus of int. acoustic meatus

Secondary spiral lamina

Scala tympani

Spiral foraminous tract

Int. acoustic meatus

Fig. 670 The left cochlear canal, viewed from above (400%). The canal has been opened in the axis of the modiolus.

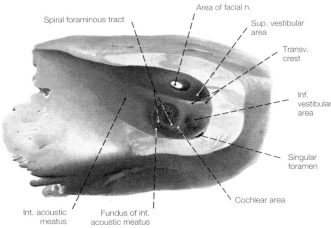

Area of facial n.

Spiral foraminous tract

Sup. vestibular area

Transv. crest

Inf. vestibular area

Singular foramen

Cochlear area

Int. acoustic meatus

Fundus of int. acoustic meatus

Fig. 671 The right internal acoustic meatus and its fundus, medial view (500%). The posterior wall has been partially removed.

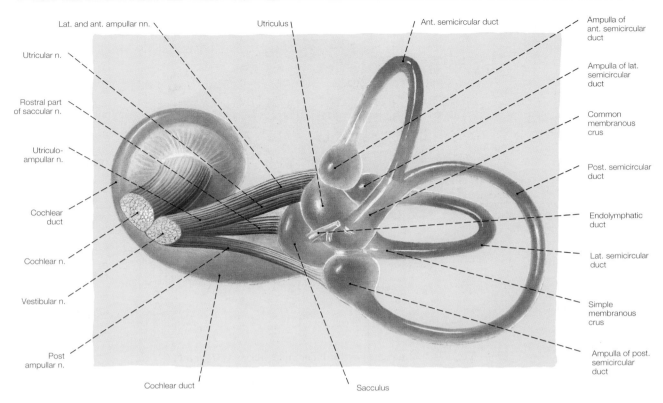

Lat. and ant. ampullar nn.

Utricular n.

Rostral part of saccular n.

Utriculo-ampullar n.

Cochlear duct

Cochlear n.

Vestibular n.

Post ampullar n.

Utriculus

Cochlear duct

Sacculus

Ant. semicircular duct

Ampulla of ant. semicircular duct

Ampulla of lat. semicircular duct

Common membranous crus

Post. semicircular duct

Endolymphatic duct

Lat. semicircular duct

Simple membranous crus

Ampulla of post. semicircular duct

Fig. 672   The right vestibulocochlear nerve (VIII) and the membranous labyrinth, posterior view (700%). Semischematic overview.

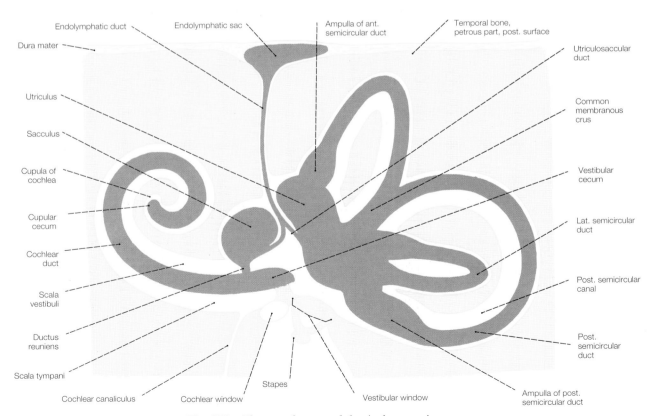

Endolymphatic duct

Dura mater

Utriculus

Sacculus

Cupula of cochlea

Cupular cecum

Cochlear duct

Scala vestibuli

Ductus reuniens

Scala tympani

Cochlear canaliculus

Endolymphatic sac

Ampulla of ant. semicircular duct

Temporal bone, petrous part, post. surface

Utriculosaccular duct

Common membranous crus

Vestibular cecum

Lat. semicircular duct

Post. semicircular canal

Post. semicircular duct

Ampulla of post. semicircular duct

Cochlear window

Stapes

Vestibular window

Fig. 673   The membranous labyrinth, overview.

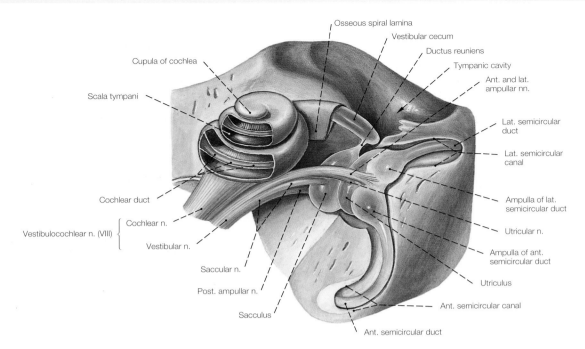

Fig. 674 The right vestibulocochlear nerve (VIII) and the membranous labyrinth, viewed from above (300%). Semischematic overview after partially stripping the outer bony shell.

Osseous spiral lamina
Vestibular cecum
Ductus reuniens
Tympanic cavity
Ant. and lat. ampullar nn.
Lat. semicircular duct
Lat. semicircular canal
Ampulla of lat. semicircular duct
Utricular n.
Ampulla of ant. semicircular duct
Utriculus
Ant. semicircular canal
Ant. semicircular duct

Cupula of cochlea
Scala tympani
Cochlear duct
Vestibulocochlear n. (VIII)
Cochlear n.
Vestibular n.
Saccular n.
Post. ampullar n.
Sacculus

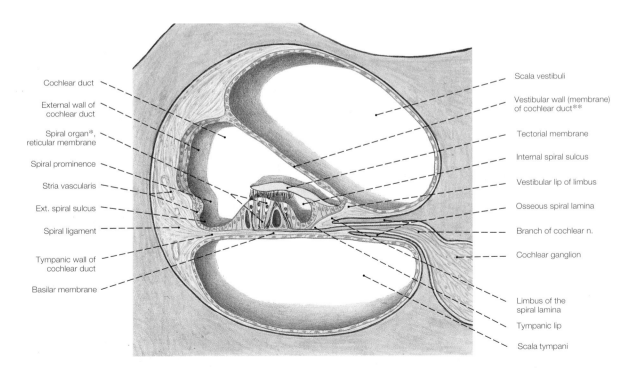

Fig. 675 The cochlea with the spiral organ. Semischematic cross section through one turn of the cochlea (2000%).

Cochlear duct
External wall of cochlear duct
Spiral organ*, reticular membrane
Spiral prominence
Stria vascularis
Ext. spiral sulcus
Spiral ligament
Tympanic wall of cochlear duct
Basilar membrane

Scala vestibuli
Vestibular wall (membrane) of cochlear duct**
Tectorial membrane
Internal spiral sulcus
Vestibular lip of limbus
Osseous spiral lamina
Branch of cochlear n.
Cochlear ganglion
Limbus of the spiral lamina
Tympanic lip
Scala tympani

* Clinical: Organ of CORTI
** Clinical: REISSNER's membrane

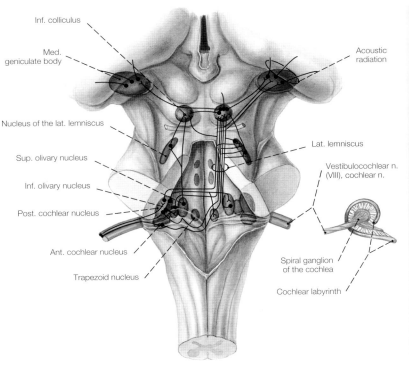

Fig. 676 The auditory pathway, overview.

Pathway for Hearing (mostly crossed)

Neuron I: Bipolar cells in the cochlear ganglion. The central processes unite to form the cochlear nerve of the vestibulocochlear nerve. Fibers from the basal cochlear parts terminate in the dorsal cochlear nucleus, those from the apical parts terminate in the ventral cochlear nucleus.

Neuron II: Multipolar ganglion cells of the cochlear nuclei. The fibers from the ventral cochlear nucleus pass mainly in the trapezoid body (relaying in part to a further neuron in the trapezoid nuclei) to the opposite side and form the lateral lemniscus, which provides a connection to the inferior colliculus. A few fibers join the lateral lemniscus of the same side. The axons of the dorsal cochlear nucleus cross superficially to the rhomboid fossa and enter the lateral lemniscus of the opposite side.

Neuron III or IV: From the inferior colliculus, connections are made with the superior colliculus, the cerebellum, and mainly with the medial geniculate body.

Neuron IV or V: The acoustic radiation connects the medial geniculate body with the transverse gyrus of HESCHL and with WERNICKE's center in the temporal lobe.

Pathway for Equilibration

Neuron I: Bipolar cells in the vestibular ganglion. The central processes form the vestibular nerve of the vestibulocochlear nerve on the floor of the internal acoustic meatus and pass to the vestibular nuclei.

Neurons II and subsequent neurons: From the lateral vestibular nucleus (DEITERS' nucleus), the fibers pass to the reticular formation, to the motor nuclei of cranial nerves III, IV and VI (via the medial longitudinal fasciculus), to the red nucleus and to the spinal cord in its anterior columns as the vestibulospinal tract.

From the medial vestibular nucleus (SCHWALB's nucleus) and from the inferior vestibular nucleus (ROLLER's nucleus), fibers contribute to the vestibulospinal tract and to connections in the reticular formation.

The superior vestibular nucleus (BECHTEREW's nucleus) sends fibers mainly to the cerebellum.

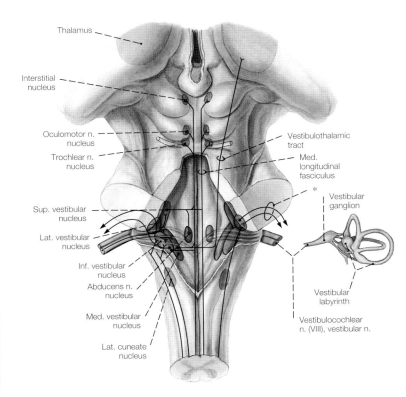

Fig. 677 The pathway for equilibration, overview.

* Connections with the cerebellum

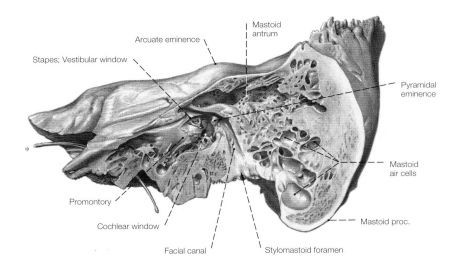

Fig. 678 Petrous portion of the left temporal
bone, anterior view. Vertical section in the
long axis.

* Probe in the carotid canal

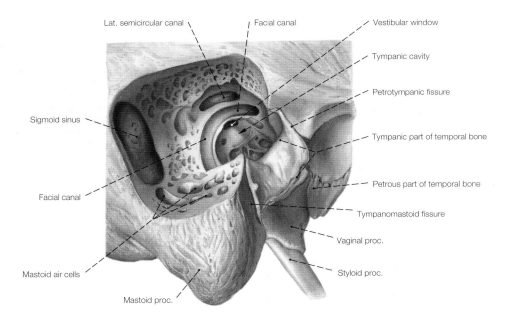

Fig. 679 The right temporal bone, lateral
view. Air cells and the sulcus of the sigmoid
sinus have been opened.

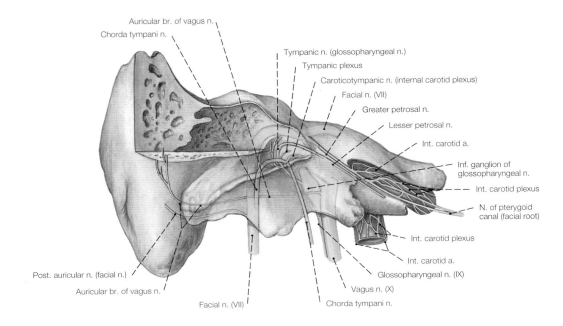

Auricular br. of vagus n.
Chorda tympani n.
Tympanic n. (glossopharyngeal n.)
Tympanic plexus
Caroticotympanic n. (internal carotid plexus)
Facial n. (VII)
Greater petrosal n.
Lesser petrosal n.
Int. carotid a.
Inf. ganglion of glossopharyngeal n.
Int. carotid plexus
N. of pterygoid canal (facial root)
Int. carotid plexus
Int. carotid a.
Glossopharyngeal n. (IX)
Vagus n. (X)
Chorda tympani n.
Facial n. (VII)
Auricular br. of vagus n.
Post. auricular n. (facial n.)

Fig. 680 The right facial (VII), glossopharyngeal (IX) and vagus (X) nerves, anterior view. The petrous portion of the temporal bone has been partially removed. The nerves are shown semitransparently.

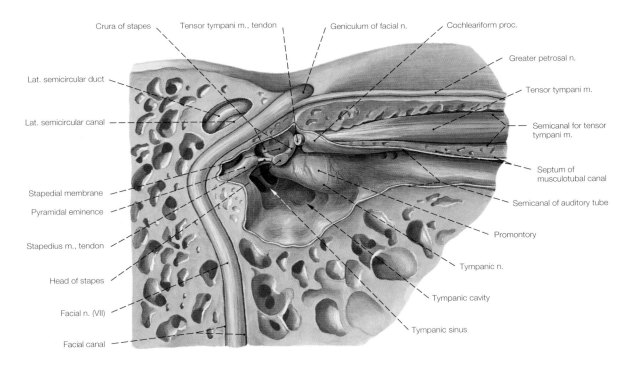

Crura of stapes
Tensor tympani m., tendon
Geniculum of facial n.
Cochleariform proc.
Greater petrosal n.
Tensor tympani m.
Lat. semicircular duct
Lat. semicircular canal
Semicanal for tensor tympani m.
Septum of musculotubal canal
Stapedial membrane
Pyramidal eminence
Semicanal of auditory tube
Promontory
Stapedius m., tendon
Tympanic n.
Head of stapes
Tympanic cavity
Facial n. (VII)
Tympanic sinus
Facial canal

Fig. 681 The left facial nerve (VII) and the tympanic cavity, anterior view. Vertical section through the long axis of the petrous portion of the temporal bone, with the facial canal opened.

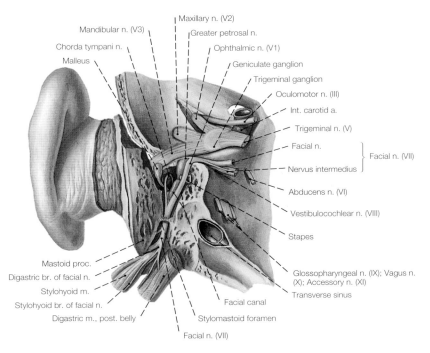

Mandibular n. (V3)
Chorda tympani n.
Malleus
Maxillary n. (V2)
Greater petrosal n.
Ophthalmic n. (V1)
Geniculate ganglion
Trigeminal ganglion
Oculomotor n. (III)
Int. carotid a.
Trigeminal n. (V)
Facial n.
Nervus intermedius
Facial n. (VII)
Abducens n. (VI)
Vestibulocochlear n. (VIII)
Stapes
Mastoid proc.
Digastric br. of facial n.
Stylohyoid m.
Stylohyoid br. of facial n.
Digastric m., post. belly
Facial n. (VII)
Facial canal
Stylomastoid foramen
Transverse sinus
Glossopharyngeal n. (IX); Vagus n. (X); Accessory n. (XI)

Fig. 682 The left facial nerve (VII) in the petrous portion of the temporal bone, posterior view. The petrous portion of the temporal bone has been partially removed and the facial canal and tympanic cavity have been opened.

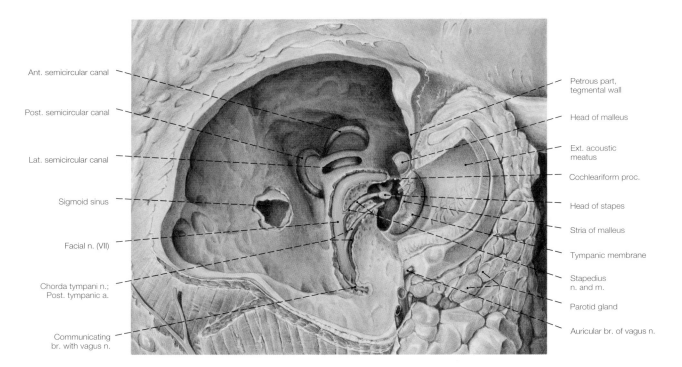

Ant. semicircular canal
Post. semicircular canal
Lat. semicircular canal
Sigmoid sinus
Facial n. (VII)
Chorda tympani n.; Post. tympanic a.
Communicating br. with vagus n.
Petrous part, tegmental wall
Head of malleus
Ext. acoustic meatus
Cochleariform proc.
Head of stapes
Stria of malleus
Tympanic membrane
Stapedius n. and m.
Parotid gland
Auricular br. of vagus n.

Fig. 683 The right tympanic cavity and the facial nerve (VII), posterolateral view. The temporal bone and external acoustic meatus have been partially removed and the facial canal has been opened.

Glossary of Anatomical Terms[a]

Abbreviations used in the Glossary:

adj.   adjective
Ar.   Arabic
dim.   diminutive
comp.   comparative
fem.   feminine
Fr.   French
fr.   from
fut.   future
G.   Greek
gen.   genitive
It.   Italian
L.   Latin
L.L.   Late Latin
masc.   masculine
Med.L.   Medieval Latin
Mod.L.   Modern Latin
myth.   mythological
ntr.   neuter
obs.   obsolete
p.   participle
pl.   plural
pp.   past participle
pr.p.   present participle
sing.   singular
superl.   superlative

Prefixes (a partial listing of frequently used general prefixes):

a-	not, without, less
ab-	from, away from, off
ad-	increase, adherence, motion toward, very
ambi-	around, on (both) sides, on all sides, both
ana-	up, toward, apart
ante-	before
anti-	against, opposing
apo-	separated from, derived from
bi-	twice, double
circum-	around
co-, col-,com-, con-	with, together, in association, very, complete
de-	away from, cessation
dia-	through, apart
di-, dif-,dir-, dis-	separation, taking apart, reversal, not, un-
e-, ex-	out of, from, away from
en-, end-,endo-	within, inner
ep-, epi-	upon, following, subsequent to
hemi-	one-half
hyper-	excessive, above normal
hypo-	beneath, diminution, deficiency, the lowest
infra-	below
in-, im-	inside
inter-	between, among
intra-, intro-	within
mes-, meso-	middle, mean, intermediacy, mesentery
meta-	after, behind, joint action, sharing
ob-, op-	against, opposite, toward
par-,para-	abnormal, involvement of two like parts
per-	through, thoroughly, intensely
peri-	around, about
post-	after, behind, posterior
prae-, pre-	anterior, before
pro-, pros-	before, forward, precursor of
quadri-	four, fourfold
re-	again, backward
retro-	backward, behind
semi-	one-half, partly
sub-	beneath, less than normal, inferior
super-, supra-	in excess, above, superior, in the upper part
sym-, syn-	together
tri-, tris-	three, three-fold

Suffixes (a partial listing of frequently used general suffixes):

-ad	toward, in the direction of, -ward
-form	in the form or shape of
-gen	producing, coming to be, precursor of
-ic	pertaining to
-ism	condition, disease, a practice, doctrine
-ite	the nature of, resembling
-logy	study of, collecting
-osis, -oses (pl.)	process, condition, state
-pod	foot, foot-shaped

abdomen (L. *abdomen,* etym. uncertain) = The part of the trunk that lies between the thorax and the pelvis; venter.

abducens (L.) = Abducting, drawing away, especially from the median plane; abducent.

abductor (L.) = A muscle that draws a part away, i.e., abducts, from the median plane.

aberrant (L. *aberrans*) = Wandering off, differing from the normal.

accessorius, -a, -um (L. fr. *ac- cedo,* pp. *-cessus,* to move toward) = Accessory; denotes certain muscles, nerves, glands, etc. that are auxiliary or supernumerary.

acetabulum, pl. **acetabula** (L., a shallow vinegar vessel or cup) = A cup-shaped depression on the external surface of the hip bone, with which the head of the femur articulates.

Achilles (G.) = Mythical Greek warrior, vulnerable only in the heel.

acoustic (G. *akoustikos,* related to hearing) = Pertaining to hearing and the perception of sound.

acromialis, -e (G.) = Acromial, relating to the acromion.

acromion (G. *acrōmion,* fr. *akron,* tip + *ōmos,* shoulder) = The lateral end of the spine of the scapula which projects as a broad flattened process overhanging the glenoid fossa.

adductor (L.) = A muscle that draws a part toward, i.e., adducts, the median plane.

adhesio, pl. **adhesiones** (L.) = Adhesion.

adipose (L.) = Fat, fatty.

aditus, pl. **aditus** (L. access, fr. *ad- eo,* pp. *-itus,* go to) = Aperture, inlet.

adminiculum, pl. **adminicula** (L. a handrest, prop, fr. *ad + manus,* hand) = That which gives support to a part.

afferens (L. fr. *af- fero,* to bring to) = Afferent, inflowing, conducting toward a center.

affixus, -a, -um (L. fr. *ad- figere*) = Fastened to.

agger, pl. **aggeres** (L. mound) = An eminence, projection, or shallow ridge.

aggregatus, -a, -um (L. *ag- grego,* pp. *-atus,* to add to, fr. *grex (greg-),* a flock) = Aggregate, to unite in a mass or cluster; the total of individual units making up a mass or cluster.

ala, gen. and pl. **alae** (L. wing) = Wing.

albicans (L.) = White.

albugineus -a, -um (L. fr. *albugo,* white spot) = A white fibrous tissue layer.

albugo, -inis (L.) = A white spot.

albus, -a, -um (L.) = White.

allantois (G. fr. *allas [allant-],* sausage + *eidos,* appearance) = A fetal membrane developing from the hindgut (or yolk sac, in humans).

alveolus, gen. and pl. **alveoli** (L. dim. of *alveus,* trough, hollow sac, cavity) = A small cell, cavity, or socket.

ambiguus, -a, -um (L. fr. *ambigo,* to wander) = Ambiguous, having more than one interpretation or direction.

amnion (G. the membrane around the fetus, fr. *amnios,* lamb) = Innermost of the extraembryonic membranes enveloping the embryo in utero and containing the amniotic fluid.

amphiarthrosis (G. *amphi-,* on both sides, about, around + *arthrōsis,* joint) = Symphysis.

amphora (L. fr. G. *amphoreus,* fr. *amphi-,* on both sides, *phoreus,* bearer) = An ancient Greek jar or vase with a large oval body, narrow, cylindrical neck, and two handles that rise almost to the level of the mouth.

ampulla, gen. and pl. **ampullae** (L. a two-handled bottle) = A saccular dilation of a canal or duct.

amygdaloideus, -a, -um (L. a tonsil, fr. G. *amygdala,* almond + G. *eidos,* appearance) = Resembling an almond or a tonsil.

[a]The terms in this glossary are taken from the 20th German edition of this atlas (*Atlas der Anatomie des Menschen/Sobotta.* Putz R. und Papst R. 20. Auflage. München: Urban & Schwarzenberg, 1993). Definitions and etymologies are based on *Stedman's Medical Dictionary* (26th edition, Williams & Wilkins, 1995). For complete definitions, the reader should refer to *Stedman's Medical Dictionary.*

analis, -e (L.) = Relating to the anus.

anastomosis, pl. **anastomoses** (G. *anastomōsis,* fr. *anastomoō,* to furnish with a mouth) = A natural communication, direct or indirect, between two blood vessels or other tubular structures.

anatomy (G. *anatomē,* dissection, fr. *ana,* apart + *tomē,* a cutting) = The morphologic structure of an organism; the science of the morphology or structure of organisms.

anconeus (G. *ankōn,* elbow) = Elbow.

angiology (G. *angeion,* a vessel or cavity of the body + *logos, treatise,* discourse) = The science concerned with the blood vessels and lymphatics in all their relations.

angulus, gen. and pl. **anguli** (L.) = Angle.

ansa, gen. and pl. **ansae** (L. loop, handle) = Any anatomical structure in the form of a loop or an arc.

ante- (L.) = Before, in front of.

antebrachium (L. *ante* + *brachium,* arm) = Forearm.

anterior (L.) = Before, ventral.

anthelix (G. *anti-* + *helix,* coil) = Antihelix.

antitragus (G. fr. *anti-,* opposite, + *tragos,* a goat, the tragus) = A projection of the cartilage of the auricle.

antrum, gen. **antri,** pl. **antra** (L. fr. G. *antron,* a cave) = Any nearly closed cavity.

anulus, pl. **anuli** (L.) = Ring.

anus, gen. **ani,** pl. **anus** (L.) = The lower opening of the digestive tract.

aorta, pl. **aortae** (Mod. L. fr. G. *aortē,* fr. *aeirō,* to lift up) = A large artery which is the main trunk of the systemic arterial system.

apertura, pl. **aperturae** (L. fr. *aperio,* pp. *apertus,* to open) = Aperture; an inlet or entrance to a cavity or channel.

apex, gen. **apicis,** pl. **apices** (L. summit or tip) = The extremity of a conical or pyramidal structure, such as the heart or the lung.

apicalis, -e (L.) = Apical.

aponeurosis, pl. **aponeuroses** (G. the end of a muscle where it becomes tendon, fr. *apo,* from, + *neuron,* sinew) = A fibrous sheet or flat, expanded tendon, giving attachment to muscular fibers and serving as the means of origin or insertion of a flat muscle.

appendix, gen. **appendicis,** pl. **appendices** (L. fr. *appendo,* to hang something on) = Appendage.

aqueductus, pl. **aqueductus** (L. fr. *aqua,* water, + *ductus,* a leading, fr. *duco,* pp. *ductus,* to lead) = Aqueduct; a conduit or canal.

arachnoidea, arachnoides (Mod. L. *arachnoideus* fr. G. *arachnē,* spider, + *eidos,* resemblance) = Arachnoid; a delicate fibrous membrane forming the middle of the three coverings of the central nervous system.

arbor, pl. **arbores** (L. tree) = In anatomy, a treelike structure with branchings.

arcuatus, -a, -um (L. bowed) = Arcuate; arcate; arciform; denoting a form that is arched or has the shape of a bow.

arcus, gen and pl. **arcus** (L. a bow) = Arch.

area, pl. **areae** (L. a courtyard) = Any circumscribed area or space; a part supplied by a given artery or nerve; a part of an organ having a special function.

areola, pl. **areolae** (L. dim. of *area*) Any small area.

arteria, gen. and pl. **arteriae** (L. fr. G. *artēria,* the windpipe, later an artery as distinct fr. a vein) = Artery.

articulatio, pl. **articulationes** (L. a forming of vines) = Joint.

arytenoideus (G. *arytainoeides,* ladleshaped, applied to cartilage of the larynx, fr. *arytaina,* a ladle, + *eidos,* resemblance) = Denoting a cartilage (arytenoid cartilage) and muscles (oblique and transverse arytenoid muscles) of the larynx.

ascendens (L.) = Ascending; going upward toward a higher position.

asper, -era, -erum (L.) = Rough, uneven.

atlas, atlantis (G. *Atlas, Atlantos,* Atlas, the mythical Titan who supported the dome of the sky on his shoulders) = First cervical vertebra (the bone that supports the head).

atrioventricular (L. fr. *atrium,* an entrance hall + *ventriculus,* dim of *venter,* belly) = Relating to both the atria and the ventricles of the heart.

atrium, pl. **atria** (L. entrance hall) = A chamber or cavity to which are connected several chambers or passageways.

auditory (L. *audio,* pp. *auditus,* to hear) = Pertaining to the sense of hearing or to the organs of hearing.

auricula, pl. **auriculae** (L. the external ear, dim. of *auris,* ear) = Auricle.

auris, pl. **aures** (L.) = Ear.

autonomicus, -a, um (L.) = Autonomic; relating to the autonomic nervous system.

avian (L. *avis,* bird) = Pertaining to birds.

axilla, gen. and pl. **axillae** (L.) = The space below the shoulder joint; armpit, axil, axillary cavity, axillary fossa, axillary space.

axis, pl. **axes** (L. axle, axis) = A straight line passing through a spherical body between its two poles, and about which the body may revolve; the second cervical vertebra.

azygos (G. *a-* priv. + *zygon,* a yoke) = An unpaired (azygous) anatomical structure.

basalis (L.) = Basal; situated nearer the base of a pyramid-shaped organ in relation to a specific reference point.

basilicus (L. fr. G. *basilikos,* royal) = Denoting a prominent or important part or structure.

basis (L. and G.) = Base.

biceps (bi- + L. *caput,* head) = A muscle with two origins or heads.

bifurcatio (bi- + L. *furca,* fork) = Bifurcation; a forking; a division into two branches.

biliferous (L. *bilis,* bile) = Rarely used term for containing or carrying bile.

bilious (L. *bilis,* bile) = Biliary.

bipartite (L.) = Consisting of two parts or divisions.

brachium (L. arm, prob. akin to G. *brachiōn*) = Arm; an anatomical structure resembling an arm.

bregma (G. the forepart of the head) = The point on the skull corresponding to the junction of the coronal and sagittal sutures.

brevis (L. short) = Brief, short.

bronchial = Relating to the bronchi.

bronchus, pl. **bronchi** (Mod. L., fr. G. *bronchos,* windpipe) = One of the two subdivisions of the trachea serving to convey air to and from the lungs.

bucca, gen. and pl. **buccae** (L.) = Cheek.

buccinator (L. *buccinare,* to blow a trumpet) = Cheek muscle, so called because employed in blowing.

buccopharyngeus, -a, -um (L.) = Buccopharyngeal; relating to both cheek or mouth and pharynx.

bulbospongiosus = Bulbocavernosus muscle.

bulbourethral (L.) = Relating to the bulbus penis and the urethra.

bulbus, gen and pl. **bulbi** (L. a plant bulb) = Bulb; any globular or fusiform structure.

bulla, gen and pl. **bullae** (L. bubble) = A bubble-like structure.

bursa, pl. **bursae** (Mediev. L., a purse) = A closed sac or envelope lined with synovial membrane and containing fluid.

calamus (L. reed, a pen) = A reed-shaped structure.

calcaneus, gen. and pl. **calcanei,** adj. **calcaneus, -a, -um** (L. *calcaneum,* the heel) = The largest of the tarsal bones; it forms the heel.

calcar (L. spur, cock's spur) = A small projection from any structure.

calix, pl. **calices** (L. fr. G. *kalyx,* the cup of a flower) = A flower-shaped or funnel-shaped structure, specifically one of the branches or recesses of the pelvis of the kidney; calyx.

calvaria, pl. **calvariae** (L. a skull) = The upper domelike portion of the skull; roof of skull; skullcap.

camera, pl. **camerae, cameras** (L. a vault) = In anatomy, any chamber or cavity, such as one of the chambers of the heart, or eye.

canaliculus, pl. **canaliculi** (L. dim. fr. *canalis,* canal) = A small canal or channel.

canalis, pl. **canales** (L.) = Canal.

canine (L. *caninus*) = Relating to a dog, i.e., canine tooth.

capitate (L. *caput,* head) = Head-shaped, having a rounded extremity.

capitulum, pl. **capitula** (L. dim. of *caput,* head) = A small head or rounded articular extremity of a bone.

capsula, gen. and pl. **capsulae** (L. dim of *capsa,* a chest or box) = An anatomical structure resembling a capsule or envelope; capsule.

caput, gen. **capitis,** pl. **capita** (L.) = The upper, anterior, or larger extremity, expanded or rounded, of any body, organ, or other anatomical structure; head.

cardia (G. *kardia,* heart) = Cardiac part of stomach.

carina, pl. **carinae** (L. the keel of a boat) = A term applied or applicable to several anatomical structures forming a projecting central ridge.

carotid (G. *karōtides,* the carotid arteries, fr. *karoō,* to put to sleep [because compression of the carotid artery results in unconsciousness]) = Pertaining to any carotid structure.

carpus, gen. and pl. **carpi** (Mod. L. fr. G. *karpos*) = Wrist.

cartilago, pl. **cartilagines** (L. gristle) = Cartilage.

caruncula, pl. **carunculae** (L. a small fleshy mass, fr. *caro,* flesh) = A small, fleshy protuberance, or any structure suggesting such a shape; caruncle.

cauda, pl. **caudae** (L. a tail) = Tail.

caudal (Mod. L. *caudalis*) = Pertaining to the tail; caudalis.

caudate = Tailed, possessing a tail.

caverna, pl. **cavernae** (L. a grotto, fr. *cavus,* hollow) = An anatomical cavity with many interconnecting chambers; cavern.

cavernosus (L.) = Relating to a cavern or a cavity; containing many cavities.

cavitas, pl. **cavitates** (Mod. L.) = Cavity.

cavum, pl. **cava** (L. ntr. of adj. *cavas*, hollow) = Cavity.

cecum, pl. **ceca** (L. ntr. of *caecus*, blind) = Blind gut, intestinum cecum, typhlon, any structure ending in a cul-de-sac.

celiac (G. *koilia*, belly) = Relating to the abdominal cavity.

centralis (L.) = Central; in the center.

cephalic (L.) = Cranial.

cerato-, **cerat**, see **kerato-, kerat-**

ceratopharyngeus = Part of middle constrictor muscle of pharynx originating from greater horn of the hyoid bone.

cerebellum, pl. **cerebella** (L. dim. of *cerebrum*, brain) = The large posterior brain mass lying dorsal to the pons and medulla and ventral to the posterior portion of the cerebrum.

cerebrum, pl. **cerebra, cerebrums** (L. brain) = The cerebral hemispheres, i.e., cerebral cortex and basal ganglia.

cerulean (L. *caeruleus*, blue, fr. *caelum*, sky) = Blue.

cervix, gen. **cervicis**, pl. **cervices** (L. neck) = Any necklike structure; collum.

chiasma, pl. **chiasmata** (G. *chiasma,* two crossing lines, fr. the letter *chi*) = A decussation or crossing.

choana, pl **choanae** (Mod. L. fr. G. *choanē*, a funnel) = The opening into the nasopharynx of the nasal cavity on either side.

choledoch (G. *cholēdochos*, containing bile, fr. *cholē*-, bile, + *dechomai*, to receive) = Common bile duct.

chondro-, chondrio- (G. *chondrion*, dim. of *chondros*, groats [coarsely ground grain], grit, gristle, cartilage) = Cartilage or cartilaginous; granular or gritty substance.

chondropharyngeus (G. chondro- + L. *pharyngeus*)= Part of the middle constrictor muscle of the pharynx originating from the lesser horn of the hyoid bone.

chorda, pl. **chordae** (L. cord) = A tendinous or a cord-like structure.

choroid (G. *choroeides*, a false reading for *chorioeides*, like a membrane) = The middle vascular tunic of the eye lying between the retina and the sclera.

chyle (G. *chylos*, juice) = A turbid white or pale yellow fluid taken up by the lacteals from the intestine during digestion and carried by the lymphatic system into the circulation.

cilium, pl. **cilia** (L. an eyelid) = Eyelash; a motile extension of a cell surface.

cinerea (L. fem of *cinereus*, ashy, fr. *cinis*, ashes) = The gray matter of the brain and other parts of the nervous system.

cingulum, gen. **cinculi**, pl. **cingula** (L. girdle, fr. *cingo*, to surround) = Girdle; a well-marked fiber bundle passing longitudinally in the white matter of the cingulate gyrus.

circle (L. *circulus*) = A ring-shaped structure or group of structures.

circumference (L. *circumferentia*, a bearing around) = The outer boundary, especially of a circular area.

circumflex (L. *circum-*, around + *flexus*, to bend) = Describing an arc of a circle or that which winds around something.

cisterna, gen. and pl. **cisternae** (L. an underground cistern for water, fr. *cista*, a box) = Any cavity or enclosed space serving as a reservoir, especially for chyle, lymph, or cerebrospinal fluid.

claustrum, pl. **claustra** (L. barrier) = A thin, vertically placed lamina of gray matter lying close to the putamen, from which it is separated by the external capsule.

clavicula, pl. **claviculae** (L. *clavicula*, a small key, fr. clavis, key) = Clavicle, collar bone.

clinoid (G. *klinē*, bed + *eidos*, resemblance) = Resembling a four-poster bed.

clitoris, pl. **clitorides** (G. *kleitoris*) = A cylindric, erectile body situated at the most anterior portion of the vulva and projecting between the laminae of the labia minora. It is the homologue of the male penis.

clivus, pl. **clivi** (L. slope) = The sloping surface from the dorsum sellae to the foramen magnum.

clunes (pl. of L. *clunis*, buttock) = Buttocks.

coccygeus (G. *kokkyx*, a cuckoo, the coccyx) = Coccygeus muscle.

cochlea, pl. **cochleae** (L. snail shell) = A cone-shaped cavity in the petrous portion of the temporal bone, forming one of the divisions of the internal ear.

cochlear = Relating to the cochlea.

colic (G. *kōlikos*, relating to the colon) = Relating to the colon; spasmodic pains in the abdomen; in young infants, paroxysms of gastrointestinal pain.

collateral = Indirect, subsidiary, or accessory to the main thing; side by side.

colliculus, pl. **colliculi** (L. mound, dim. of *collis*, hill) = A small elevation above the surrounding parts.

collis = Hill, see colliculus above.

collum, pl. **colla** (L.) = Neck; a constricted or necklike portion of any organ or anatomical structure; cervix.

colon (G. *kolon*) = The portion of the large intestine extending from the cecum to the rectum.

columna, gen. and pl. **columnae** (L.) = Column.

comitant = Concomitant.

commissura, gen. and pl. **commissurae** (L. a joining together, seam, fr. *com- mitto*, to send together, combine) = Commissure; angle or corner of the eye, lips or labia; a bundle of nerve fibers passing from one side to the other in the brain or spinal cord.

communicans, pl. **communicantes** (L. pres. p. of *communico*, pp. *-atus*, to share with someone, make common) = Communicating, connecting or joining.

communis (L.) = Denotes a structure serving several branches.

compages (L.) = A joining together or that which is joined together.

concha, pl. **conchae** (L. a shell) = A structure comparable to a shell in shape, as the pinna of the ear or the turbinate bones of the nose.

condylar (L. fr. G. *kondylos*, knuckle, the knuckle of any joint) = Relating to a condyle.

condylus (L.)= Condyle; a rounded articular surface at the extremity of a bone.

condyloid (G. *kondylōdēs*, like a knuckle, fr. *kondylos*, condyle, + *eidos*, resemblance) = Relating to or resembling a condyle.

confluence (L. *confluens*) = A flowing together; a joining of two or more streams; confluens.

conic, conical (G. fr. *kōnos,* cone) = Relating to a cone.

coniotomy = Cricothyrotomy.

conjugate (L. *con- jugo*, pp. *-jugatus*, to join together) = Conjugate; conjugate diameters of the pelvis.

conjunctiva, pl. **conjunctivae** (L. fem. of *conjunctivus*, fr. *conjungo*, pp. *-junctus*, to bind together) = The mucous membrane investing the anterior surface of the eyeball and the posterior surface of the lids.

connexus (L.) = Connection.

conoid (G. *kōnoeidēs*, cone-shaped) = A cone-shaped structure.

constrictor (L. fr. *constringo*, to draw together) = Anything that binds or squeezes a part.

conus, pl. **coni** (L. fr. G. *kōnos*, cone) = Cone.

cor, gen. **cordis** (L.) = Heart.

coracobrachialis (L.) = Relating to the coracoid process of the scapula and the arm.

coracoid (G. *korakōdēs*, like a crow's beak, fr. *korax*, raven, + *eidos*, appearance) = Shaped like a crow's beak, denoting a process of the scapula.

corium, pl. **coria** (L. skin, hide, leather) = Dermis.

cornea (L. fem. of *corneus,* horny) = The transparent tissue constituting the anterior sixth of the outer wall of the eye.

corniculate (L. *corniculatus*, horned) = Resembling a horn; having horns or horn-shaped appendages.

corona, pl. **coronae** (L. garland, crown, fr. G. *korōnē*) = Crown.

corpus, gen. **corporis**, pl. **corpora**, (L. body) = Body; any body or mass.

corrugator (L. cor- rugo [conr-], pp. -atus, to wrinkle, fr. *ruga*, a wrinkle) = A muscle that draws together the skin, causing it to wrinkle.

cortex, gen. **corticis**, pl. **cortices** (L. bark) = The outer portion of an organ.

costa, gen. and pl. **costae** (L.) = Rib.

costophrenic = Pertaining to the ribs and diaphragm.

costosternal = Pertaining to the ribs and the sternum.

coxa, gen. and pl. **coxae** (L.) = Hip bone; hip joint.

cranialis (L.) = Cranial; relating to the cranium or head.

cranium, pl. **crania** (Mediev. L. fr. G. *kranion*) = Skull.

crassus, -a, -um (L.) = Thick, dense, solid.

cremaster (G. *kremastēr*, a suspender, in pl. the muscles by which the testicles are retracted, fr. *kremannymi*, to hand) = Cremaster muscle.

crenate, crenated (L. *crena*, a notch) = Indented.

cribriform (L. *cribrum*, a sieve, + *forma*, form) = Sievelike; containing many perforations, cribrate.

cricoarytenoid (L.) = Relating to the cricoid and arytenoid cartilages.

cricoid (L. *cricoideus*, fr. G. *krikos*, a ring, *eidos*, form) = Ring-shaped; denoting the cricoid cartilage.

cricopharyngeal (L.) = Relating to the cricoid cartilage and the pharynx.

cricothyroid (L.) = Relating to the cricoid and thyroid cartilages.

cricotracheotomy (L.) = Incision of the cricoid cartilage and trachea.

crista, pl. **cristae** (L. crest) = Crest.

cruciate (L. *cruciatus*) = Shaped like, or resembling, a cross.

cruciform (L. *crux*, cross, + *forma*, form) = Shaped like a cross.

crus, gen. **cruris**, pl. **crura** (L.) = Leg; any anatomical structure resembling a leg; usually (in the plural) a pair of diverging bands or elongated masses.

cubitus, gen. and pl. **cubiti** (L. elbow) = Elbow.

cuboid, cuboidal (G. *kybos*, cube, + *eidos*, resemblance) = Resembling a cube in shape.

culmen, pl. **culmina** (L. summit) = The anterior prominent portion of the vermis of the cerebellum.

cumulus, pl. **cumuli** (L. a heap) = A collection or heap of cells.

cuneiform (L.) = Wedge-shaped.

cuneus, pl. **cunei** (L. wedge) = The region of the medial aspect of the occipital lobe of each cerebral hemisphere bounded by the parieto-occipital fissure and calcarine fissure.

cupula, pl. **cupulae** (L. dim. of *cupa*, a tub) = Cupola; a cup-shaped or domelike structure.

curvature (L. *curvatura*, fr. *curvo*, pp. *-atus*, to bend, curve) = A bending or flexure.

cuspis, pl. **cuspides** (L. a point) = Cusp.

cutaneous (L. *cutis*, skin) = Relating to the skin.

cutis (L.) = Skin.

cymba conchae (G. *kymbē*, the hollow of a vessel, a cup, bowl, a boat) = The upper, smaller part of the external ear lying above the crus helicis.

cystic (G. *kystis*, bladder) = Relating to the urinary bladder or gallbladder; relating to a cyst; containing cysts.

dartos (G. skinned or flayed, fr. *derō*, to skin) = A layer of smooth muscular tissue in the integument of the scrotum.

decidua (L. *deciduus*, falling off) = Deciduous membrane.

declive (L. *declivis*, sloping downward, fr. *clivus*, a slope) = The posterior sloping portion of the vermis of the cerebellum.

decussate (L. *decusso*, pp. *-atus*, to make in the form of an X, fr. *decussis*, a large, bronze Roman [2nd c. BC], 10-unit coin marked with an X to indicate its denomination) = To cross; crossed like the arms of an X.

decussation (L. *decussatio*) = Any crossing over or intersection of parts.

deferent (L. *deferens*, pres. p. of *defero*, to carry away) = Carrying away.

deltoid (G. *deltoeidēs*, shaped like the letter *delta*) = Resembling the Greek letter delta; triangular; deltoid muscle.

deltoideopectoralis, -e (L. fr. G.) = Pertaining to the deltoid muscle and the pectoralis muscles.

dens, pl. **dentes** (L.) = Tooth.

dental (L. *dens*, tooth) = Relating to the teeth.

dentate (L. *dentatus*, toothed) = Notched; toothed; cogged.

denticulate, denticulated (L. *denticulus*, a small tooth) = Finely dentated, notched, or serrated; having small teeth.

dentinum (L. *dens*, tooth) = Dentin.

depel (L. fr. *depellare*) = To drive away, expel.

depressor (L. *de- primo*, pp. *-pressus*, to press down) = A muscle that flattens or lowers a part.

descending (L. *de- scendo*, pp. *-scensus*, to come down, fr. *scando*, to climb) = Running downward or toward the periphery; descendens.

dexter (L. fr. *dextra*, ntr. dextrum) = Located on or relating to the right side.

diagonal (L. *diagonalis*, fr. G. *diagonios*, fr. angle to angle) = A line passing obliquely from the vertical.

diameter (G. *diametros*, fr. *dia*, through, + *metron*, measure) = A straight line connecting two opposite points on the surface of a more or less spherical or cylindrical body.

diaphragm (G. *diaphragma*) = The musculomembranous partition between the abdominal and thoracic cavities.

diaphysis, pl. **diaphyses** (G. a growing between) = Shaft.

diarthrosis, pl. **diarthroses** (G. articulation) = Synovial joint.

diencephalon, pl. **diencephala** (G. *dia*, through, + *enkephalos*, brain) = That part of the prosencephalon composed of the epithalamus, dorsal thalamus, subthalamus, and hypothalamus.

digastric (G. *di-*, two, + *gastēr*, belly) = Having two bellies; denoting especially a muscle with two fleshy parts separated by an intervening tendinous part.

digital (L. *digitus*) = Relating to or resembling a digit or digits, i.e., finger(s) or toe(s), or an impression made by them.

digitate (L. *digitatus*, having fingers, fr. *digitus*, finger) = Marked by a number of finger-like processes or impressions.

digitation (Mod. L. *digitatio*) = A process resembling a finger.

dilator (L. *dilato*, to spread out, dilate) = Dilatator; an instrument, muscle or substance that enlarges an orifice.

diploë (G. *diploë*, fem. of *diplous*, double) = The central layer of spongy bone between the two layers of compact bone of the flat cranial bone.

diploic = Relating to the diploë.

discus, pl. **disci** (L. fr. G. *diskos*, a quoit, disk) = Lamella; disc.

distal (L. *distalis*) = Situated away from the center of the body, or from the point of origin.

diverticulum, pl. **diverticula** (L. *deverticulum* (or *di-*), a by-road, fr. *de-verto*, to turn aside) = A pouch or sac opening from a tubular or saccular organ.

dorsal (Mediev. L. *dorsalis*, fr. dorsum, back) = Pertaining to the back or any dorsum; posterior.

dorsum, gen. **dorsi**, pl. **dorsa** (L. back) = The upper or posterior surface, or the back, of any part.

ductus, gen. and pl. **ductus** (L. a leading, fr. *duco*, pp. *ductus*, to lead) = Duct.

duodenum, gen. **duodeni**, pl. **duodena** (Mediev. L. fr. L. *duodeni*, twelve) = The first division of the small intestine, about 12 fingerbreadths in length.

dura (L. fem. of *durus*, hard) = Hard; syn. dura mater, a tough fibrous membrane forming the outer covering of the central nervous system.

efferent (L. *efferens*, fr. *effero*, to bring out) = Conducting outward from a given organ or part thereof.

ejaculation (L. *e-iaculo*, pp. *-atus*, to shoot out) = Emission of seminal fluid.

elastic (G. *elastreō*, epic form of *elaunō*, drive, push) = Having the property of returning to the original shape after being compressed, bent, or otherwise distorted.

emboliform (G. *embolos*, plug [embolus] + L. *forma*, form) = Shaped like an embolus.

eminentia, pl. **eminentiae** (L. prominence, fr. *e- mineo*, to stand out, project) = Eminence; a circumscribed area raised above the general level of the surrounding surface.

emissarium (L. an outlet, fr. *e- mitto*, pp. *-missus*, to send out) = An outlet or drain; vena emissaria.

enamelum (L.) = Enamel; the hard glistening substance covering the exposed portion of a tooth.

encephalic (G.) = Relating to the brain, or to the structures within the cranium.

encephalon, pl. **encephala** (G. *enkephalos*, brain, fr. *en*, in, + *kephalē*, head) = Brain; that portion of the central nervous system contained within the cranium.

endocardium, pl. **endocardia** (G. *endon*, within, + *kardia*, heart) = The innermost tunic of the heart.

endolympha (G. *endon*, within, + L. *lympha*, a clear fluid) = Endolymph; the fluid contained within the membranous labyrinth of the inner ear.

endometrium, pl. **endometria** (G. *endon*, within, + *metra*, uterus) = The mucous membrane comprising the inner layer of the uterine wall.

enteric (G. *enterikos*, fr. *entera*, bowels) = Relating to the intestine.

ependyma (G. *ependyma*, an upper garment) = The cellular membrane lining the central canal of the spinal cord and the ventricles.

epicardium (G. *epi*, upon, + *kardia*, heart) = The layer of pericardium on the surface of the heart; visceral layer.

epicondylus, pl. **epicondyli** (L.) = Epicondyle; a projection from a long bone near the articular extremity above or upon the condyle.

epicranium (G. *epi*, upon, + *kranion*, skull) = The muscle, aponeurosis, and skin covering the cranium.

epidermis, pl. **epidermides** (G. *epidermis*, the outer skin, fr. *epi*, upon, + *derma*, skin) = Cuticle; the outer epithelial portion of the skin.

epididymis, gen. **epididymidis**, pl. **epididymides** (Mod. L. fr. G. *epididymis*, fr. *epi*, upon, + *didymos*, twin, in pl. testes) = An elongated structure connected to the posterior surface of the testis.

epidural (G.) = Peridural; upon or outside the dura mater.

epigastric (G.) = Relating to the epigastrium.

epigastrium (G. *epigastrion*) = Epigastric region.

epiglottic, epiglottidean (G.) = Relating to the epiglottis.

epiglottis (G. *epiglōttis*, fr. *epi*, upon + *glōttis*, the mouth of the windpipe) = A leaf-shaped plate of elastic cartilage covered with mucous membrane at the root of the tongue.

epipharynx (G. *epi*, upon, over + pharynx) = The nasopharynx.

epiphysis, pl. **epiphyses** (G. an excrescence, fr. *epi*, upon + *physis*, growth) = A part of a long bone developed from a center of ossification distinct from that of the shaft and separated at first from the latter by a layer of cartilage.

epiploic (G. *epiploon*, omentum) = Omental.

episcleral (G. *epi*, upon, + *skleros*, hard) = Upon the sclera; relating to the episclera (the connective tissue between the sclera and the conjunctiva).

epistropheus (G. the pivot) = Axis.

epithalamus (G. *epi*, upon, + *thalamos*, a bed, bedroom) = A small dorsomedial area of the thalamus corresponding to the habenula, the stria medullaris and the pineal gland.

epitympanic (G.) = Above, or in the upper part of the tympanic cavity or membrane.

eponychium (G. *epi*, upon, + *onyx* [*onych*-], nail) = Epionychium; perionychium; nail skin, the epidermis forming the ungual wall behind and at the sides of the nail.

epoöphoron (G. *epi*, upon, + *oophoros*, egg-bearing) = A collection of rudimentary tubules in the mesosalpinx between the ovary and the uterine tube.

equator (Mediev. L. *aequator,* fr. L. *aequo*, to make equal) = The periphery of a plane cutting a sphere at the midpoint of, and at right angles to, its axis.

equine (L. *equinus*, fr. *equus*, horse) = Relating to, derived from, or resembling the horse, mule, ass.

erector (Mod. L.) = One who or that which raises or makes erect.

esophagus, pl. **esophagi** (G. *oisophagos*, gullet) = The portion of the digestive canal between the pharynx and stomach.

ethmoidal (G. *ēthmos*, sieve, + *eidos*, resemblance) = Resembling a sieve; ethmoid.

excavation (L. fr. *ex- cavo*, pp. *-cavatus*, to hollow out, fr. *ex*, out, + *cavus*, hollow) = Excavatio; a cavity, pouch, or recess.

excretorius, -a, -um (L. *ex- cerno*, pp. *-cretus*, to separate) = Relating to excretion (the process whereby a material product of a tissue or organ is passed out of the body).

extensor (L. one who stretches, fr. *extendo*, to stretch out) = A muscle the contraction of which tends to straighten a limb.

external (L. *externus*) = Exterior; on the outside or further from the center.

extremitas (L. fr. *extremus*, last, outermost) = Extremity; one of the ends of an elongated or pointed structure.

facialis (L.) = Facial; relating to the face.

facies, pl. **facies** (L.) = Face; surface; expression.

falciform (L. *falx*, sickle, + *forma*, form) = Falcate; having a crescentic or sickle shape.

falx, pl. **falces** (L. sickle) = A sickle-shaped structure.

fascia, pl. **fasciae** (L. a band or fillet) = A sheet of fibrous tissue that envelops the body beneath the skin and encloses muscles.

fasciculus, gen. and pl. **fasciculi** (L. dim. of *fascis*, bundle) = Fascicle; a band or bundle of fibers.

fasciola, pl. **fasciolae** (L. dim. of *fascia*, band, fillet) = A small band or group of fibers.

fastigium (L. top, as of a gable; a pointed extremity) = Apex of the roof of the fourth ventricle of the brain.

fauces, gen. **faucium** (L. the throat) = The space between the cavity of the mouth and the pharynx.

fel, gen. **fellis** (L.) = The bile.

femoral (L.) = Relating to the femur or thigh.

femur, gen. **femoris**, pl. **femora** (L. thigh) = The thigh.

fenestra, pl. **fenestrae** (L. window) = An anatomical aperture.

ferruginous (L. *ferrugineus*, iron rust, rust-colored) = Iron-bearing; associated with or containing iron; of the color of iron rust.

fetus, pl. **fetuses** (L. offspring) = In man, the product of conception from the end of the eighth week to the moment of birth.

fiber (L. *fibra*, a slender thread or filament) = Extracellular filamentous structures; the nerve cell axon; elongated threadlike cells.

fibrinoid (L. *fibra*, fiber + G. *eidos*, resemblance) = Resembling fibrin; an homogenous, refractile, proteinaceous material formed in the walls of blood vessels and in connective tissue under certain conditions.

fibrocartilage (L.) = Fibrocartilago; appears as a transition between tendons or ligaments or bones.

fibrous (L.) = Composed of or containing fibroblasts, and the fibrils and fibers formed by such cells.

fibula (L. *fibula*, [contr. fr. *figibula*,] that which fastens, a clasp, buckle, fr. *figo*, to fix, fasten) = The lateral and smaller of the two bones of the leg; calf bone.

filiform (L. *filum*, thread) = Filamentous.

filum, pl. **fila** (L. thread) = A structure of filamentous or threadlike appearance.

fimbria, pl. **fimbriae** (L. fringe) = Any fringe-like structure.

fimbriate, fimbriated (L.) = Having fimbriae or fringes.

fissura, pl. **fissurae** (L. fr. *findo*, to cleave) = Fissure; a deep furrow, cleft, or slit.

flaccid (L. *flaccidus*) = Relaxed, flabby, or without tone.

flexor (L. *flecto*, pp. *flexus*, to bend) = A muscle the action of which is to flex a joint.

flexure (L. *flexura*) A bend, as in an organ or structure.

flocculus, pl. **flocculi** (Mod. L. dim. of *floccus*, a tuft of wool) = A tuft or shred of cotton or wool or anything resembling it; a small lobe of the cerebellum; floccule.

flumen, pl. **flumina** (L.) A flowing, or stream; sym. stream.

foliate (L. *folium*, a leaf) = Pertaining to or resembling a leaf or leaflet; foliaceous, foliar, foliose.

folliculus, pl. **folliculi** (L. a small sac, dim. of *follis*, bellows) = Follicle.

fonticulus, pl. **fonticuli** (L. dim of *fons* (*font*-), fountain, spring) = Fontanel.

foramen, pl. **foramina** (L. an aperture, fr. *foro*, to pierce) = An aperture or perforation through a bone or a membranous structure.

forceps (L. a pair of tongs) = An instrument for seizing a structure; in anatomy, bands of white fibers in the brain.

formatio, pl. **formationes** (L. fr. *formo*, pp. *-atus*, to form) = Formation; a structure of definite shape or cellular arrangement.

fornix, gen. **fornices**, pl. **fornices** (arch, vault) = An arch shaped structure; often the arch-shaped roof (or roof portion) of an anatomical space.

fossa, gen. and pl. **fossae** (L. a trench or ditch) = A depression usually more or less longitudinal in shape below the level of the surface of a part.

fossula, pl. **fossulae** (L. dim of *fossa*, ditch) = A small fossa; a minor fissure or slight depression on the surface of the cerebrum.

fovea, pl. **foveae** (L. a pit) = A relatively small cup-shaped depression or pit.

frenulum, pl. **frenula** (Mod. L. dim. of L. *frenum*, bridle) = A small frenum or bridle; habenula.

frons, gen. **frontis** (L.) = Forehead.

frontalis (L.) = Frontal; in front; relating to the anterior part of a body.

fundiform (L. *funda*, a sling, + *forma*, shape) = Looped; sling-shaped.

fundus, pl. **fundi** (L. bottom) = The bottom or lowest part of a sac or hollow organ.

fungiform (L. *fungus*, a mushroom) = Shaped like a fungus or mushroom; fungilliform.

funiculus, pl. **funiculi** (L. dim. of *funis*, a cord) = Cord.

galea (L. a helmet) = A structure shaped like a helmet; epicranial aponeurosis.

Gallus (L. a cock) = A genus of gallinaceous birds, including the domestic chicken.

ganglion, pl. **ganglia, ganglions** (G. a swelling or knot) = An aggregation of nerve cell bodies located in the peripheral nervous system; a cyst.

gaster (G. *gastē*, belly) = Stomach.

gastricus (L.) = Relating to the stomach; gastric.

gastrocnemius (G. *gastroknēmia*, calf of the leg, fr. *gaster* (*gastr*-), belly, + *knēmē*, leg) = Calf of the leg; gastrocnemius muscle.

gelatinous (L. *gelo*, pp. *gelatus*, to freeze, congeal) = Jelly-like or resembling gelatin.

gemellus (L. dim. of *geminus*, twin) = Inferior or superior gemellus muscle.

geniculum, pl. **genicula** (L. dim of *genu*, knee) = A small genu or angular kneelike structure; a knotlike structure.

genioglossus (G. *geneion*, chin, + *glōssa*, tongue) = Genioglossus muscle.

geniohyoideus (G. *geneion*, chin, + *hyoeidēs*, shaped like the letter upsilon) = Geniohyoid muscle.

genital (L. *genitalis*, pertaining to reproduction, fr. *gigno*, to bring forth) = Relating to reproduction or generation; relating to the primary female or male sex organs or genitals.

genitofemoral (L.) = Relating to the genitalia and the thigh; the genitofemoral nerve.

genu, gen. **genus**, pl. **genua** (L.) = Knee; any structure of angular shape resembling a flexed knee.

gingiva, gen. and pl. **gingivae** (L.) = Gum.

glabella (L. *glabellus*, hairless, smooth, dim. of *glaber*) = A smooth prominence on the frontal bone above the root of the nose.

glandula, pl. **glandulae** (L. gland, dim of *glans*, acorn) = Gland.

glia (G. glue) = Neuroglia.

globus, pl. **globi** (L.) = A round body; ball; globe.

glomus, pl. **glomera** (L. *glomus*, a ball) = A small globular body; a highly organized arteriolovenular anastomosis forming a tiny nodular focus in many organs of the body.

glomerulus, pl. **glomeruli** (Mod. L. dim. of L. *glomus*, a ball of yarn) = A plexus of capillaries; the twisted secretory portion of a sweat gland; a cluster of dendritic ramifications and axon terminals.

glossoepiglottic, glossoepiglottidean (G. *glōssa*, tongue + Mod L. (Fr. G.) *pharyngeus*, pharynx) = Relating to the tongue and the epiglottis.

glossopharyngeal (G. *glossa*, tongue) = Relating to the tongue and the pharynx.

glossal (G.) = Lingual; relating to the tongue.

gluteal (G. *gloutos*, buttock) = Relating to the buttocks.

gracilis (L.) = Slender; denoting a thin or slender structure.

granulatio, pl. **granulationes** (L.) = Granulation; formation into grains or granules; the state of being granular.

granule (L. *granulum*, dim. of *granum*, grain) = A grain-like particle; a granulation.

griseus (L.) = Gray.

gubernaculum (L. a helm) = A fibrous cord connecting two structures; gubernaculum testis.

gustatory (L. *gustatio*, fr. *gusto*, pp. *-atus*, to taste) = Relating to gustation, or taste.

gyrus, gen. and pl. **gyri** (L. fr. G. *gyros*, circle) = One of the prominent rounded elevations that form the cerebral hemispheres.

habenula, pl. **habenulae** (L.) = Frenulum; the circumscript cell mass in the dorsomedial thalamus below the pineal gland.

hallux, pl. **halluces** (a Mod. L. form for L. *hallex* [*hallic*-], great toe) = The great toe.

hamatum (L. ntr. of *hamatus*, hooked, fr. *hamus*, a hook) = Hamate bone.

hamulus, gen. and pl. **hamuli** (L. dim. of *hamus*, hook) = Any hooklike structure.

haustrum, pl. **haustra** (L. a machine for drawing water, fr. *haurio*, pp. *haustus*, to draw up, drink up) = One of a series of saccules or pouches, so called because of a fancied resemblance to the buckets on a water wheel.

helicine (G. *helix*, a coil) = Coiled; helical.

helicotrema (G. *helix*, a spiral, + *trēma*, a hole) = A semilunar opening at the apex of the cochlea.

hemiazygos (G. *hemi*, half + *a-*, priv. + *zygon*, a yoke) = Hemiazygos vein. An unpaired anatomical structure.

hemisphere (hemi + G. *sphaira*, ball, globe) = Half of a spherical structure; hemispherium.

hemorrhoidal (G. fr. *haima*, blood + *rhoia*, a flow) = Relating to hemorrhoids.

hepar, gen. **hepatis** (L. borrowed fr. G. *hēpar*, the liver) = Liver.

hepatic (G. *hēpatikos*) = Relating to the liver.

hernia (L. rupture) = Protrusion of a part or structure through the tissues normally containing it.

hiatus, pl. **hiatus** (L. an aperture, fr. *hio*, pp. *hiatus*, to yawn) = An aperture, opening, or foramen.

hilum, pl. **hila** (L. a small bit or trifle) = The part of an organ where the nerves and vessels enter and leave; porta.

hippocampus (G. *hippocampos*, seahorse) = The complex, internally convoluted structure that forms the medial of the cortical mantle of the cerebral hemisphere.

hircus, gen. and pl. **hirci** (L. he-goat) = The odor of the axillae; one of the hairs growing in the axillae.

horizontalis (L.) = Horizontal, referring to the plane of the body, perpendicular to the vertical plane.

humerus, gen. and pl. **humeri** (L. shoulder) = The bone of the arm.

hyaloid (G. *hyalos*, glass, + *eidos*, resemblance) = Hyaline; of a glassy, homogeneous, translucent appearance.

hymen (G. *hymēn*, membrane) = Virginal membrane.

hyo (G. *hyoeides*, shaped like the letter upsilon) = Combining form meaning U-shaped, or hyoid.

hyoepiglottic (G.) = Hyoepiglottidean; relating to the hyoid bone and the epiglottis.

hyoid (G. *hyoeidēs*, shaped like the letter upsilon) = U-shaped or V-shaped; denoting the hyoid bone.

hyothyroid (G.) = Relating to the hyoid bone and the thyroid; thyrohyoid membrane.

hypochondrium, pl. **hypochondria** (L. fr. G. *hypochondrion*, abdomen, belly, fr. *hypo*, under, + *chondros*, cartilage [of ribs]) = Hypochondriac region.

hypochondriac (L. fr. G.) = Hypochondriacal; beneath the ribs; relating to the hypochondrium.

hypogastric (G. *hypogastrion*, lower belly, fr. *hypo*, under, + *gaster*, belly) = Relating to the hypogastrium.

hypogastrium (G. *hypogastrion*, lower belly, fr. *hypo*, under, + *gaster*, belly) = Pubic region.

hypoglossal (L. *hypoglossus*, fr. *hypo*, under, + *glossus*, tongue) = Subglossal; below the tongue.

hyponychium (hypo- + G. *onyx*, nail) = The epithelium of the nail bed.

hypopharynx (G.) = Laryngeal part of pharynx.

hypophysis (G. an undergrowth) = Pituitary gland.

hypothalamus (L. hypo- + thalamus) The ventral and medial region of the diencephalon forming the walls of the ventral half of the third ventricle.

hypothenar (hypo- + G. *thenar*, the palm) = The fleshy mass at the medial side of the palm; denoting any structure in relation with this part.

ileocecal (L. fr. G.) = Relating to both ileum and cecum.

ileum (L. fr. G. eileō, to roll up, twist) = The third portion of the small intestine.

iliac (L.) = Relating to the ilium.

ilium, pl. **ilia** (L. groin, flank) = Ilium (a bone).

impression (L. *impressio*, fr. *im- primo*, pp. *-pressus*, to press upon) = Impressio; an imprint or negative likeness.

imus (L.) = Lowest; the most inferior or caudal of several similar structures.

incisive (L. fr. *incido*, to cut into) = Cutting; relating to the incisor teeth.

incisura, pl. **incisurae** (L. a cutting into) = Incisure; notch.

inclination (L. *inclinatio*, a leaning) = A leaning or sloping.

incus, gen. **incudis**, pl. **incudes** (L. anvil) = Anvil; ambos; the middle of the three ossicles in the middle ear.

index, gen. **indicis**, pl. **indices** or **indexes**

(L. one that points out, an informer, the forefinger, an index, fr. *in- dico*, pp. *-atus*, to declare) = Forefinger; index finger; a guide, standard, indicator, symbol, or number denoting the relation in respect to size, capacity, or function, of one part or thing to another.

indusium, pl. **indusia** (L. a woman's undergarment, fr. *induo*, to put on) = A membranous layer or covering; the amnion.

inferior (L. lower) = Situated below or directed downward.

infundibulum, pl. **infundibula** (L. a funnel) = A funnel or funnel-shaped structure or passage.

inguen (L.) = The inguinal region.

inguinal (L. *inguen* (*inguin*-), groin) = Relating to the groin.

inscription (L. *inscriptio*) = Inscriptio; a mark, band or line.

insertion (L. *insertio*, a planting in, fr. *inserto*, *-sertus*, to plant in) = A putting in; the attachment of a muscle to the more movable part of the skeleton, as distinguished from origin.

insula, gen. and pl. **insulae** (L. island) = Island; any circumscribed body or patch on the skin; Insular cortex.

integument (L. *integumentum*, a covering, fr. *in- tego*, to cover) = The rind, capsule or covering of any body, or part.

internus, -a, -um (L.) = Internal.

intersection (L. *intersectio*) = The site of crossing of two structures.

intestinum, pl. **intestina** (L. *intestinus*, internal, ntr. as noun, the entrails, fr. *intus*, within) = Intestine, gut, bowel.

intima (L. fem. of *intimus*, inmost) = Innermost; inner coat of a vessel.

intumescence (L. *in-tumesco*, to swell up, fr. *tumeo*, to swell) = Intumescentia; the process of enlarging or swelling.

iridial, iridian, iridic (G. *iris* [*irid*-], rainbow) = Iridal; relating to the iris.

iris, pl. **irides** (G. rainbow) = The iris of the eye.

ischiadic (L.) = Ischial or sciatic.

ischioanal (G. *ischion*, hip-joint, haunch [*ischium*]) = Relating to the ischium and the anus.

ischiocavernous (G.) = Relating to the ischium and the corpus cavernosum.

ischium, gen. **ischii**, pl. **ischia** (Mod. L. fr. G. *ischion*, hip) = Hip bone.

isthmus, pl. **isthmi, isthmuses** (G. *isthmos*) = A constriction connecting two larger parts of an organ or other anatomical structure.

jejunal (L.) = Relating to the jejunum.

jejunum (L. *jejunus*, empty) = The portion of small intestine between the duodenum and the ileum.

jugular (L. *jugulum*, throat) = Relating to the throat or neck; relating to the jugular veins.

jugulum (L.) = Throat.

junctura, pl. **juncturae** (L. a joining) = Junction, juncture, joint; the point, line, or surface of union of two parts.

kerato-, kerat- (G. *keras*, horn) = Horny tissue or cells; the cornea.

labium, gen. **labii**, pl. **labia** (L.) = Lip; any lip-shaped structure.

labyrinthus (L. fr. G. *labyrinthos*, labyrinth) = Any of several anatomical structures with numerous intercommunicating cells or canals.

lacerated (L. *lacero*, to tear to pieces, fr.

lacer, mangled) = Torn; rent; having a ragged edge.

lacinia (L. fringe) = Fimbria.

lacrimal (L. *lacrima,* a tear) = Relating to the tears, their secretion, the secretory glands, and the drainage apparatus.

lactiferous (L. *lacti* fr. *lac, lactis,* milk + *fero,* to bear) = Yielding milk.

lacuna, pl. **lacunae** (L. a pit, dim. of *lacus,* a hollow, a lake) = A small space, cavity or depression; a gap or defect.

lacus, pl. **lacus** (L. lake) = A small collection of fluid.

lambdoid (G. *lambda + eidos,* resemblance) = Resembling the Greek letter *lambda,* as does the lambdoid suture.

lamella, pl. **lamellae** (L. dim. of *lamina,* plate, leaf) = A thin sheet or layer.

lamina, pl. **laminae** (L.) = Thin plate or flat layer.

lanugo (L. down, wooliness, fr. *lana,* wool) = Fine, soft, lightly pigmented fetal hair.

laryngotomy (G. *larynx + tomē,* incision) = A surgical incision of the larynx.

larynx, pl. **larynges** (Mod. L. fr. G.) = The organ of voice production; the portion of the respiratory tract between the pharynx and the trachea.

lateral (L. *lateralis,* lateral, fr. *latus,* side) = On the side.

latissimus (L. broad) = The broadest.

latus, -a, -um (L. broad) = Broad.

latus, gen. **lateris,** pl. **latera** (L. broad) = Flank; the side of the body between the pelvis and the ribs.

lemniscus, pl. **lemnisci** (L. fr. G. *lēmniskos,* ribbon or fillet) = A bundle of nerve fibers ascending from sensory relay nuclei to the thalamus.

lens (L. a lentil) = The transparent biconvex cellular refractive structure lying between the iris and the vitreous humor.

lenticular (L. *lenticula,* a lentil) = Relating to or resembling a lens of any kind; of the shape of a lentil.

lentiform (L.) = Lens-shaped.

leptomeninges, sing. **leptomeninx** (G. *leptos,* slender, delicate, weak, + *mēninx,* pl. *mēninges,* membrane) = The two delicate layers of the meninges, the arachnoid mater and pia mater, considered together.

levator (L. a lifter, fr. *levo,* pp. *-atus,* to lift, fr. *levis,* light) = One of several muscles whose action is to raise the part into which it is inserted.

liber, -era, -erum (L.) = Free.

lien (L.) = Spleen.

ligamentous (L.) = Relating to or of the form or structure of a ligament.

ligamentum, pl. **ligamenta** (L. a band, tie, fr. *ligo,* to bind) = Ligament; a band or sheet of fibrous tissue connecting two or more structures.

limbus, pl. **limbi** (L. a border) = The edge, border, or fringe of a part.

limen, pl. **limina** (L.) = Threshold; entrance, the external opening of a canal or space.

limit (L. *limes,* boundary) = A boundary or end.

linea, gen. and pl. **lineae** (L.) = Line; a long narrow mark, strip, or streak.

lingua, gen. and pl. **linguae** (L. tongue) = Tongue.

lingula, pl. **lingulae** (L. dim. of *lingua,* tongue) = A term applied to several tongue-shaped processes.

liquor, gen. **liquoris,** pl. **liquores** (L.) = Any liquid or fluid.

lobar (G.) = Relating to any lobe.

lobular (L.) = Relating to a lobule.

lobulus, gen. and pl. **lobuli** (Mod. L. dim. of *lobus,* lobe) = Lobule; a small lobe or subdivision of a lobe.

lobus, gen. and pl. **lobi** (LL. fr. G. *lobos*) = Lobe; one of the subdivisions of an organ or other part; a rounded projecting part.

locus, pl. **loci** (L.,) = A place; a specific site.

longitudinal (L. *longitudo,* length) = Running lengthwise; in the direction of the long axis of the body or any of its parts; studied over a period of time.

longus, -a, -um (L.) = Long.

longissimus, -a, -um (L.) = Longest.

lucid (L. *lucidus,* clear) = Clear, not obscured or confused.

lumbar (L. *lumbus,* a loin) = Relating to the loins, or the part of the back and sides between the ribs and the pelvis.

lunate (L.) = Lunar; relating to the moon or to a month; resembling the moon in shape.

lunula, pl. **lunulae** (L. dim. of *luna,* moon) = The pale arched area at the proximal portion of the nail plate; a small semilunar structure.

luteal (L. *luteus,* saffron-yellow) = Relating to the corpus luteum.

lymph (L. *lympha,* clear spring water) = A clear, transparent, sometimes faintly yellow and slightly opalescent fluid that is collected from the tissues throughout the body.

lymphatic (L. *lymphaticus,* frenzied) = Pertaining to lymph; a vascular channel that transports lymph.

macula, pl. **maculae** (L. a spot) = A small spot, different in color from the surrounding tissue.

macular, maculate (L.) = Relating to or marked by macules; denoting the central retina.

magnus, -a, -um (L.) = Large; great.

major (L. comp. of *magnus,* great) = Larger or greater in size of two similar structures.

mala (L. cheek bone) = Cheek; zygomatic bone.

malar (L.) = Relating to the mala, the cheek or cheek bones.

malleable (L. *malleus,* a hammer) = Capable of being shaped by being beaten or by pressure.

malleolar (L.) = Relating to one or both malleoli.

malleolus, pl. **malleoli** (L. dim. of *malleus,* hammer) = A rounded bony prominence such as those on either side of the ankle joint.

mamilla, pl. **mamillae** (L. nipple) = A small rounded elevation resembling the female breast; nipple.

mamillothalamic (L.) = A tract connecting the mamillary bodies with the thalamus.

mamma, gen. and pl. **mammae** (L.) = Breast.

mandibula, pl. **mandibulae** (L. a jaw, fr. *mando,* pp. *mansus,* to chew) = Mandible.

manubrium, pl. **manubria** (L. handle) = The portion of the sternum or of the malleus that represents the handle.

manus, gen. and pl. **manus** (L.) = Hand.

margo, gen. **marginis,** pl. **margines** (L.) = Margin, border.

masculine (L. *masculus,* male, fr. *mas,* male) = Relating to or marked by the characteristics of the male sex or gender.

massa, gen. and pl. **massae** (L.) = Mass.

masseter (G. *masētēr,* masticator) = The masseter muscle.

masticate (L. *mastico,* pp. *-atus,* to chew) = To chew; to perform mastication.

mastoid (G. *mastos,* breast, + *eidos,* resemblance) = Resembling a mamma; breast-shaped; relating to the mastoid process, antrum, cells, etc.; mastoidal.

mater (L. mother) = The "sheltering" coverings of the central nervous system.

matrix, pl. **matrices** (L. womb; female breeding animal) = The formative portion or a tooth or a nail; the intercellular substance of a tissue; a surrounding substance within which something is contained or embedded.

maxilla, gen. and pl. **maxillae** (L. jawbone) = Upper jaw bone, upper jaw.

maximum (L. ntr. of maximus, greatest) = The greatest amount, value, or degree attained or attainable.

meatus, pl. **meatus** (L. a going, a passage, fr. *meo,* pp. *meatus,* to go, pass) = A passage or channel, especially the external opening of a canal.

medial (L. *medialis,* middle) = Relating to the middle or center.

median (L. *medianus,* middle) = Central, middle; lying in the midline.

mediastinum (Mod. L. a middle septum, fr. Mediev. L. *mediastinus,* medial, fr. L. *mediastimus,* a lower servant, fr. *medius,* middle) = A septum between two parts of an organ or a cavity; the median partition of the thoracic cavity.

medius (L.) = Middle.

medulla, pl. **medullae** (L. marrow, fr. *medius,* middle) = Any soft marrow-like structure, especially in the center of a part.

membrane (L. *membrana,* a skin or membrane that covers parts of the body, fr. *membrum,* a member) = A thin sheet or layer of pliable tissue, serving as a covering or envelope of a part, as the lining of cavity, as a partition or septum, or to connect two structures.

meningeal (G.) = Relating to the meninges.

meninx, gen. **meningis,** pl. **meninges** (Mod. L. fr. G. *mēninx,* membrane) = Any membrane; specifically, one of the membranous coverings of the brain and spinal cord.

meniscus, pl. **menisci** (G. *mēniskos,* crescent) = A crescent-shaped structure.

mental (L. *mens (ment-),* mind; *mentum,* chin) = Relating to the mind; relating to the chin.

mentum, gen. **menti** (L.) = Chin.

mesencephalon (G. *mesos,* middle, *enkephalos,* brain) = Midbrain.

mesentery (Mod. L. *mesenterium,* fr. G. *mesenterion,* fr. G. *mesos,* middle, + *enteron,* intestine) = A double layer of peritoneum attached to the abdominal wall and enclosing in its fold a portion or all of one of the abdominal viscera, conveying to it its vessels and nerves.

metacarpal (G.) = Relating to the metacarpus.

metacarpus, pl. **metacarpi** (G. *meta,* after, between, + *karpos,* wrist) = The five bones of the hand between the carpus and the phalanges.

metatarsal (G.) = Relating to the metatarsus or to one of the metatarsal bones.

metatarsus, pl. **metatarsi** (G. *meta*, after, between, + *tarsos*, tarsus) = The distal portion of the foot between the instep and toes.

metencephalon (G. *meta*, after, between, + *enkephalos*, brain) = The anterior of the two major subdivisions of the rhombencephalon, composed of the pons and the cerebellum.

minor (L.) = Smaller; lesser.

mitral (L. *mitra*, a coif or turban) = Relating to the mitral or bicuspid valve; shaped like a bishop's miter.

modiolus, pl. **modioli** (L. the nave of a wheel) = The central cone-shaped core of spongy bone about which turns the spiral canal of the cochlea.

molar (L. *molaris*, relating to a mill, millstone) = Denoting a grinding, abrading, or wearing away; molar tooth.

mollities (L. *mollis*, soft = Characterized by a soft consistency; malacia.

mons, gen. **montis**, pl. **montes** (L. a mountain) = An anatomical prominence of slight elevation above the general level of the surface.

motor (L. a mover, fr. *moveo*, to move) = Denoting those neural structures which by the impulses generated and transmitted by them cause muscle fibers or pigment cells to contract, or glands to secrete.

mucous (L. *mucosus*, mucous, fr. *mucus*) = Relating to mucus or a mucous membrane.

multifid (L. *multifidus*, fr. *multus*, much, + *findo*, to cleave) = Divided into many clefts or segments.

muscular (L.) = Relating to a muscle or the muscles.

musculocutaneous (L.) = Relating to both muscle and skin.

musculus, gen. and pl. **musculi** (L. a little mouse, a muscle, fr. *mus* [*mur*-], a mouse) = Muscle.

myelencephalon (G. *myelos*, medulla, marrow, *enkephalos*, brain) = Medulla oblongata.

myenteric (G. *mys*, muscle, + *enteron*, intestine) = Relating to the myenteron, the muscular coat of the intestine.

mylohyoid (G. *mylē*, a mill, in pl. *mylai*, molar teeth) = Relating to the molar teeth, or posterior portion of the lower jaw, and to the hyoid bone.

myo- (G. *mys*, muscle) = Muscle.

myocardium, pl. **myocardia** (G. *myo* + *kardia*, heart) = The middle layer of the heart, consisting of cardiac muscle.

myology (G. *myo* + *logos*, study) = The branch of science concerned with the muscles and their accessory parts.

myometrium (G. *myo* + *mētra*, uterus) = The muscular wall of the uterus.

naris, pl. **nares** (L.) = Nostril.

nasal (L. *nasus*, nose) = Relating to the nose; rhinal.

nasus (L.) = Nose.

navicular (L. *navicularis*, relating to shipping) = Scaphoid.

neonate (G. *neo*, *neos*, new, recent + L. *natus*, born, fr. *nascor*, to be born) = A neonatal infant; newborn.

nervous (L. *nervosus*) = Relating to a nerve or the nerves.

nervus, gen. and pl. **nervi** (L.) = Nerve.

nidus, pl. **nidi** (L. nest) = A nest; the nucleus or central point of origin of a nerve; a focus of infection.

nigra (L. fr. *niger*, black) = The substantia nigra.

nodulus, pl. **noduli** (L. dim. of *nodus*) = Nodule; a small node.

nodus, pl. **nodi** (L. a knot) = Node; a circumscribed mass of tissue.

norma, pl. **normae** (L. a carpenter's square) = Profile.

nucha (Fr. *nuque*) = The back of the neck; nape.

nucleus, pl. **nuclei** (L. a little nut, the kernel, stone of fruits, the inside of a thing, dim. of *nux*, nut) = A central point, group, or mass about which gathering, contraction, or accretion takes place.

nutritive (L. fr. *nutrio*, to nourish) = Pertaining to nutrition; capable of nourishing.

obex (L. barrier) = The point on the midline of the dorsal surface of the medulla oblongata that marks the caudal angle of the fourth ventricle.

oblique (L. *obliquus*) = Slanting; deviating from the perpendicular, horizontal, sagittal, or coronal plane of the body.

oblongata (L. fem. of *oblongatus*, fr. *oblongus*, rather long) = Medulla oblongata.

oblongus (L.) = Rather long.

obtund (L. *ob- tundo*, pp. *-tusus*, to beat against, blunt) = To dull or blunt, especially to blunt sensation or deaden pain.

obturation (L.) = Obstruction or occlusion.

obturator (L. *obturo*, pp. *-atus*, to occlude or stop up) = Any structure that occludes an opening (see obturation).

occipital (L.) = Occipitalis; relating to the occiput, referring to the occipital bone or to the back of the head.

occiput, gen. **occipitis** (L.) = The back of the head.

octavus (L.) = Eighth; Vestibulocochlear nerve, the eighth cranial nerve.

oculomotor (L. *oculomotorius*, fr. *oculo-* + *motorius*, moving) = Pertaining to the oculomotor cranial nerve.

oculus, gen. and pl. **oculi** (L.) = Eye.

olecranon (G. the head or point of the elbow, fr. *ōlene*, ulna, + *kranion*, skull, head) = The prominent curved proximal extremity of the ulna; elbow bone; olecranon process.

olfactory (L. *ol- facio*, pp. *-factus*, to smell) = Relating to the sense of smell; osmatic.

oliva, pl. **olivae** (L.) = A smooth oval prominence of the ventrolateral surface of the medulla oblongata; olive.

omentum, pl. **omenta** (L. the membrane that encloses the bowels) = A fold of peritoneum passing from the stomach to another abdominal organ.

omental (L. *omentalis*) = Relating to the omentum; epiploic.

omoclavicular (G. *ōmos*, shoulder, + clavicle) = Relating to the shoulder and the clavicle.

omohyoid (G.) = Relating to the shoulder and the hyoid bone; omohyoid muscle.

omphaloenteric (G. *omphalos*, naval [umbilicus]) = Relating to the umbilicus and the intestine.

oophor-, **oophoro** (Mod. L. *oophoron*, ovary, fr. G. *ōophoros*, egg-bearing) = The ovary.

opercular (L.) = Relating to an operculum.

operculum, gen. **operculi**, pl. **opercula** (L. cover or lid, fr. *operio*, pp. *opertus*, to cover) = Anything resembling a lid or a cover; the portions of the frontal, parietal, and temporal lobes bordering the lateral sulcus and covering the insula.

ophthalmic (G. *ophthalamikos*) = Relating to the eye; ocular.

opponens (L. *op- pono* [*obp*-], pres. p. *-ens*, to place against, oppose) = The name given to several muscles of the fingers or toes, by the action of which these digits are opposed to the others.

optic, **optical** (G. *optikos*) = Relating to the eye, vision, or optics.

ora, pl. **orae** (L.) = An edge or a margin; plural of L. *os*, the mouth.

orbicular (L. *orbiculus*, a small disk, dim. of *orbis*, circle) = Similar in form to an orb; circular in form.

orbit (L. *orbita*, wheel-track, fr. *orbis*, circle) = Eye socket, orbital cavity.

orifice (L. *orificium* = Any aperture or opening.

os, gen. **oris**, pl. **ora** (L. mouth) = The mouth; an opening into a hollow organ or canal.

os, gen. **ossis**, pl. **ossa** (L. bone) = Bone.

osteology (G. *osteon*, bone, + *logos*, study) = The anatomy of the bones; the science concerned with the bones and their structure.

ostium, pl. **ostia** (L. door, entrance, mouth) = A small opening, especially one of entrance into a hollow organ or canal.

otic (G. *otikos*, fr. *ous*, ear) = Relating to the ear.

oval (L.) = Relating to an ovum; egg-shaped.

ovarium, pl. **ovaria** (Mod. L. fr. *ovum*, egg) = Ovary.

ovum, gen. **ovi**, pl. **ova** (L. egg) = The female sex cell.

pachymeninx (G. *pachys*, thick, + *meninx*, membrane) = The dura mater.

palatal (L.) = Relating to the palate; palatine.

palato- (L. *palatum*, palate) = Palate.

palatum, pl. **palati** (L.) = Palate.

pallid (L. *pallidus*) = Pale.

pallium (L. cloak) = The cerebral cortex; brain mantle; mantle.

palm (L. *palma*) = The flat of the hand.

palmar (L. *palmaris*, fr. *palma*) = Referring to the palm of the hand; volar.

palmate, **palmated** (L.) = Resembling a hand with the fingers spread.

palpebra, pl. **palpebrae** (L.) = Eyelid.

pampiniform (L. *pampinius*, a tendril, + *forma*, form) = Having the shape of a tendril; denoting a vinelike structure.

pancreas, pl. **pancreata** (G. *pankreas*, the sweetbread, fr. *pas* (*pan*), all, + *kreas*, flesh) = Salivary gland of abdomen.

panniculus, pl. **panniculi** (L. dim. of *pannus*, cloth) = A sheet or layer of tissue.

papilla, pl. **papillae** (L. a nipple, dim. of *papula*, a pimple) = Any small nipple-like process.

paradidymis, pl. **paradidymides** (G. *para-*, alongside of, near, + *didymos*, twin, in pl. *didymoi*, testes) = Parepididymis; a small body sometimes attached to the front of the lower part of the spermatic cord above the head of the epididymis.

parametrium, pl. **parametria** (G. *para-* +

mētra, uterus) = The connective tissue of the pelvic floor.

parenchyma (G. anything poured in beside, fr. *parencheō*, to pour in beside) = The distinguishing or specific cells of a gland or organ, contained in and supported by the connective tissue framework.

paries, gen. **parietis**, pl. **parietes** (L. wall) = A wall, as of the chest, abdomen, or any hollow organ.

parietal (L.) = Relating to the wall of any cavity.

paroophoron (G. *para-* + *ōophoron*, ovary) = Remnants of the lower part of the wolffian body appearing as a few scattered tubules in the broad ligament.

parotic (G. *para*, beside, + *ous* (*ot-*), ear) = Near or beside the ear.

parotid (G. *parōtis* (*parōtid-*), the gland beside the ear, fr. *para*, beside, + *ous* (*ot-*), ear) = Parotid salivary gland.

pars, pl. **partes** (L. *pars* (*part-*), a part) = A part; a portion.

parvus (L.) = Small.

patella, gen. and pl. **patellae** (L. a small plate, the kneecap, dim. of *patina*, a shallow disk, fr. *pateo*, to lie open) = Kneecap.

pecten (L. comb) = A structure with comblike processes or projections.

pectinate (L.) = Pectiniform; combed; comb-shaped.

pectoral (L. *pectoralis*, fr. *pectus*, breast bone) = Relating to the chest.

pectus, gen. **pectoris**, pl. **pectora** (L.) = The anterior wall of the chest or thorax; the breast.

pedunculus, pl. **pedunculi** (Mod. L. dim of *pes*, foot) = Peduncle; a stalk or stem.

pellucid (L. *pellucidus*) = Allowing the passage of light.

pelvic = Relating to the pelvis.

pelvis, pl. **pelves** (L. basin) = The cup-shaped ring of bone, with its ligaments, at the lower end of the trunk; any basin-like or cup-shaped cavity.

penis (L. tail) = The organ of copulation in the male.

perforans (L. perforating) = A term applied to several muscles or nerves which, in their course, perforate other structure.

perforated (L. *perforatus*, fr. *per- foro*, pp. *-atus*, to bore through) = Pierced with one or more holes.

pericardium, pl. **pericardia** (L. fr. G. *pericardion*, the membrane around the heart) = The closed sac containing the heart, consisting of a visceral and a parietal layer of connective tissue.

perilympha (G. *peri*, around, about, + L. *lympha*, a clear fluid) = Perilymph; the fluid contained within the osseous labyrinth.

perimetrium, pl. **perimetria** (G. *peri-*, around, + *mētra*, uterus) = The serous coat of the uterus.

perineal = Relating to the perineum.

perineum, pl. **perinea** (L. fr. G. *perineon*, *perinaion*) = The area between the thighs extending from the coccyx to the pubis and lying below the diaphragm.

periodontium, pl. **periodontia** (L. fr. *peri*, + *odous*, tooth) = Alveolodental or peridental membrane; the tissues that surround and support the teeth.

periorbita (peri- + L. *orbita*, orbit) = Periorbit; orbital fascia.

periorchitis (peri- + G. *orchis*, testis, + *-itis*, inflammation) = Inflammation of the tunica vaginalis testis.

periosteum, pl. **periostea** (Mod. L. fr. G. *peri*, around, + *osteon*, bone) = The fibrous membrane covering the entire surface of a bone except its articular cartilage.

peritoneum, pl. **peritonea** (Mod. L. fr. G. *peritonaion*, fr. *periteinō*, to stretch over) = The serous sac that lines the abdominal cavity and covers most of the viscera contained therein.

permanent (L. fr. *per-* throughout + *manere*, to remain) = Continuing or enduring without marked change; stable.

peroneal (L. *peroneus*, fr. G. *peronē*, fibula) = Relating to the fibula.

perpendicular (L. *per-*, through, + *pendere*, to hang) = A line at right angles to the plane of the horizon or to another line or surface.

pes, gen. **pedis**, pl. **pedes** (L.) = Foot.

petiolus (L. dim. of *pes*, the stalk of a fruit) = Petiole; a stem or pedicle.

petrosphenoid = Relating to the petrous portion of the temporal bone and the sphenoid bone.

petrous (L. *petrosus*, fr. *petra*, a rock) = Of stony hardness; petrosal.

phalanx, gen. **phalangis**, pl. **phalanges** (L. fr. G. *phalanx* [*-ang*], line of soldiers, bone between two joints of the fingers and toes) = One of the long bones of the digits.

pharyngeal (Mod. L. pharyngeus) = Relating to the pharynx.

pharynx, gen. **pharyngis**, pl. **pharynges** (Mod. L. fr. G. *pharynx* [*pharyng-*], the throat, the joint opening of the gullet and windpipe) = The upper expanded portion of the digestive tube.

philtrum, pl. **philtra** (L. fr. G. *philtron*, a love-charm, depression on upper lip, fr. *phileō*, to love) = The infranasal depression; the groove in the midline of the upper lip.

phrenic (G. *phrēn*, the diaphragm, mind, heart) = Relating to the diaphragm; relating to the mind.

pia (L. fem. adj.). = Tender; pia mater

pigment (L. *pigmentum*, paint) = Any coloring matter.

pilus, pl. **pili** (L.) = Hair.

pineal (L. *pineus*, relating to the pine, *pinus*) = The pineal gland.

piriform (L. *pirum*, pear, + *forma*, form) = Pear-shaped.

pisiform (L. *pisum*, pea, + *forma*, appearance) = Pea-shaped.

pituitary (L. *pituita*, phlegm or thick mucous secretion) = Relating to the pituitary gland.

pius, -a, -um (L.) = Tender.

placenta (L. a cake) = Organ of metabolic interchange between fetus and mother.

planta, gen. and pl. **plantae** (L.) = Sole (of foot).

planum, pl. **plana** (L. plane) = A plane or flat surface.

planus (L.) = Flat.

platysma, pl. **platysmas, platysmata** (G. *platysma*, a flat plate) = Platysma muscle.

pleura, gen. and pl. **pleurae** (G. *pleura*, a rib, pl. the side) = The membrane enveloping the lungs and lining the walls of the pleural cavity.

plexus, pl. **plexus, plexuses** (L. a braid) = A network or interjoining of nerves and blood vessels or of lymphatic vessels.

plica, gen. and pl. **plicae** (Mod. L. a plait or fold) = One of several anatomical structures in which there is a folding over of the parts.

pollex, gen. **pollicis**, pl. **pollices** (L.) = Thumb.

pons, pl. **pontes** (L. bridge) = Any bridge-like formation connecting two more or less disjoined parts of the same structure or organ; pons cerebelli.

pontile, pontine (L. bridge) = Relating to a pons.

poples (L. the ham of the knee) = Popliteal fossa.

popliteal (L.) = Relating to the popliteal fossa; popliteus.

porta, pl. **portae** (L. gate) = Hilum; porta hepatis.

portio, pl. **portiones** (L. portion) = A part.

porus, pl. **pori** (L. fr. G. *poros*, passageway) = Opening; sweat pore.

postcentral (L. *post*, after, behind, posterior) = The postcentral gyrus.

posterior (L. comp. of *posterus*, following) = After, in relation to time or space; denoting the back surface of the body.

posterolateral = Behind and to one side.

precentral (L. *prae*, anterior, before) = Precentral gyrus.

preputium, pl. **preputia** (L. *praeputium*, foreskin) = Prepuce.

princeps, pl. **principes** (L. chief, fr. *primus*, first, + *capio*, to take, choose) = Principal.

procerus (L. long, stretched out) = Procerus muscle.

process (L. *processus*, an advance, progress, process, fr. *pro-cedo*, pp. *-cessus*, to go forward) = A method or mode of action; a projection or outgrowth.

profundus (L.) = Deep.

prominence (L. *prominentia*) = Tissues or parts that project beyond a surface.

promontorium, pl. **promontoria** (L. a mountain ridge, a headland, fr. *promineo*, to jut out) = Promontory; an eminence or projection.

pronator (L.) = A muscle which turns a part into the prone position.

pronephros, pl. **pronephroi** (L. and G. *pro*, before, forward, + G. *nephros*, kidney) = Primordial kidney; forekidney.

prone (L. *pronus*, bending down or forward) = The body or a part thereof when lying face downward.

proprius (L.) = One's own.

prosencephalon (G. *prosō*, forward, + *enkephalos*, brain) = Forebrain.

prostata (Mod. L. fr. G. *prostatōs*, one standing before, protects) = Prostate gland; a chestnut-shaped body, surrounding the beginning of the urethra in the male.

prostatic = Relating to the prostate.

protuberance (Mod. L. *protuberantia*, fr. *protubero*, to swell out, fr. *tuber*, swelling) = A swelling or knoblike outgrowth.

proximal (Mod. L. *proximalis*, fr. *proximus*, nearest, next) = Nearest the trunk or the point of origin; mesial.

psoas (G. *psoa*, the muscles of the loins) = Psoas major and minor muscles.

pterygoid (G. *pteryx* [*pteryg-*], wing, + *eidos*, resemblance) = Wing-shaped; resembling a wing.

pudendum, pl. **pudenda** (L. ntr. of *pudendus*, particip. adj. of *pudeo*, to feel ashamed) = The external genitals, especially the female genitals.

pulmo, gen. **pulmonis**, pl. **pulmones** (L.) = Lung.

pulmonary (L. *pulmonarius*, fr. *pulmo*, lung) = Relating to the lungs.

pulpa (L. flesh) = Pulp; a soft, moist, coherent solid.

pulvinar (L. a couch made fr. cushions, fr. *pulvinus*, cushion) = The expanded posterior extremity of the thalamus which forms a cushion-like prominence overlying the geniculate bodies.

pupil (L. *pupilla*, dim. of *pupa*, a girl or doll) = The circular orifice in the center of the iris through which light rays enter the eye.

putamen (L. that which falls off in pruning, fr. *puto*, to prune) = The outer, larger, and darker gray of the three portions into which the lenticular nucleus is divided.

pyelo-, pyel- (G. *pyelos*, trough, tub, vat) = Pelvis, usually the renal pelvis.

pyloric = Relating to the pylorus.

pylorus, pl. **pylori** (L. fr. G. *pylōros*, a gate-keeper, the pylorus, fr. *pylē*, gate, *ouros*, a warder) = A muscular device to open and to close an orifice or the lumen of an organ.

pyramidal = Of the shape of a pyramid.

pyramid (G. *pyramis* [*pyramid-*], a pyramid) = A term applied to a number of anatomical structures have a more or less pyramidal shape; pyramis.

quadrangular (L. *quadrangularis*, fr. *quadrangulum*, quadrangle) = Having four angles.

quadrate (L. *quadratus*, square) = Having four equal sides; square.

quadriceps (L. fr. *quadri-*, four, + *caput*, head) = Having four heads; denoting a muscle of the thigh and one of the calf.

radial (L. *radialis*, fr. *radius*, ray, lateral bone of the forearm) = Relating to the radius bone of the forearm; relating to any radius; radiating.

radiatio, pl. **radiationes** (L. fr. *radius*, ray, beam) = Radiation; a term applied to any one of the thalamocortical fiber systems that together compose the corona radiata of the cerebral hemisphere's white matter.

radicular (L. *radicula*, dim. of *radix*, root) = Relating to a radicle; pertaining to the root of a tooth.

radius gen. and pl. **radii** (L. spoke of a wheel, rod, ray) = A straight line passing from the center to the periphery of a circle; the lateral and shorter of the two bones of the forearm.

radix, gen. **radicis**, pl. **radices** (L.) = Root; the primary or beginning portion of any part.

ramus, pl. **rami** (L.) = A branch.

raphe (G. *rhaphē*, suture, seam) = The line of union of two contiguous, bilaterally symmetrical structures.

recessus, pl. **recessus** (L. a withdrawing, a receding) = Recess; a small hollow or indentation.

rectum, pl. **rectums** or **recta** (L. *rectus*, straight, pp. of *rego*, to make straight) = The terminal portion of the digestive tube.

rectus (L.) = Straight.

recurrent (L. *re-curro*, to run back, recur) = Turning back on itself; denoting symptoms or lesions reappearing after an intermission.

regio, gen. **regionis**, pl. **regiones** (L.) =

Region; a portion of the body or an organ having a special function or special nervous or vascular supply.

ren, gen. **renis**, pl. **renes** (L.) = Kidney.

renal (L.) = Nephric.

respiratory (L. *respiratio*, fr. *re-spiro*, pp. *-atus*, to exhale, breathe) = Relating to respiration.

rete, pl. **retia** (L. a net) = A network of nerve fibers or small vessels.

retina (Mediev. L. prob. fr. L. *rete*, a net) = The nervous tunic of the eyeball.

retinaculum, gen. **retinaculi**, pl. **retinacula** (L. a band, a halter, fr. *retineo*, to hold back) = A frenum, or a retaining band or ligament.

retroperitoneal (L.) = Behind, external or posterior to the peritoneum.

rhinencephalon (G. fr. *rhis*, nose, + *enkephalos*, brain) = Collective term denoting the parts of the cerebral hemisphere directly related to the sense of smell.

rhombencephalon (G. fr. *rhombos*, a rhomb or rhombus, + *enkephalos*, brain) = Hindbrain.

rhomboid, rhomboidal (G. *rhombos*, + *eidos*, appearance) = Resembling a rhomb, i.e., an oblique parallelogram with unequal sides.

rima, gen. and pl. **rimae** (L. a slit) = A slit or fissure or narrow elongated opening between two symmetrical parts.

risorius (L. *risor*, a laughter, fr. *rideo*, pp. *risus*, to laugh) = Risorius muscle.

rostral (L. *rostralis*, fr. *rostrum*, beak) = Relating to any rostrum or structure resembling a beak.

rostrum, pl. **rostra, rostrums** (L. a beak) = Any beak-shaped structure.

rotator (L. *rotatio*, fr. *roto*, pp. *rotatus*, to revolve, rotate) = A muscle by which a part can be turned circularly.

rotund (L. *rotundus*) = Marked by roundness; rounded.

ruber (L.) = Red.

ruga, pl. **rugae** (L. a wrinkle) = A fold, ridge, or crease; a wrinkle.

saccus, pl. **sacci** (L. a bag, sack) = A sac.

sacrum, pl. **sacra** (L. [lit. sacred bone], ntr. of *sacer* (*sacr-*), sacred) = The sacrum.

sacral (L.) = Relating to or in the neighborhood of the sacrum.

sagittal (L. *sagitta*, an arrow) = Resembling an arrow; in the line of an arrow shot from a bow; referring to a plane or direction.

saliva (L. akin to G. *sialon*) = Spittle; a clear, tasteless, odorless, slightly acid viscid fluid consisting of the secretion from the salivary glands and the mucous glands of the oral cavity.

salpinx, pl. **salpinges** (G. a trumpet [tube]) = Official alternate term for the uterine tube.

saphenous (Med. L. attributed by some as derived fr. Ar. *safin*, standing; by others, fr. G. saphēnēs, manifest, clearly visible) = Relating to or associated with a saphenous vein; denoting a number of structures in the leg.

sartorius (L. *sartor*, a tailor, the muscle being used in crossing the legs in the tailor's position, fr. *sarcio*, pp. *sartus*, to patch, mend) = Sartorius muscle.

scala, pl. **scalae** (L. a stairway) = Scale; one of the cavities of the cochlea; a small thin plate of horny epithelium.

scalene (G. *skalēnos*, uneven) = A trian-

gle having sides of unequal length; the scalene muscles.

scapha (L. fr. G. *skaphē*, skiff) = A boat-shaped structure; the longitudinal furrow between the helix and the antihelix of the auricle.

scaphoid (G.) = Navicular; boat-shaped; hollowed.

sclera, pl. **scleras, sclerae** (Med. L. fr. *skle;amros*, hard) = Sclerotic coat of eye; white of eye.

scriptorius (L. fr. *scribere*, to write) = As in calamus scriptorius (L. a writing pen) = The narrow lower end of the fourth ventricle.

scrotal = Relating to the scrotum.

scrotum, pl. **scrota, scrotums** (L.) = A musculocutaneous sac containing the testes.

secund (L. *secundus*, following) = Unilateral.

segment (L. *segmentum*, fr. *seco*, to cut) = A section; a territory of an organ having independent function, supply, or drainage.

segmental = Relating to a segment.

sella (L. saddle) = Saddle.

semicanal (L. *semis*, half) = A half canal.

semicircular (L.) = Forming a half circle or an incomplete circle.

semilunar (L. *semi-* + *luna*, moon) = Half moon; lunar.

semimembranous (L.) = Consisting partly of membrane; denoting the semimembranosus muscle.

seminal (L.) = Relating to the semen; original or influential of future developments.

semioval (L.) = Half oval.

semispinal (L.) = Half spinal; denoting muscles attached in part to the spinous processes of the vertebrae.

semitendinous (L.) = Composed in part of tendon; denoting the semitendinosus muscle.

septal (L.) = Relating to a septum.

septum, gen. **septi**, pl. **septa** (L. *saeptum*, a partition) = A thin wall dividing two cavities or masses of softer tissue.

serrate, serrated (L. *serratus*, fr. *serra*, a saw) = Toothed.

sesamoid (G. *sēsamoeidēs*, like sesame) = Resembling in size or shape a grain of sesame; denoting a sesamoid bone.

sigmoid (G. *sigma*, the letter S, + *eidos*, resemblance) = Resembling in outline the letter S or one of the forms of the Greek sigma.

simple (L. *simplex*) = Not complex or compound; composed of a minimum number of parts.

sinister (L.) = Left.

sinuatrial (L.) = Relating to the sinus venosus and the right atrium of the heart; sinoatrial.

sinus, pl. **sinus, sinuses** (L. *sinus*, cavity, channel, hollow) = A channel for the passage of blood or lymph; a cavity or hollow space in bone or other tissue; a dilatation in a blood vessel.

soleus (Mod. L. fr. L. *solea*, a sandal, sole of the foot [of animals], fr. *solum*, bottom, floor, ground) = Soleus muscle.

solitary (L. *solitarius*) = Standing alone; not grouped with others.

spatium, pl. **spatia** (L.) = Space.

spermatic (G. *sperma*, seed) = Relating to the sperm or semen.

sphenoid (G. *spheēnoeidēs*, fr. *sphēn*,

wedge, + *eidos*, resemblance) = Sphenoidal; wedge-shaped; relating to the sphenoid bone.

sphincter (G. *sphinktēr*, a band or lace) = A muscle that encircles a duct, tube or orifice in such a way that its contraction constricts the lumen or orifice.

spine (L. *spina*, a thorn, the backbone) = Vertebral column.

spinal (L. *spinalis*) = Relating to any spine or spinous process; relating to the vertebral column.

spinocostalis (L.) = The superior and inferior serratus posterior muscles regarded as one.

spiral (Mediev. L. *spiralis*, fr. G. *speira*, a coil) = Coiled; a structure in the shape of a coil.

splanchnic (G. *splanchnon*, viscus) = Visceral.

splanchnology (G. *splanchno-* + *logos*, study) = The branch of medical science dealing with the viscera.

spleen (G. *splēn*) = Splen; lien; a large vascular lymphatic organ lying in the upper part of the abdominal cavity on the left side between the stomach and diaphragm.

splenium, pl. **splenia** (Mod. L. fr. G. *splēnion*, bandage) = A compress or bandage; a structure resembling a bandaged part.

splenius (Mod. L. fr. G. *splēnion*, a bandage) = Splenius muscle of head or neck.

spongiose (L. *spongiosus*) = Resembling or characteristic of a sponge.

squama, pl. **squamae** (L. a scale) = A thin plate of bone; an epidermal scale.

squamous (L. *squamosus*) = Relating to or covered with scales; scaly, squamate.

stapedius, pl. **stapedii** (Mod. L.) = Stapedius muscle.

stapes, pl. **stapes, stapedes** (Mod. L. stirrup) = The smallest of the three auditory ossicles.

stellate (L. *stella*, a star) = Star-shaped.

sternal (L.) = Relating to the sternum.

sternoclavicular (L.) = Relating to the sternum and clavicle.

sternocleidomastoid (Mod. L.) = Relating to the sternum, clavicle, and mastoid process.

sternocostal (L. *costa*, rib) = Relating to the sternum and the ribs.

sternohyoid (L.) = Relating to the sternum and the hyoid bone.

sternothyroid (L.) = Relating to the sternum and the thyroid cartilage.

sternum, gen. **sterni**, pl. **sterna** (Mod. L. fr. G. *sternon*, the chest) = A long flat bone articulating with the cartilages of the first seven ribs and the clavicle, forming the middle part of the anterior wall of the thorax.

stratum, gen. **strati**, pl. **strata** (L. *sterno*, pp. *stratus*, to spread out, strew, ntr. of pp. as noun, *stratum*, a bed cover, layer) = One of the layers of differentiated tissue, the aggregate of which forms any given structure; layer; lamina.

stria, gen. and pl. **striae** (L. channel, furrow) = A strip, band, streak or line, distinguished by color, texture, depression, or elevation from the tissue in which it is found.

striate (L. *striatus*, furrowed) = Striped; marked by striae.

styloglossus (G.) = Relating to the styloid process of the temporal bone and the tongue.

stylohyoid (G.) = Relating to the styloid process of the temporal bone and the hyoid bone.

styloid (G. *stylos*, pillar, post) = The styloid process of the temporal bone.

stylomastoid (G.) = Relating to the styloid and the mastoid processes of the temporal bone.

stylopharyngeus (G.) = The stylopharyngeus muscle.

submucous (L.) = Beneath a mucous membrane.

substance (L. *substantia*, essence, material, fr. *sub- sto*, to stand under, be present) = Stuff; material; matter.

sulcus, gen. **sulci** (L. a furrow or ditch) = One of the grooves or furrows on the surface of the brain; any long narrow groove, furrow, or slight depression.

supercilium, pl. **supercilia** (L. fr. *super*, above, + *cilium*, eyelid) = Eyebrow; an individual hair of the eyebrow.

superficial (L. *superficialis*, fr. *superficies*, surface) = Cursory; pertaining to or situated near the surface.

superior (L. comp. of *superus*, above) = Situated above or directed upward; opposite of inferior; cranial.

supinator (L. *supino*, to bend backwards, place on back, fr. *supinus*, supine) = A muscle that produces supination of the forearm.

supreme (L. *supremus*, superl. of *superius*) = The highest; uppermost.

sural (L.) = Relating to the calf of the leg.

suspensory (L. *suspensio*, fr. *sus- pendo*, to hang up, suspend) = Suspending; supporting.

sustentaculum, pl. **sustentacula** (L. a prop. fr. *sustento*, to hold upright) = A structure that serves as a stay or support to another.

suture (L. *sutura*, a sewing, a suture, fr. *suo*, to sew) = A form of fibrous joint in which two bones are united by a fibrous membrane continuous with the periosteum; to unite two surfaces by sewing.

sympathetic (G. *sympathetikos*, fr. *sympatheo*, to feel with, sympathize, fr. *syn*, with, + *pathos*, suffering) = Denoting the sympathetic part of the autonomic nervous system; sympathic.

symphysis, gen. **symphyses** (G. a growing together) = Form of cartilaginous joint in which union between two bones is effected by fibrocartilage; amphiarthrosis; a union, meeting point, or commissure of any two structures.

synarthrosis, pl. **synarthroses** (G. fr. *syn*, together, + *arthrōsis*, articulation) = Fibrous and cartilaginous joints.

synchondrosis, pl. **synchondroses** (Mod. L. fr. G. *syn*, together, + *chondros*, cartilage, + *-osis*, condition) = A union between two bones formed either by hyaline cartilage or fibrocartilage.

syndesmosis, pl. **syndesmoses** (G. *syndesmos*, a fastening, fr. *syndeō*, to bind, + *-osis*, condition) = A form of fibrous joint in which opposing surfaces that are relatively far apart are united by ligaments.

synostosis (G. *syn* + *osteon*, bone, *-osis*, condition) = Osseous union between the bones forming a joint.

synovia (Mod. L., a word coined by Paracelsus, fr. G. *syn*, together, + *ōmon* [L. *ovum*], egg) = Synovial fluid.

taenia (L. fr. G. *tainia*, band, tape, a tapeworm) = A coiled bandlike anatomical structure.

talar (L.) = Relating to the talus.

talocalcaneal (L.) = Relating to the talus and the calcaneus.

talocrural (L.) = Relating to the talus and the bones of the leg; denoting the ankle joint.

talonavicular (L.) = Relating to the talus and the navicular bone.

talus, gen. **tali** (L. ankle bone, heel) = The bone of the foot that articulates with the tibia and fibula to form the ankle joint.

tapetum, pl. **tapeta** (L. *tapeta*, a carpet) = Any membranous layer or covering.

tarsal (G.) = Relating to a tarsus in any sense.

tarsometatarsal (G.) = Relating to the tarsal and metatarsal bones.

tarsus, gen. and pl. **tarsi** (G. *tarsos*, a flat surface, sole of the foot, edge of eyelid) = The seven tarsal bones of the instep; the fibrous plates giving solidity and form to the edges of the eyelids.

tectorium (L. an overlaying surface [plaster, stucco] fr. *tego*, to cover) = An overlaying structure; tectorial membrane of cochlear duct.

tectum, pl. **tecta** (L. roof, roofed structure, fr. *tego*, to cover) = Any rooflike covering or structure.

tegmen, gen. **tegminis**, pl. **tegmina** (L. a covering, fr. *tego*, to cover) = A structure that covers or roofs over a part.

tegmentum, pl. **tegmenta** (L. a covering structure, fr. *tego*, to cover) = A covering structure; mesencephalic tegmentum.

tela, gen. and pl. **telae** (L. a web) = Any thin weblike structure; a delicate tissue.

telencephalon (G. *telos*, end, + *enkephalos*, brain) = The anterior division of the prosencephalon; endbrain.

temporalis (L.) = Temporal; relating to the temple; temporalis muscle.

tempus, gen. **temporis**, pl. **tempora** (L. time) = The temple.

tendinous (L.) = Relating to, composed of, or resembling a tendon.

tendo, gen. **tendinis**, pl. **tendines** (Mediev. L. fr. L. *tendo*, to stretch out, extend) = Tendon.

tensor, pl. **tensores** (Mod. L. fr. L. *tendo*, to stretch) = A muscle the function of which is to render a part firm and tense.

tentorium, pl. **tentoria** (L. tent, fr. *tendo*, to stretch) = A membranous cover or horizontal partition.

tenuis (L.) = Thin, fine, slight, slender.

teres, gen. **teretis**, pl. **teretes** (L. round, smooth, fr. *tero*, to rub) = Round and long; denoting certain muscles and ligaments.

terminal (L. *terminus*, a boundary, limit) = Relating to the end, final; relating to the extremity or end of any body.

testicular (L.) = Relating to the testes.

testis, pl. **testes** (L.) = One of the two male reproductive glands, located in the cavity of the scrotum.

thalamic (G.) = Relating to the thalamus.

thalamus, pl. **thalami** (G. *thalamos*, a bed, a bedroom) = The large, ovoid mass of gray matter that forms the larger dorsal subdivision of the diencephalon.

theca, pl. **thecae** (G. *thēkē*, a box) = A sheath or capsule.

thenar (G. the palm of the hand) = Thenar eminence.

thoracic (G.) = Relating to the thorax.

thoracoacromial (G.) = Relating to the acromion and the thorax; thoracoacromial artery.

thoracolumbar (G.) = Relating to the thoracic and lumbar portions of the vertebral column; relating to the origins of the sympathetic division of the autonomic nervous system.

thorax, gen. **thoracis**, pl. **thoraces** (L. fr. G. thōrax, breastplate, the chest, fr. thōrēssō, to arm) = The upper part of the trunk between the neck and the abdomen.

thymic (G.) = Relating to the thymus gland.

thymus, pl. **thymi**, **thymuses** (G. thymos, excrescence, sweetbread) = A primary lymphoid organ located in the superior mediastinum and lower part of the neck.

thyroarytenoid (G.) = Relating to the thyroid and arytenoid cartilages; thyroarytenoid muscle.

thyroepiglottic (G.) = Relating to the thyroid cartilage and the epiglottis.

thyrohyoid (G.) = Relating to the thyroid cartilage and the hyoid bone; the thyrohyoid muscle.

thyroid (G. thyreoeidēs, fr. thyreos, an oblong shield, + eidos, form) = Resembling a shield; denoting the thyroid gland and the thyroid cartilage of the larynx.

thyropharyngeal (G.) = Denoting the thyropharyngeal portion of the inferior pharyngeal constrictor muscle.

tibia, gen. and pl. **tibiae** (L. the large shinbone) = The medial and larger of the two bones of the leg.

tibial (L. tibialis) = Relating to the tibia or to any structure named fr. it.; denoting the medial or tibial aspect of the lower limb.

tonsil (L. tonsilla, a stake, in pl. the tonsils) = Any collection of lymphoid tissue.

torus, pl. **tori** (L. swelling, knot, bulge) = A rounded swelling, such as that caused by a contracting muscle.

trabecula, gen. and pl. **trabeculae** (L. dim. of trabs, a beam) = One of the supporting bundles of fibers traversing the substance of a structure; a small piece of spongy substance of bone.

trachea, pl. **tracheae** (G. tracheia artēria, rough artery) = The air tube extending from the larynx into the thorax; windpipe.

tracheobronchial (G.) = Relating to both trachea and bronchi, denoting a set of lymph nodes.

tract (L. tractus, a drawing out) = An elongated area, e.g., path, track, way.

tragus, pl. **tragi** (G. tragos, goat, in allusion to the hairs growing on the part, like a goatee) = A tonguelike projection of the cartilage of the auricle in the front of the opening of the external acoustic meatus.

transverse (L. transversus, fr. trans, across, + verto, to turn) = Crosswise; lying across the long axis of the body or of a part.

trapezoid (G. trapeza, table, + eidos, resemblance) = Resembling a trapezium; trapezoid bone.

triangular (L. triangulum, fr. tri-, three, + angulus, angle = Three-sided.

triceps (L. fr. tri-, three, + caput, head) = Three-headed.

tricuspid, tricuspidal, tricuspidate (L.) = Having three points, prongs, or cusps.

trigeminal (L. trigeminus, threefold, fr. tri- + geminus, twin) = Relating to the fifth cranial or trigeminal nerve.

trigone (L. trigonum, fr. G. trigōnon, triangle) = Any triangular area.

tripod (G. tripous, fr. tri- + pous, foot) = Three-legged; a stand having three legs or supports.

triquetrous (L. triquetrus, three-cornered) = Triangular.

triticeous (L. triticeus, fr. triticum, a grain of wheat) = Resembling or shaped like a grain of wheat.

trochanter (G. trochantēr, a runner, fr. trechō, to run) = One of the bony prominences near the upper extremity of the femur.

trochlea, pl. **trochleae** (L. pulley, fr. G. trochileia, a pulley, fr. trechō, to run) = A structure serving as a pulley.

trunk (L. truncus, stem) = The body, excluding the head and extremities; a primary nerve, vessel or collection of tissue before its division.

tuba, gen. and pl. **tubae** (L. a straight trumpet) = Tube.

tubarius (L.) = Tubal; relating to a tube.

tuber, pl. **tubera** (L. protuberance, swelling) = A localized swelling, a knob.

tubercle (L. tuberculum, dim. of tuber, a swelling) = A nodule; a circumscribed, rounded, solid elevation on the skin, mucous membrane, or surface of an organ; a slight elevation from the surface of a bone giving attachment to a muscle or ligament.

tuberosity (L.) = A large tubercle or rounded elevation, especially from the surface of a bone.

tunic (L. tunica, a coat) = Coat or covering; one of the enveloping layers of a part.

turcica (Mod. L.) = Turkish.

tympanic (G.) = Relating to the tympanic cavity or membrane.

tympanum, pl. **tympana**, **tympanums** (L. fr. G. tympanon, a drum) = Tympanic cavity.

ulna, gen. and pl. **ulnae** (L. elbow, arm, fr. G. ōlenē) = The medial and larger of the two bones of the forearm.

umbilical (L.) = Relating to the umbilicus.

umbilicus, pl. **umbilici** (L. navel) = The pit in the center of the abdominal wall marking the point where the umbilical cord entered in the fetus; belly button, navel.

umbo, gen. **umbonis**, pl. **umbones** (L. boss of a shield, a knob) = A projecting point of a surface.

uncinate (L. uncinatus) = Hooklike or hook-shaped.

uncus, pl. **unci** (L. a hook, fr. G. onkos) = Any hook-shaped process or structure.

unguiculate (L.) = Having nails or claws, as distinguished from hooves.

unguis, pl. **ungues** (L.) = Nail.

urachus (G. ourachos, the urinary canal of a fetus) = That portion of the reduced allantoic stalk between the bladder and the umbilicus which is normally a fibrous cord postnatally.

ureter (G. ourētēr, urinary canal) = The thick-walled tube that conducts the urine from the kidney to the bladder.

urethra (G. ourēthra) = A canal leading from the bladder, discharging the urine externally; urogenital canal.

urethral (G.) = Relating to the urethra.

urine (L. urina; G. ouron) = The fluid and dissolved substances excreted by the kidney.

urogenital (L.; G.) = Relating to the organs of reproduction and urination; genitourinary.

uterine (L.) = Relating to the uterus.

uterus, pl. **uteri** (L.) = The hollow muscular organ in which the impregnated ovum is developed into the child; womb.

utriculus, pl. **utriculi** (L. dim. of uter, leather bag) = Utricle; the larger of the two membranous sacs in the vestibule of the labyrinth.

uvula, pl. **uvuli** (Mod. L. dim. of L. uva, a grape, the uvula) = An appendant fleshy mass.

vagina, gen. and pl. **vaginae** (L. sheath, the vagina) = The genital canal in the female; sheath.

vagus, gen. and pl. **vagi** (L. wandering, so-called because of the wide distribution of the nerve) = The vagus nerve.

vallate (L. vallo, pp. -atus, to surround with, fr. vallum, a rampart) = Bordered with an elevation, as a cupped structure.

vallecula, pl. **valleculae** (L. dim. of vallis, valley) = A crevice or depression on any surface.

valvula, pl. **valvulae** (Mod. L. dim. of valva, one leaf of a double door) = Valvule; a small valve.

vas, gen. **vasis**, pl. **vasa**, gen. and pl. **vasorum** (L. a vessel, dish) = A duct or canal conveying any liquid.

vascular (L. vasculum, a small vessel, dim. of vas) = Relating to or containing blood vessels.

vastus (L.) = Great.

velum, pl. **vela** (L. veil, sail) = Any structure resembling a veil or curtain; any serous membrane or membranous envelope or covering.

vena, gen. and pl. **venae** (L.) = Vein.

venter (L. venter [ventr-], belly) = Abdomen; belly.

ventral (L. ventralis) = Pertaining to the belly or to any venter; anterior.

ventricle (L. ventriculus, dim. of venter, belly) = A normal cavity.

vermiform (L. dim. of vermis, worm, + forma, form) = Worm-shaped; resembling a worm in form.

vermis, pl. **vermes** (L. worm) = Any structure or part resembling a worm in shape; the narrow middle zone between the two hemispheres of the cerebellum.

vertebra, gen. and pl. **vertebrae** (L. joint, fr. verto, to turn) = One of the segments of the spinal column.

vertical (L.) = Relating to the vertex; perpendicular; denoting any plane or line that passes longitudinally through the body in the anatomical position.

vesica, gen. and pl. **vesicae** (L.) = Bladder; any hollow structure or sac containing a serous fluid.

vesical (L.) = Relating to any bladder, but usually the urinary bladder.

vesicle (L. vesicula, a blister, dim of vesica, bladder) = A small circumscribed elevation of the skin containing fluid; blister.

vestibular (L.) = Relating to a vestibule.

vestibule (L. vestibulum) = A small cavity or a space at the entrance of a canal.

vestibulocochlear (L.) = Relating to the vestibule and cochlea of the ear.

vibrissa, gen. and pl. **vibrissae** (L. found only in pl. vibrissae, fr. vibro, to quiver) = One of the hairs growing at the nares or vestibule of the nose.

villous (L.) = Relating to villi; shaggy; covered with villi.

villus, pl. **villi** (L. a shaggy hair [of beasts]) = A projection from the surface, especially of a mucous membrane; an elongated dermal papilla.

vinculum, pl. **vincula** (L. a fetter, fr. *vincio,* to bind) = A frenum, frenulum, or ligament.

visceral (L.) = Relating to the viscera.

viscus, pl. viscera (L. the soft parts, internal organs) = An organ of the digestive, respiratory, urogenital, and endocrine systems as well as the spleen, the heart, and great vessels.

vitreous (L. *vitreus,* glassy, fr. *vitrum,* glass) = Glassy; resembling glass.

vocal (L. *vocalis*) = Pertaining to the voice or the organs of speech.

vomer, gen. **vomeris** (L. ploughshare) = A flat bone of trapezoidal shape forming the interior and posterior portion of the nasal septum.

vomeronasal (L.) = Relating to the vomer and the nasal bone.

vulva, pl. **vulvae** (L. a wrapper or covering, seed covering, womb, fr. *volvo,* to roll) = The external genitalia of the female.

xiphoid (G. *xiphos,* sword, + *eidos,* appearance) = Sword-shaped; the xiphoid process.

zona, pl. **zonae** (L. fr. G. *zōnē,* a girdle, one of the zones of the sphere) = Zone; a segment; any encircling or beltlike structure.

zonule (L. *zonula,* dim. of *zona,* zone) = A small zone.

zygomatic (G. a bar, bolt, the os jugale, fr. *zygon,* yoke) = Relating to the zygomatic bone.

Index

Page numbers followed by *t* denote Tables.